navigating your hormones on the journey to menopause

peri menopause power.

maisie hill

GREEN TREE
LONDON • OXFORD • NEW YORK • NEW DELHI • SY

GREEN TREE
Bloomsbury Publishing Plc
50 Bedford Square, London, WC1B 3DP, UK
29 Earlsfort Terrace Dublin 2, Ireland

First published in Great Britain 2021

A catalogue record for this book is available from the British Library

Library of Congress Cataloguing-in-Publication data has been applied for

ISBN: TPB: 978-1-4729-7886-8; ePub: 978-1-4729-7887-5;
ePDF: 978-1-4729-7889-9

6 8 10 9 7 5

Typeset in Minion Pro by Deanta Global Publishing Services, Chennai, India
Printed and bound in Great Britain by CPI Group (UK) Ltd, Croydon, CR0 4YY

To find out more about our authors and books visit www.bloomsbury.com
and sign up for our newsletters

To every single one of you who read *Period Power* and sent me
a message or left a comment asking me 'What happens next?'
– this book is for you and thanks to you.
And to my ovaries, for doing an outstanding job.

HOW TO USE THIS BOOK

My clients come to me wanting help. They want strategies that will make a difference to their symptoms and their lives, and I assume that it's the same for you. So, if you've got a particular symptom that's bothering you, such as hot flushes or changes to your mental health, you can head straight to the relevant chapter(s). Get the information you need as soon as possible.

What also helps my clients is understanding why they're having their particular experience because knowledge alone can have a profound effect. Seeing my clients' faces as it all starts to make sense to them always brings a smile to mine, which is why I've explained the science behind perimenopause and postmenopause in this book. But I appreciate that scientific language can be confusing – that's why there's a glossary at the back (see pages 288–292) that you can refer to, if and when you need it.

This is a book that you can come back to as you journey through perimenopause and enter your postmenopausal years. Some of it will apply now, some will become more relevant later on, but, ultimately, having an overall sense of the menopause transition will help you to be prepared and to have a positive experience, which is what I want for all of us.

Language and Inclusivity

Perimenopause is a process that happens to those born with 'female' reproductive organs, but I appreciate that not everyone who reads this book will be female – some of you will be non-binary or trans. It's with this consideration in mind that I've tried to be inclusive in my choice of language, referring to women either because that's the language used in the research papers I reference, or to make a point about patriarchy.

CONTENTS

INTRODUCTION

You might wonder what a 40-year-old is doing writing a book about menopause. I mean, that's something that happens in your fifties, right? Not quite.

Whilst the average age of menopause is 51, menopause itself only lasts for one day, because it simply marks the one-year anniversary of your last period. Perimenopause, on the other hand, refers to the period of time in which you'll have cycles, but start to experience 'menopausal' symptoms. When most of us are talking about menopause, what we actually mean is perimenopause. Perimenopause is most likely to start in your forties, but for some it will begin in your thirties. It can last as little as two years or as long as 12, and if more of us were aware of the subtleties of this transition, we'd recognise the hallmark signs of our hormones shifting far sooner and actually be able to do something about it.

To begin with you might notice that your periods roll around quicker than they used to and that you need to up your game in order to manage blood loss. Symptoms such as night sweats, insomnia, headaches, migraines and breast tenderness may appear in the days surrounding the start of your period. These are the early signs that your hormonal landscape is shifting and that you're entering your perimenopausal years. With time, those signs will become increasingly prevalent, and in the later stage of perimenopause, your periods will become less frequent and other symptoms, such as vaginal dryness, joint pain and bladder changes, will become more likely.

You may be someone who glides through perimenopause without any significant issues. You might hurtle into it unexpectedly and feel rocked to your core. You might be comfortable managing your experience without help. You might want to do things 'naturally' and feel confident that you can. You could be up for taking hormone replacement therapy (HRT) and whatever else modern medicine has to offer. You could also find that somewhere along the line your thoughts and feelings about how you'll manage 'the change', change. What works well for you at first may not do the same further down the line, and one form of treatment might work wonders for your best mate, but not for you.

Whilst we're on the subject, just as there are no prizes handed out for birthing a child without pain relief, there is no prize for going through the menopause transition without using HRT. Whatever your thoughts on how best to navigate the menopause transition are, you'll find explanations and strategies that will help you in this book.

Your needs are likely to change throughout this process – and it's okay to change your mind about how you support your health and wellbeing. I don't want you to judge yourself, or anyone else, for the choices you make. Whatever course of action you decide upon, I want you to feel good about it. My hope is that this book will help you to make decisions about your medical care and your life, because indecision is exhausting. Going back and forth worrying about the 'right' course of action takes up mental space that quite frankly, in this stage of life, you don't have. Not to mention preventing and interrupting your sleep, which you could certainly do without.

By the end of this book, you'll have a chunky toolkit of tips and techniques that you can use to improve your experience of perimenopause as well as your postmenopausal years. To begin with, the decisions you make are likely to be about managing your symptoms, but as you'll discover, the decisions you make now will impact the decades that follow. Perimenopause is often described as a window of opportunity and that's what I'd like you to consider it as.

Perimenopausal symptoms include (but certainly aren't limited to):

- More frequent or further-apart periods (or a thoroughly unpredictable combination of the two)
- Changes to menstrual flow – heavier, longer, shorter, lighter
- Increased PMS
- ALL THE RAGE, ALL THE TIME
- Sleep disturbances
- Fatigue
- Breast tenderness
- Headaches and migraines
- Brain fog
- Poor memory
- Bloating

- Hot flushes
- Night sweats
- Dry mouth
- Joint and muscle pain
- Mood changes such as anxiety and depression
- Panic attacks
- Vaginal dryness
- Pain during penetrative sex
- Reduced sexual desire
- Increased sexual desire (yes, really)
- Bladder changes – leakage, urgency, needing to pee in the night
- Skin changes – acne, dry skin, oily skin, loss of plumpness and elasticity
- Itchy skin
- Hair loss, or thinning
- Diarrhoea or constipation, or both.

Perimenopause is more than just physical symptoms, though. In the Autumn phase of life, we are confronted with thoughts and feelings that may have been supressed for years; creative and sexual desires that suddenly emerge or disappear; a greater need for self-expression; and a deep longing to walk away from life as we know it. And then there's going about your daily life feeling like a tinderbox that's ready to ignite, thanks to the irritability, impatience and red-hot rage that course through your body. Perimenopause is a baptism of fire that forces you to face yourself, your history and your future. There is an intensity to perimenopause that we are rarely prepared for, but desperately need to be, because rather than it be something that happens to us, we can have a sense of agency over our experience and find our power.

The Current State of Affairs

In the last three years there's been a 37 per cent increase in online searching for information about the menopause and it's hardly surprising given that, according to independent Nuffield Health group, 13 million women in the UK are currently perimenopausal or postmenopausal, and, because of the increase in population size that came from the first- and second-wave baby boomers, it's estimated that more than 50 million women and those assigned female at birth in the US have now reached the average

age of menopause. By 2050, this figure is expected to quadruple. Yet the sheer volume and range of symptoms and needs of those who are peri- and postmenopausal is not reflected in the research, public health education and spending. If the tables were turned and men were the ones who were wide awake drenched in sweat at 1am, if their cognitive function changed and their penises shrivelled up, how much money do you reckon would be coughed up to help them? There certainly wouldn't be a worldwide shortage of HRT, as there currently is. After menopause we still have a third of our lives left and the impact of the hormone shifts during the menopause transition echoes throughout those decades, but there simply isn't enough research being done to reflect this fact.

As discussion around topics such as periods and miscarriage has come to the fore in recent years, menopause is only just starting to get some attention. Stars such as Michelle Obama, Ulrika Jonsson, Meg Mathews, Louise Minchin and Michelle Heaton have opened up about their experiences of menopause and received an outpouring of praise and public support for doing so. Psychologist and menopause expert Diane Danzebrink is the founder of the not-for-profit organisation Menopause Support and the driving force behind the #makemenopausematter campaign, which seeks to improve menopause education among GPs, include menopause in the PSHE curriculum for teenagers and raise awareness in the workplace. It also recommends that employers create menopause guidelines, so that they can support their employees. This work is needed. Those who do speak to their GP about their symptoms (many don't) are often supplied with outdated advice as the majority of doctors lack sufficient training in how to identify and manage menopausal symptoms, with most receiving little to no training in the reproductive health of women beyond their childbearing years. One would be forgiven for thinking that our wombs are only worthy of attention when they're incubating other humans. The British Menopause Society estimates that over one third of women will spend half their lives as postmenopausal women, yet their needs are not being addressed by health professionals.

All of this comes at a high cost. Marriages can rapidly deteriorate, work performance declines and 10 per cent of women consider giving up work altogether due to their symptoms. Health risks increase and the risk of suicide goes up. The average age of menopause is 51 and the Samaritans reports that the age group with the highest suicide rate for women is 50 to 54. Menopause is not a disease, it is natural and normal, and it is also a stage of life in which we need evidence-based guidance and helpful support, and it's thanks to the passion and tireless work of women like Diane that we are finally seeing progress.

Why Me?

Who am I to write a book about perimenopause when I haven't gone through it yet? It's a question I've asked myself repeatedly. I considered waiting a few years until I was on the other side of it – and I know that there will be people who think that I should have waited. My decision to write this book was based on the countless comments, DMs and emails I received from people who read *Period Power* and wanted to know more about what happens to our hormones during perimenopause – so many of you asked me 'What happens next?' that I even considered it as a title for this book. All those messages had an impact, because your urgent need for more information became my urgent need to get that information to you, so that you can understand what's going on and that there are lots of things that can be done to improve your experience. I'm grateful to all the perimenopausal and postmenopausal clients that I've had over the last 15 years for putting their trust in me as their practitioner and coach, and for allowing me to share their stories with you throughout this book. It's thanks to their questions and pursuit of a different experience of perimenopause that this book is in your hands.

I'm sure that this book would be very different if I had waited, but would it be more helpful to you? I'm not so sure. I spent 10 years supporting hundreds of families as a birth doula before I experienced pregnancy and birth and, in all honesty, I was a better doula before I became a mother. Once I had my son, I tried to prevent my own experiences from muddying the waters as I helped my clients navigate their choices and make informed decisions, but they still hovered around in the background, whereas the decade I spent doula-ing before I became a parent was without the prejudice of my own experience. My clients benefitted from that and I hope you'll feel the same way as you read *Perimenopause Power*. I've pulled information from different quarters, done some hefty research so you don't have to, and woven it together with my clinical experience so that you're able to make informed decisions about your health and hormones during the menopause transition.

I like to be ahead of the curve, and I want to prepare myself and my family for the next phase of my life as best I can. I remember what it was like living with a perimenopausal mother whilst I went through my teen years, and I want a different experience for my son and partner. One where there is dialogue, awareness and understanding that there are times when I need to walk out the door and stomp my way along the coast or up the hills. I wanted to know what options will be available to me when the time comes and writing this book has allowed me to do that. I've been able to make some decisions ahead of time, some of which have surprised me. I'm also being confronted by the challenges of midlife. I'm learning to wield the power of my hormones and quietly relishing the radical overhaul that they are demanding of me.

If nothing else, I hope that this book addresses the almighty cock-up caused by the flawed findings of the Women's Health Initiative study – the piece of research that's led to 20 years of largely unfounded and scary headlines (more on this on pages 79–80).

So, shall we do this?

Let's go.

1

WTF is happening?

Throughout our reproductive years we get used to what's normal for us – whatever our individual experience of our cycle has been. Amidst any cycle-related symptoms such as pain, heavy flow, PMS, breast tenderness and bloating, and changes to your energy, mood and behaviour, there's a degree of knowing what to expect. Your cycle may have resembled the stunning highs and plummeting lows of a hair-raising rollercoaster, but at least you had an idea of what to expect on your particular rollercoaster.

In perimenopause the ride changes. Subtly at first and then with full force. Instead of being on the same rollercoaster ride every cycle, it feels like you're always on a different one, especially once you start oscillating between shorter and longer cycles, rarely with any kind of predictability. Yep, it's time to say goodbye to regular cycles – if you ever had them, as some people experience lifelong irregularity.

Clients who come to me are often unsure whether they're perimenopausal. They tell me that their cycle has gone off-piste in some way; either the length of their cycle has shifted or their period has changed. Perhaps some new symptoms have appeared or existing ones have gotten worse. Changes such as these are often (but not always) due to perimenopause, but because they don't fit the picture we have in our minds of a menopausal woman who's hot and sweaty, and leaning against an open freezer, my clients don't necessarily identify the cause as perimenopause. The hot flushes we all associate with menopause can come further down the line.

Others come to me because they're experiencing a vast array of symptoms that indicate they're going through perimenopause, but they're unaware that's what's going on. It's rare for anyone to talk about perimenopause until they're well and truly in it, and years of subtle, even obvious, signs and symptoms may precede the hot and sweaty phase without being categorised as perimenopause. This, by the way, is not something that I judge. It does enrage me that so many of us don't have a clue about what our hormones and reproductive organs get up to, but I don't blame anyone for not knowing. Patriarchy is responsible for that.

And then there are those who absolutely know and are in need of help.

Regardless of where you're at (because I'm hoping that some of you are reading this waaaaay in advance of perimenopause), I want to kick things off with understanding what perimenopause is and when it starts, because if you're anything like me, you want a nice clear-cut description; a black and white way of knowing if you're in the club or not.

The Shouting Stage

According to the staging system developed by a group of scientists from five countries and multiple disciplines at the Stages of Reproductive Aging Workshop (STRAW) in 2001, early perimenopause begins when the length of your cycle varies by seven or more days in consecutive cycles. They also noted that during the late reproductive phase of life, subtle changes to flow and length may take place. But I've worked with many women who I would classify as experiencing the hormonal shifts of perimenopause who don't meet these criteria.

In my professional experience, symptoms do appear before getting to a seven-day variation in cycle length and I don't think you need to wait until you reach this official point to describe your experience as perimenopause. These symptoms include a shortened cycle, changes to menstrual flow, night sweats before and around the time of your period, the appearance of blinding headaches and debilitating migraines, breast swelling and tenderness that leaves you fearful of being hugged, and rage that could fuel a country.

This is also my personal experience. In the last year, my cycle has shortened to 24 to 25 days, with an occasional 'normal-for-me' length cycle somewhere between 28 and 32 days. I started struggling to fall asleep in the days before I started bleeding and this was accompanied by premenstrual night sweats, which at least served as notice that my period would be early. But the first major shift was that my premenstrual mood changes ramped the fuck up. Sound familiar? I know I'm not the only one. Over the years, clients have reported similar experiences to me.

This is a life phase that the Centre for Menstrual Cycle and Ovulation Research (CeMCOR, www.cemcor.ubc.ca) has described as 'very early perimenopause'. CeMCOR is thankfully bucking the trend in terms of what defines the start of perimenopause, because it places the emphasis on our changing experiences which, better than regular cycles, indicate changes in our hormone levels. How refreshing. On its website, CeMCOR states that 'if our experiences have changed, if our hormone levels have changed – the scientific evidence is that perimenopausal oestrogen levels are higher, more variable and unpredictable, ovulation is less frequent and progesterone levels are lower, then perimenopause has started, even if our cycles are regular and normal in length'. CeMCOR has published a series of *experience changes*, any three of which can be used to define the start of perimenopause in those with regular, normal-length menstrual cycles:

- New heavy and/or longer menstrual flow
- Shorter menstrual cycle lengths (≤ 25 days)
- New sore, swollen, and/or lumpy breasts
- New or increased menstrual cramps
- New mid-sleep wakening
- Onset of night sweats, especially around flow
- New or markedly increased migraine headaches
- New or increased premenstrual mood swings
- Notable weight gain without changes in exercise or food intake.

So many of us are starting to dance with perimenopause, but we have no idea. We miss out on opportunities to do something about it – time where we could be proactive and positively impact our experience of perimenopause and life beyond menopause. This is what I want to change.

When Will It Happen?

Most of us will experience natural menopause – when periods stop – between the ages of 45 and 55. The average age is 51, though this figure varies slightly depending on which country you live in. You'd be forgiven for thinking that 'natural' menopause refers to going through it without HRT, as if there will be an award for doing so. (There isn't.) It's a term that defines the age at which you go through menopause naturally versus entering menopause as a result of medical treatments or surgical intervention, such as the use of radiation or surgical removal of the ovaries.

Perimenopause – where you still have a cycle, but begin to experience 'menopausal' symptoms – lasts on average for four years, but can be as long as 10 to 15 years. The first subtle sign that change is afoot is often a shortened menstrual cycle and, along with a varying cycle length, hormone levels fluctuate, often wildly. Although menopause is thought of as a time of hormone deficiency, specifically the withdrawal of oestrogen, perimenopause is more often a time when oestrogen remains high. The peak oestrogen level in a 20-year-old will be around 500–1,000 pmol/L, but during perimenopause oestrogen can be as high as 5,000 pmol/L – hardly a deficiency. (It doesn't matter if you aren't familiar with the unit of measurement here, which is picamoles per litre or pmol/l, the point is the contrast.) Eventually, oestrogen does decline, and you may switch between cycles where oestrogen is high and cycles where it is low, but progesterone is the hormone that takes a bow first. During the time when oestrogen is high and progesterone is low, symptoms such as shorter cycles, heavy and/or longer periods, period pain, premenstrual spotting, bloating, headaches and migraines, sleep issues, anxiety, depression, irritability AND ALL THE RAGE appear.

The gradual and erratic decrease of oestrogen secretion that's a feature of the late stage of perimenopause, in the run-up to menopause itself, sees your periods becoming further apart and the emergence of symptoms such as hot flushes, night sweats and vaginal dryness. Once oestrogen declines, changes to your genito-urinary system take place, and the risk of cardiovascular diseases, diabetes and osteoporosis goes up.

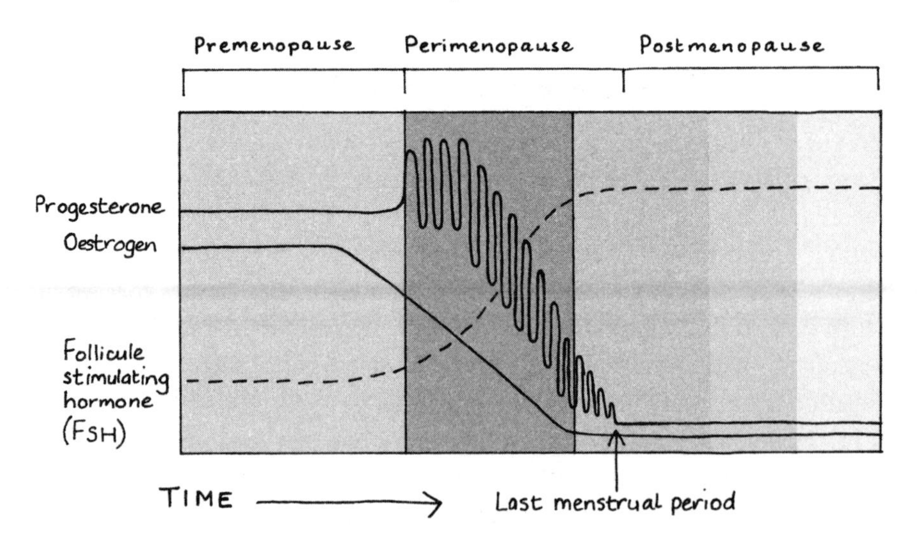

Defining Menopause

Premenopause is the years in which you experience a menstrual cycle.

Perimenopause is the period of time in which you still have periods, although they're likely to be irregular, and experience 'menopausal' symptoms. This can be further defined as:

Very early menopause: Cycle length may be the same or slightly shorter, new symptoms appear and/or existing ones worsen. Oestrogen is often high in relation to progesterone.
Early perimenopause: Cycle length becomes shorter. Oestrogen is often high in relation to progesterone.
Late perimenopause: Cycle length becomes longer, symptoms such as hot flushes, night sweats and vaginal dryness may emerge. Oestrogen becomes low.

Menopause itself is only one day long and marks the one-year anniversary since your last menstrual period.

Postmenopause is when periods have stopped and hot flushes are more likely, as are increasing symptoms such as vaginal dryness and urinary tract infections. We spend a third of our lives in this phase.

It's Called 'the Change' for a Reason

Although there is research on the age of natural menopause and the factors underlying it, when it comes to the timing and duration of perimenopause, the research – like most areas of female reproductive health – is frustratingly limited. Some people will have a positive experience of perimenopause. It is, after all, a life event not a disease or disorder. For others it will be confusing, overwhelming and have a huge impact on the quality of their lives.

There is no one-size-fits-all approach to this process. Your experience of perimenopause and the years that follow will be unique to you. And it really is a process. Just as you get used to a particular symptom or way of feeling, things change, and then change again, and again. No wonder it's referred to as 'the change'. It's unpredictable and it can suck. But it's also a window of opportunity and that's what I encourage you to focus on (Chapter 6 will help you to figure out how to do so).

Will a Test Tell Me if I'm Perimenopausal?

Perimenopause is not a disease, but diagnosis is usually made based on signs and symptoms. Blood tests for hormones aren't a reliable determinant of perimenopause as hormone levels can vary cycle to cycle, tend to bounce around all over the place during perimenopause and, in some cases, they will be in the range of someone who's *pre*menopausal. That being said, if you start to experience symptoms before the age of 45, you should have the blood tests as you may be experiencing early menopause or premature ovarian insufficiency (POI – see page 291).

But if it's not perimenopause, then what is it?

- Pregnancy (it happens more than we realise).
- Thyroid dysfunction becomes more common as we age and it can occur alongside perimenopause, but it can also occur on its own and, because it mirrors some of the symptoms of perimenopause, some people will be misdiagnosed. I've had clients who experienced weight gain, depressed mood, changes to their periods and other cycle irregularities, who were convinced that they were perimenopausal, but their thyroid turned out to be the problem.
- High prolactin levels can interfere with the normal production of other hormones and ovulation. Your GP will usually test your prolactin levels alongside other hormonal checks in order to rule it out or identify it as the cause of irregular cycles. If prolactin is high, you'll need a pregnancy test to rule out the most obvious cause, have your thyroid function checked, and be referred for a brain scan (MRI) as a common cause of high prolactin is the presence of a non-cancerous tumour on the pituitary gland called a prolactinoma (these often shrink during menopause).

- Amenorrhoea (missing periods) because of undereating, over-exercising and stress.
- Stress has a massive impact on the cycle, something everyone is waking up to since lockdown life started in 2020. If your cycle has become shorter or longer, stress could be the reason why and it could be causing a whole host of other symptoms too.

Running Out of Eggs

In the past it was assumed that menopause took place when you ran out of eggs, the pool of ovarian follicles dwindling to the point of no return. Changes to the relationship between two glands in your head – the hypothalamus and pituitary – were thought to take place as a consequence of declining ovarian function. But an increasing body of evidence suggests that is not the case. Instead, multiple factors lead to a gradual dampening and loss of synchronisation in the way your hormones communicate with each other and with your reproductive system. This takes place in addition to, and independently of, what your ovaries are up to (or *not* up to, as the case may be).

The communication circuits which run between your brain, the pituitary and the hypothalamus glands in your head and your reproductive system go through significant changes during the menopause transition, but before we get onto that, let's travel back in time to your teen years.

Unlike teenagers today, you probably didn't have a mobile phone as a teenager. But you were keen to talk to your mates. So keen that you'd hang around your landline family phone, waiting for it to be 6pm when off-peak charges would start. You'd have plenty to chat about, so did your mate, and sometimes another friend would be trying to get through to you too. If your mum was on the phone, then you'd search for some change to take to the phone box at the end of your road, because you couldn't possibly wait to communicate. I realise that this recollection ages me like nothing else, but this is exactly what was going on with your hormonal and reproductive system at that point in your life too – the various components were keen to communicate and they were highly responsive to one another.

Let's move onto what happened as you reached adulthood. For most of your reproductive years, communication between your brain and hormonal glands has been tightly orchestrated and responsive, like when you got your first mobile phone. Back in the Nokia days, it was easy to get hold of friends because we weren't up to much. Instead of using up precious minutes of your plan you'd use missed calls to send signals and receiving a text was so novel that you always replied immediately. But as we enter perimenopause, we forget to make calls, even ones that are important. You might go back and forth with calls all day with someone, but fail to catch each other at a mutually convenient time. Or your friend might spot your message, but not reply instantly, because, let's be honest, they can't be bothered. Communication between your brain, hormones and reproductive system is not what it used to be – messages aren't sent out and picked up as they ought to be or the timing is off.

It's the significant changes to these circuits of communication that are the hallmark of perimenopause and they appear to take place independently of declining ovarian function. As such, perimenopause mirrors puberty in that it is a process mediated by the hypothalamus. Menopause doesn't simply happen when you run out of eggs.

After menopause, your ovaries still contain some remaining follicles – intact follicles have been found in the ovaries of 70-year-olds! But whilst they can undergo a degree of hormonal activity, for the majority of the time, it's not enough to cause the changes to the lining of your uterus which would result in an episode of bleeding. Though at age 52, 4.5 per cent of us will have a period after a year of having none, and whilst that may be down to what a few remaining follicles are getting up to, you need to tell your GP about *any* postmenopausal bleeding. Do not assume that postmenopausal bleeding is down to lurking follicles trying to do their thing. Any episode of postmenopausal bleeding should be reported as it is a red flag for endometrial cancer (see page 222).

Menopause marks the permanent end of your cycling years and on average we spend three decades in postmenopause, so now is the time for you to consider what you want the next 30-plus years to be like.

Anatomical Changes During Perimenopause

It's not just your external appearance that changes with age; your reproductive system undergoes a progressive ageing process too.

WTF is happening?

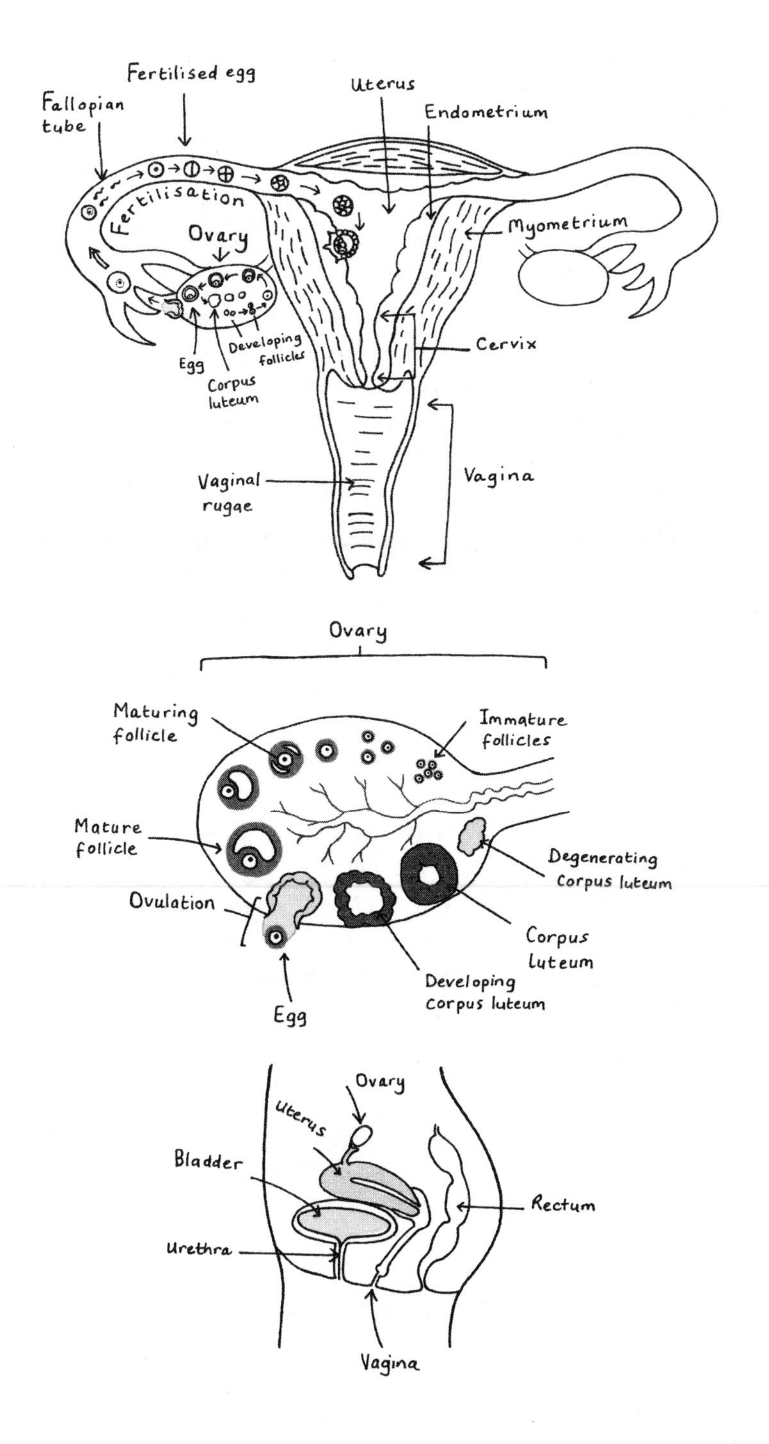

Vulva

When most people talk about the *vagina*, they're actually talking about the *vulva*. If you're confused about what's what, you're in the majority, and there's certainly no need to feel any shame about not knowing – we've been made to feel shame about our bodies for a long time so let's lessen that burden right now. That being said, it's good to know the names of your body parts because a) it's your body and b) it's important that you can talk about any genito-urinary symptoms with health professionals.

Your vulva is all of your external genitalia, including your mons pubis (that's the mound of fatty tissue on top of your pubic bone that's populated with pubic hair), labia minora (inner lips) and majora (outer lips), your clitoris and its hood, as well as your perineum (the area between your vulva and anus) and the external openings of your vagina and urethra (the hole that you pee from). Your vagina is the internal tube which connects your external genitalia – your vulva – with your uterus and it is only the opening to the vagina that can be seen once the labia are parted.

Your vulva thins during the menopause transition, and so does your vagina. Yes, you can get wrinkles down there too. The labia majora lose some of the subcutaneous fat, so you might notice that they're less plump than they used to be. The mons pubis can become more obvious, either because of changes to your pubic bone (pubic symphysis) or, and you're going to love this, because the fat that was originally around your lower abdomen has now descended to the start of your vulva. And to top it all off, pubic hair becomes sparser, thins, loses its coarseness, becomes wispier … and turns grey or white.

The entrance to your vagina – known scientifically as the vaginal introitus – becomes tighter, which can make tampon use (if you're still menstruating) and penetration painful. In postmenopause, the vulva also experiences a reduction in blood flow and your vulval skin can be particularly irritated by excessive washing and wiping, and unnecessary 'cleansers' and creams that contain propylene glycol, parabens and fragrances can cause further irritation.

Vagina

Your vagina cannot be seen externally. It runs at a 45-degree angle pointing backwards towards your bum and the front of it (the anterior wall) is slightly shorter than the back of it (the posterior wall). Your bladder sits in front of your vagina and uterus, and your rectum (the last section of your large intestine) sits behind it. The chances of having pelvic organ prolapse – where an organ's position changes – increase after the age of 50, when declining oestrogen levels impact the anatomy and function of the pelvic floor.

Though we tend to think of the vagina as a hole, largely because of how it's depicted as being something that is there to be filled, most of the time the walls of your vagina are in contact with each other. When something is inside your vagina, such as a tampon, menstrual cup, sex toy, penis or baby as it's being born, it expands in order to accommodate what's inside it. The vagina is able to do this thanks to the presence of ridges called rugae, which make it highly elastic and capable of expanding, producing the so-called tenting effect that lifts your cervix higher when you're aroused and stimulated. When oestrogen is circulating throughout your reproductive years, the lining of your vagina is thicker and you have plenty of rugae. In the years around the time of your last menstrual period and in postmenopause, when oestrogen becomes deficient, the vaginal lining thins and there are fewer folds. The consequence of this is that the vagina becomes less elastic and accommodating.

The walls of the vagina also dry and atrophy (that's the lovely medical term for 'waste away'), and become pale and more prone to irritation. The normal vaginal secretions which help to maintain a healthy pH reduce, leaving you feeling less lubricated and increasing the risk of tears, bleeding and infection.

In the same way that your gut has its own unique ecosystem of friendly bacteria called the microbiome, so does your vagina, and when it's out of balance you can end up with recurrent bouts of yeast infections and bacterial vaginosis. The vagina does not need to be cleaned or rinsed out, and using vaginal cleaning products or douching can upset the balance of bacteria and cause harm. It's thought that a lack of a healthy vaginal microbiome can result in pelvic inflammatory disease, bacterial vaginosis, sexually transmitted infections (STIs), miscarriage, ectopic pregnancy, premature birth and cervical cancer.

During the menopause transition, less oestrogen causes the pH of the vagina to become less acidic, altering the vaginal microbiome. In premenopause, healthy bacteria called lactobacilli rule the roost. They produce lactic acid and hydrogen peroxide, which maintain the acidic environment of your vagina in order to protect against infection. In postmenopause there are far fewer lactobacilli and the pH is less acidic, which means you're more prone to infections and it can also exacerbate the genito-urinary syndrome of menopause. In some cases, hormone therapy, such as taking oestrogen, can increase the number of lactobacilli and acidity of the vagina.

Genito-urinary Syndrome of Menopause (GSM)

Genito-urinary syndrome of menopause describes the menopausal signs and symptoms of the vulva, vagina and lower urinary tract (your bladder, urethra – the tube that takes wee from your bladder to the hole just above your vagina – and the sphincters, which open and close in order to wee). GSM encompasses the signs and symptoms associated with the loss of oestrogen at the time of menopause, which can involve:

- Genital symptoms such as burning, dryness and irritation
- Sexual symptoms such as lack of lubrication, discomfort and pain
- Urinary symptoms such as urgency, increased frequency, painful or difficult urination and urinary tract infections (UTIs).

Cervix

The top of your vagina is where your cervix is found. Sometimes the cervix is referred to as the neck of the womb, because it's actually the lowest and narrowest part of the uterus. Your cervix is a bit like a gate, in that for most of your life its job is to stay shut, only opening at ovulation to allow sperm in, at menstruation to allow blood out and during childbirth to allow a baby out.

After menopause it becomes thinner and loses some of its strength. The transformation zone – the area of the cervix that is most likely to become cancerous and that is assessed during cervical screenings – moves up a bit, which can make a visual examination of the cervix, called a colposcopy, slightly more difficult, but this shouldn't impact on your experience of having a cervical screening. The main reason cervical screening can be more uncomfortable during and after menopause is down to hormonal changes that affect the vagina, but your nurse can use a smaller speculum and lubricant to help this. You may also find that lying on your side is a more comfortable position for you to be in. Please don't worry about asking your nurse to help you figure it out. I promise that they've heard it all before, and they can help you to feel comfortable and in control.

After menopause, lack of oestrogen results in a reduction, or absence, of cervical fluid. This is because of changes to the junctions between the cells that line the cervix and because of reduced blood flow to the cervix.

Uterus

During your cycling years your uterus resembles the size and shape of an upside-down pear. After menopause it reduces by around 20 per cent. Changes to the ligaments, muscles and other tissues that support the uterus also take place and these can cause it to drop down. This is known as a prolapse and, no, it isn't something that you should accept as being part of the ageing process. There's a lot that can be done to prevent and treat prolapse, which we'll explore in Chapter 2.

Abnormal uterine bleeding is common during perimenopause and there are many reasons why it can happen, as well as ways of improving or resolving it without resorting to having it removed surgically in what's known as a hysterectomy (see page 208). Hysterectomies are often performed because the uterus is seen to have done all it can do – once the reproductive years are over, it may as well come out. And there are times when its removal is appropriate and helpful, but recent research suggests that the uterus has a role beyond carrying children: researchers have discovered that, in animal studies, hysterectomies impair some types of short-term memory, suggesting that the uterus and ovaries are part of a system that communicates with the brain and is involved in cognitive function. They concluded that common gynaecological surgeries may disrupt this communication system and lead to alterations in brain functioning.

Ovaries

The ovaries are two pearl-coloured glands which sit on either side of the uterus just beneath the end of each fallopian tube. Ligaments which attach to the uterus and pelvic wall hold them in place. They have two roles: to produce a mature egg in each menstrual cycle that will be released at ovulation; and producing hormones such as oestradiol (the form of oestrogen we're most familiar with), testosterone, progesterone and inhibin, all of which play a part in the hormonal ebb and flow of your menstrual cycle, as well as your overall health and wellbeing.

Unlike sperm, which is continually produced across the reproductive years, your follicles are finite. You were born with all the eggs you'll ever have and what you've got left is what you've got left. As your follicles decline, so does the ability of your cells to make oestrogen (oestradiol), progesterone, testosterone and some of the 'mother' hormone dehydroepiandrosterone (DHEA), which several other hormones are made from. Progesterone often declines more rapidly than the others, because its production relies upon ovulation taking place and, as well as producing less as a result of ovulation as we age, during menopause, we have more anovulatory cycles – cycles where we don't ovulate and therefore don't produce progesterone.

It's likely that as we age follicular cells also become less sensitive to signals from the hypothalamus-pituitary-ovarian (HPO) axis. So, whilst we can bang on about declining ovarian function, we can't forget about the role of your central nervous system, aka that beautiful brain of yours.

Your ovaries also shrink. Before menopause they were the size of unshelled almonds – 3 to 4cm in size. After menopause they shrink to the size of a blueberry – 0.5 to 1cm. The older you get, the smaller they get, but that doesn't mean that they eventually disappear. Nor does it mean that they don't serve a purpose after menopause. Your ovaries continue to pack a punch after you stop ovulating. During postmenopause, they continue to secrete testosterone and androstenedione, which can be converted into oestrogens – your ovaries produce androgens for up to 10 years after menopause – so unless there's a clear medical reason to have your ovaries removed, you wanna hang on to them.

And as if all that wasn't enough, the muscles which make up your pelvic floor can also lose tone, which can make your vagina, uterus or bladder fall out of their usual position in what's described as a prolapse. I realise that all this sounds dire, but I want you to know that there is a lot that can be done to improve many of these uncomfortable symptoms, which I'll share with you in the relevant chapters. Now that we've covered what happens with your anatomy, let's move onto what happens to your hormones.

Hormones of the Cycle

You're probably aware that your hormones have great influence over your energy levels and mood. You might know that there are times of the month when you feel 'hormonal'. And there might be times of the month where you don't think about it all, because you feel great and you're busy living your best life. But the truth is, the hormones of the menstrual cycle have a massive influence on energy, mood and behaviour. How these hormones fluctuate during perimenopause will greatly impact your experience – as will your mindset and life circumstances. Meet the main players of your cycle.

The Miranda Priestly

Gonadotropin-releasing hormone (GnRH) is the boss of your cycle and small amounts of it are regularly released in pulses by a gland in your head called the hypothalamus. These pulses are picked up by a neighbouring gland called the pituitary and, in turn, stimulate it to release two other hormones: follicle stimulating hormone (FSH) and luteinising hormone (LH). The amount of each hormone is dependent on the frequency and magnitude that GnRH is pulsed at. Slow pulses seem to get FSH going, whereas LH responds to higher frequencies. Think of GnRH as Meryl Streep's character in *The Devil Wears Prada*; her presence is felt everywhere and nothing happens without her saying so – but it's her minions that do the actual work.

As we age, the co-ordination and pattern of GnRH pulses alter. The pace slows, instructions aren't always sent out and messages don't always arrive. It's these changes in GnRH pulses that provide evidence that menopause isn't solely about diminishing egg quality and quantity. It's also because Miranda's lost her commanding presence.

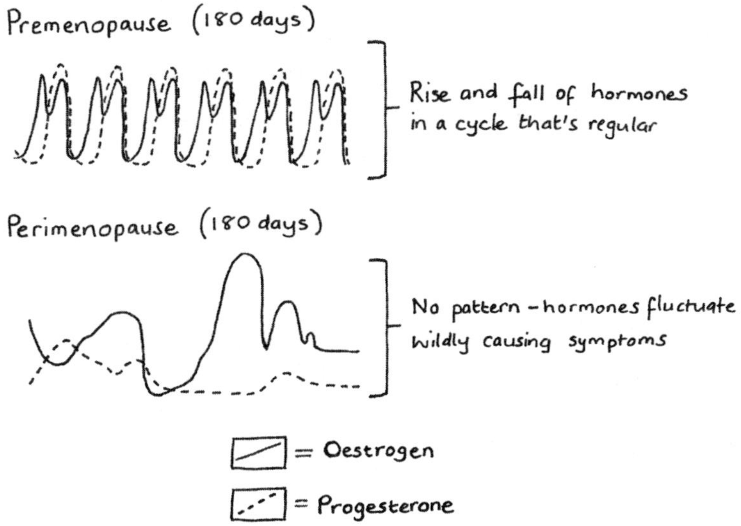

The Tyra

Follicle stimulating hormone (FSH) does exactly what it says on the tin – it stimulates the follicles in your ovaries to grow and mature, and eventually release an egg at ovulation. Towards the end of each cycle, just before your period starts, it recruits a group of follicles from your ovaries, one of which will end up being selected for ovulation. Then, at the start of the cycle, it stimulates your follicles further and, once one outshines the others, it stands down because another hormone, called inhibin-B, sends a signal to say no more follicles are needed for that cycle. Then, later on in the cycle, just before ovulation, it arrives back on the scene, along with another hormone, called luteinising hormone (LH), and they take turns egging each other on, and once they peak, ovulation occurs. Imagine Tyra Banks in *America's Next Top Model*. She's there at the start praising all the contestants, making them feel good, then she steps back, waits to see who will outperform the others, and then shows up to award the winner with their prize.

In perimenopause your brain has to shout louder to get the message to your ovaries. To do this, it produces more FSH. More follicle stimulation causes the development of one follicle, or multiple follicles, to be accelerated. Remember how Tyra retreats once the group of contestants has been assembled? Around the age of 35, secretion of the hormone that inhibits FSH – inhibin – begins to decline and this accelerates once you land in your forties. That means that there's nobody telling Tyra she's not needed right now. Instead, she stays in the room egging the contestants on. This increases the amount of oestrogen secreted by the follicles and the threshold of oestrogen required to trigger LH happens sooner, bringing forward the moment of ovulation and shortening the length of your cycle.

Increased levels of FSH means that more follicles are stimulated. This can result in an 'overshooting' effect, where more than one follicle, or contestant, will be recruited. Although most of these will die off, it's the rise in FSH that is thought to be behind the rate of non-identical twins. Non-identical, or dizygotic, twins are produced when each twin develops from a separate egg and sperm cell, rather than the one fertilised egg dividing and producing identical twins. In other words, non-identical twins are created as a result of multiple ovulation, which is more common as we age in an apparent last-ditch attempt to use what we've got.

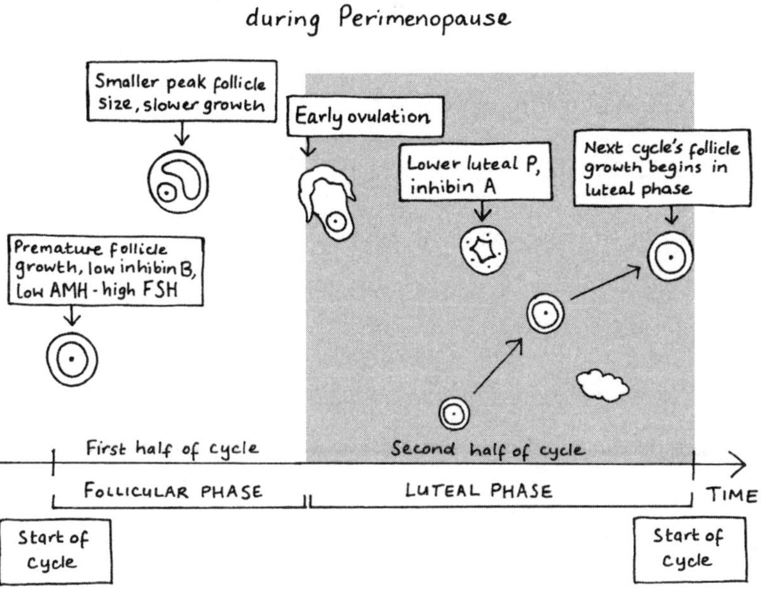

The Beyoncé

Oestrogen is the hormone which reigns over the first half of your cycle – the follicular phase. It's secreted by your developing follicles and causes the lining of your uterus to plump up in anticipation of a fertilised egg potentially implanting in the second half of your cycle – your luteal phase. Oestrogen can make you feel confident, alluring and sensual. It can clear up your skin and even make your features more symmetrical. It helps us to learn new skills and feel on top of the world. Oestrogen is your Beyoncé hormone.

Menopause is usually thought of as a time of declining levels of oestrogen; symptoms such as vaginal dryness and painful joints are all associated with low levels of oestrogen, after all. But although there is an eventual withdrawal of oestrogen in the later stages of menopause transition, once your periods begin to spread out and eventually stop, during perimenopause *oestrogen is usually the highest it's ever been.* And whilst getting all the Beyoncé you can may sound good, this is definitely a case of too much of a good thing, because it can result in symptoms such as heavy periods, irritability, bloating and breast/chest tenderness.

We talk and think about oestrogen as being one hormone, but there's actually more than one type of oestrogen:

- Oestrone (E1) is produced in the ovaries and by the conversion of androgens ('male' hormones) in the fat cells around the body. It's the predominant circulating oestrogen in postmenopause, although it's weaker compared to oestradiol.
- Oestradiol (E2) is the most potent form of oestrogen: 10 times as potent as oestrone and 100 times more potent than oestriol. It's produced by your ovaries during your reproductive years and is responsible for the development of sexual development characteristics such as breast development and widening of the hips, as well as the development and maintenance of the reproductive system. Oestradiol rises and falls throughout the menstrual cycle and also plays a role in the health of your brain, breasts, bones and cardiovascular system. This form of oestrogen plays over 300 roles in the body, which is why, once it does a runner, you really feel it.
- Oestriol (E3) is found at almost undetectable levels unless you're pregnant and, like oestrone, it's a weak form of oestrogen. During pregnancy the placenta produces vast amounts of it.
- Oestetrol (E4) is only produced by the liver of a developing baby during pregnancy.

Oestrogen is actually made from the conversion of androgen hormones such as testosterone and androstenedione. This conversion is possible because of an enzyme called aromatase. Enzymes help with thousands of bodily processes such as digesting food, building muscle and destroying toxins, by speeding up the chemical reactions involved in them. Without enzymes, we wouldn't be able to sustain life – they're a big deal! The enzyme aromatase hangs out in oestrogen-producing cells around your body such as your ovaries, blood vessels, brain, skin, bone and fat cells, where it converts androgens (aka 'male' hormones) into oestrogen. Once the production of oestrogen from your ovaries dwindles, aromatase activity increases in fat and muscle around your body to produce oestrone (E1). This is the shift in oestrogen production from oestradiol (E2), the type of oestrogen you've known throughout your cycling years, to its less potent sister, oestrone (E1).

The Solange

Luteinising hormone shows up just before ovulation, as oestrogen reaches its peak. LH delivers the power and strength that results in ovulation, and also lays the foundation for progesterone production in the second half of the cycle. So, although it seems like Beyoncé (oestrogen) is the star of the show, it's Solange – the surge in LH – that triggers ovulation.

Unlike FSH and oestrogen, secretions of LH remain pretty stable during perimenopause and only increase when cycles are close to ending. As GnRH secretion becomes less co-ordinated, the timing of the LH surge just before ovulation becomes impaired; the pulses of LH become broader and less frequent. All of which has a knock-on effect in terms of how responsive your ovaries are.

The Serena

Testosterone is not a male hormone; it is produced by all humans. It peaks around the time of ovulation, at the same time as oestrogen and LH peak. It's active, ambitious, sexy and competitive – the Serena Williams of hormones. Testosterone strengthens our bones and muscles, and contributes to an increase in sexual desire around ovulation.

In those of us born as females, testosterone is made in two locations: the adrenal glands, which sit on top of your kidneys produce DHEA (the mother hormone, which several other hormones are made from) and androstenedione, which can be converted into testosterone; and your ovaries, which also produce testosterone.

Testosterone production decreases after menopause, but most of the time your ovaries produce more testosterone in the first five years after menopause than they did during premenopause. But how can we have a decrease in production if the ovaries are producing more? It's because the big shift is in what happens to the primary source of testosterone: the conversion of androstenedione, from your adrenal glands, to testosterone is reduced.

When testosterone is low, you can get symptoms such as mood swings, belly fat, low energy, brain fog, low sexual desire, low muscle mass and bone loss. High testosterone, on the other hand, can cause acne, an increase in body and facial hair, a loss of scalp hair and aggression.

The Kristen Stewart

Progesterone is produced as a result of ovulation and it dominates the second half of your cycle. It develops and maintains the lining of your womb so that it's ready for a fertilised egg to implant, if one comes along. Progesterone is essential for conceiving and sustaining a pregnancy. It's the Kristen Stewart of hormones – progesterone is edgy, doesn't want to be the centre of attention, and prefers to stay at home eating apple pie and enjoying the company of women.

But this isn't its only role. Progesterone is crucial for bone health and preventing breast and uterine cancer. It has to be used as a component in HRT as without it the lining of the uterus can thicken up, which is a risk factor for uterine cancer. In most people, progesterone soothes mood and aids sleep, because it's converted into allopregnanolone (ALLO) which calms the receptors in your brain that help you to calm the fuck down. For a small percentage of people, though, such as those with premenstrual dysphoric disorder (PMDD), the response to ALLO is different thanks to dysfunctional receptors, so instead of feeling calm, we experience mood disturbances, anxiety, depression, irritability and intrusive thoughts.

As we age, progesterone production declines, which impacts fertility as well as your experience of your menstrual cycle. Declining production of progesterone during perimenopause is associated with a reduction in the levels of ALLO, which is a potential cause of the mood changes which can take place during perimenopause. Signs and symptoms of low progesterone include:

- Premenstrual spotting
- Breakthrough bleeding in the second half of your cycle
- Difficulty getting pregnant
- Difficulty staying pregnant
- PMS
- Cyclical headaches
- Heavy menstrual flow
- Irregular cycles or more frequent cycles
- Bloating and/or water retention
- Swollen breasts, accompanied by tenderness or pain
- Clumsiness or poor co-ordination
- Itchy or restless legs, particularly at night
- Difficulty sleeping
- Ovarian cysts, breast cysts or endometrial cysts (polyps).

Progesterone also keeps oestrogen in check, so once it becomes lower, oestrogen gets higher and you get symptoms associated with excess oestrogen too. Progesterone is the forgotten-about hormone at all ages and stages of reproductive health, only seen as important if you're trying to conceive, but it's important throughout our reproductive and post-reproductive years. During perimenopause, it's the balancing act between oestrogen and progesterone that we must pay attention to, because, to begin with, oestrogen is usually high and progesterone is low.

DHEA

Dehydroepiandrosterone (DHEA), one of the precursor hormones from which other hormones are made, doesn't actually do much biologically, but it becomes potent when it's converted into other hormones, such as testosterone and oestrogen. DHEA is mainly made from cholesterol in your adrenal glands, though your ovaries are able to make small amounts too. DHEA is important because during your cycling years, it produces 75 per cent of your oestrogen and, after menopause, it becomes the sole source of oestrogen and testosterone.

Cycle 101

Your menstrual cycle is controlled by a circuit of communication that runs between those two glands in your head – the hypothalamus and the pituitary – and your ovaries. This circuit is known as the hypothalamic-pituitary-ovarian (HPO) axis and it's responsible for a largely predictable chain of events, and the ebb and flow of hormones in each menstrual cycle. Once we enter perimenopause, though, the hormones and events of the cycle become increasingly erratic. I want you to know what's going on so that you can make sense of your experience – the good, the bad and the ugly.

First of all, when I say cycle, I don't mean your period. Your period is the point in your cycle when you're bleeding. Your cycle refers to the whole 28 days or however long your cycle might be. As little as 12.4 per cent of us actually have a 'textbook' 28-day cycle and perimenopause is certainly a time when cycle length varies.

Oestrogen is the hormone that reigns over the first half of your cycle – the follicular phase. Its job is to prepare you for pregnancy, whether that's something you're up for or not. In the first half of the cycle, oestrogen causes the lining of your uterus – the endometrium – to plump up and it also increases production of cervical fluid, which is essential for the survival and movement of sperm. Oestrogen also drives behaviour in the first half of the cycle. If you've noticed that you're chattier, up for going out, attracted to people and interested in sex in the run-up to ovulation that's oestrogen (and testosterone) trying to take care of business.

After ovulation, progesterone is produced in order to support implantation and pregnancy, if they're to take place. Progesterone alters and maintains your endometrium so that it's suitable for a fertilised egg to nestle into. In the same way that oestrogen primed you for mating in the first half of the cycle, progesterone seeks to nourish and protect you in the second half. Progesterone slows you down; you might be more introverted and less interested in going out, or only with close friends. This is progesterone's way of keeping you safe. Your digestive system even slows down so that your body can extract more nutrients from food and nourish a developing embryo.

Not everyone will experience their cycle in this way and you don't have to be a slave to your hormones, but I'm guessing that knowing this will help you to understand the basics of what your hormones are trying to achieve.

Phases of the Cycle

Now you've got the short version of events, let's take a deeper dive into what happens in each phase of the cycle and how they change during perimenopause.

Follicular Phase: Menstruation to Ovulation

The follicular phase runs from the first day of your period until the moment you ovulate. It's your follicular phase that largely determines the length of your cycle. The luteal phase is relatively stable at around 14 days in length, though this is likely to become shorter as you progress through perimenopause and, as cycles where you don't ovulate become more common, you'll have fewer and fewer luteal phases. Your follicular phase, on the other hand, might be 14 days or it could be nine or 44. If you ovulate on the early side, your period will be early. Ovulate later and your period will be late. When we talk about a delayed period, what we really mean is delayed ovulation.

The follicular phase can be further divided into the time when you're bleeding and the time when your body is preparing for ovulation.

Menstruation

Day 1 of your cycle is the first day you experience significant bleeding. It doesn't matter what time of day it happens. Any spotting counts as the end of the previous cycle, even if it continues for several days. Premenstrual spotting indicates that progesterone may be low, which is common as we age and during perimenopause. When progesterone is low, the endometrium doesn't receive the support it needs to be maintained and it starts shedding early.

The bleeding process is initiated when, in the absence of conception, progesterone and oestrogen levels fall towards the end of the cycle. This hormonal drop-off, which you might feel acutely mood-wise, triggers the release of hormone-like substances called prostaglandins. Prostaglandins cause the blood vessels in your endometrium to constrict and spiral, which deprives the endometrial cells of oxygen and they die. Prostaglandins also stimulate the muscular middle layer of your uterus to contract in order to expel blood and the dead cells that need to be transported out of you. It's this contracting effect that can cause menstrual cramps and period poos too. Non-steroidal anti-inflammatories like ibuprofen work well for period pain and heavy periods, because they block the enzymes that produce prostaglandins, which is why ibuprofen is often more helpful than taking paracetamol. It's also why curcumin, an active ingredient in turmeric, can be so helpful for period pain and heavy periods, because it inhibits these enzymes too.

Heavy periods and periods that are more drawn-out become more prevalent during perimenopause when circulating oestrogen is higher and progesterone – which has a lightening effect on periods – declines. Progesterone production diminishes because you have fewer cycles where you ovulate (and you need to ovulate to produce progesterone) and, even when you do ovulate, the amount you produce isn't what it used to be, which is why the second half of your cycle can shorten and premenstrual spotting becomes more of an issue, not to mention increased premenstrual anxiety, sleep issues, breast tenderness, and premenstrual headaches and migraines.

After a couple of days of bleeding, your endometrium is ready to rebuild. By day 3, oestrogen and progesterone receptors are present, providing the lock that the keys (oestrogen and progesterone) will find and attach to, so that they can do their respective jobs of thickening and maintaining it. By day 6, your endometrium has been rebuilt and it's around 4 to 7mm thick. Now it's time to gear up for the main event of your cycle: ovulation.

Period Pain (dysmenorrhoea)

Period pain may be common but that doesn't mean it's normal or that you should accept it. A small amount of mild abdominal cramping can be expected but it shouldn't be to the degree that you're reliant on pain medication to get through the day.

You're probably wondering why it exists, especially if it feels like your uterus is raging a war every time you menstruate. Just before you start a period, the lining of your uterus breaks down and it releases prostaglandins which make it contract and relax in order to aid the physical process of bleeding. But if you release higher levels of prostaglandins then you can experience severe and painful cramping. Prostaglandins prime the nervous system for pain and heighten the pain response, and they're responsible for any nausea and vomiting that you experience around the time of your period. They're also what cause period poos because they can cause your bowels to contract. Strong uterine contractions result in an increase in intrauterine pressure which means less oxygen can get to the contracting muscles, which leads to more pain.

I experienced debilitating period pain for years, so I completely get the need for pain relief and if you're someone who has heavy flow – which is common during perimenopause – then consider using non-steroidal anti-inflammatories (NSAIDs) such as ibuprofen and naproxen, as they lower your production of prostaglandins and help with pain and blood loss. Other ways to improve period pain include:

- Reduce inflammation by cutting out or limiting your intake of sugar, alcohol and dairy, particularly in the second half of your cycle. Since my first book, *Period Power*, came out, I've received so many DMs from people telling me that cutting out cow dairy has got rid of their period pain.

- Consider if you have histamine intolerance (see page 262).
- Acupuncture, herbs and physical therapies such as physiotherapy, reflexology and the Arvigo Techniques of Maya Abdominal Therapy (see page 259) can all be a real saviour when it comes to period pain.
- Supplements such as magnesium, B-vitamins, omega-3 fatty acids (such as fish oil) and curcumin are all known for their ability to reduce period pain.
- Heat therapy, the fancy description for a hot bath or water bottle, can improve blood flow and relieve pain, and data from two clinical trials concluded that it can be as effective as treatment with an NSAID.
- Castor oil packs on your lower abdomen can be used to improve flow through the pelvis and reduce period pain. You can find instructions on how to do them on my website www.maisiehill.com/perimenopausepower
- Stop smoking. Active and passive smoking are related to menstrual pain.
- Orgasms release pain-relieving endorphins and oxytocin and many of my clients use masturbation and/or sex in their self-care plan for when they're bleeding.
- Try taking cannabidiol (CBD) oil (see page 150). If your cycle is somewhat regular, then take it 7-10 days before your period is due and during the first few days of your period. If you have no idea if you're coming or going then you're probably experiencing other symptoms that CBD can help with and may benefit from more regular use.
- Rest and exercise can both improve period pain. Some of my clients find that movement whilst they're bleeding helps with pain, and for others it's a total no go, so experiment and see what helps you. Exercise throughout the menstrual cycle can help with lots of cycle-related symptoms, and it's great for your bones and mental health too.
- Some people are sensitive to nightshade vegetables such as white potatoes, aubergine, peppers and tomatoes, and eating them can result in inflammation and pain.

Period pain is common in those with conditions such as endometriosis and adenomyosis, which we'll cover in more detail in Chapter 9.

Pre-ovulation

Okay, I kind of lied when I told you that this is the point in the cycle where your body gears up for ovulation. It's true that a lot happens in this final week or so, but it's really the home straight of a *very* long race. One that started when you were in your mum's uterus.

When your mum was pregnant with you, you had the most ovarian follicles you've ever had – 7 million – but from week 24 of her pregnancy, they started dying off in huge numbers, so that by the time you were born, only 1 million remained. Once you entered puberty, 400,000 were left. At that point, a few follicles commenced growth every day, so that throughout your reproductive years there would be a continual supply of follicles ready to be recruited as contenders for ovulation. But most never get called up. In fact, only around 400 or so end up being released as a mature egg at ovulation, accounting for the average number of periods you're likely to have. The ones that don't make the grade deteriorate and are absorbed by the body.

Around six months before a follicle releases its egg at ovulation it develops a blood supply and moves through several stages of development. Towards the end of each menstrual cycle, these follicles get the nod from follicle stimulating hormone (FSH) that their time has come and a group of them is recruited. Despite all that's happened before this, these follicles are still considered to be immature. And they're about to be put through their paces. Under the influence of FSH they mature and start to produce oestrogen, which is why, from day 3 or so in your cycle, you might notice an increase in energy and positivity. By day 6, one follicle outshines the rest in both maturity and size, and it secretes increasing amounts of oestrogen. In combination with the other ovarian hormone, inhibin, oestrogen sends a signal to the pituitary gland in your head to produce less FSH. It's how your ovaries communicate that they've got the follicle for this cycle – there's no need to keep searching for a candidate and FSH can stand down.

During the early stage of perimenopause, this process shifts a bit. For a start, there are fewer follicles left to recruit. Your brain is also having to work harder at communicating with your ovaries, so FSH is higher. More FSH means that follicles grow earlier in the cycle than they used to and they also grow more rapidly. Research which compared the follicle size of women under the age of 34 to those who were 45 years old and over found that although follicle growth was initially more substantial in the older group thanks to increased FSH early on in the cycle, the peak diameter of the follicle just before ovulation was less than that of the younger women. As you might expect, the maturation process of a dominant follicle was also less likely to succeed in the older women, resulting in anovulatory cycles (see the box below).

A study of 511 premenopausal and perimenopausal women found that 10 years before the final period took place, most cycles were ones where ovulation took place. Ovulatory cycles slowly became less frequent until four to five years before the final period, at which point the number of ovulatory cycles rapidly declined along with progesterone production. In the final year, only 22.8 per cent of cycles showed evidence of ovulation.

Can You Have a Period Without Ovulating?

Yes.

When we talk about the menstrual cycle, we're actually talking about what scientists call the ovulatory cycle. That's because ovulation takes place roughly two weeks before you have a period. But there are times when you don't ovulate and have an *anovulatory cycle.*

In an ovulatory cycle, it's the rapid withdrawal of oestrogen and progesterone at the end of the luteal phase that stimulates menstruation. In an anovulatory cycle you don't have a luteal phase or period, because without ovulation, you don't produce progesterone. Instead, you're in a prolonged follicular phase where you'll produce varying levels of oestrogen and, at some point, you'll experience anovulatory bleeding (aka breakthrough bleeding).

It's common to experience occasional anovulatory cycles throughout our cycling years, often in response to stress, undereating and disordered eating, over-exercising and whilst recovering from using hormonal birth control. They're also common in those with polycystic ovarian syndrome (PCOS). There are times in life when they are more prevalent too, such as during the teen years and perimenopause. In fact, anovulatory cycles are one reason why you *and* your teenager could both be struggling with periods that are long and heavy. (Side-note: be kind to each other.) This is because progesterone inhibits the growth of the endometrium and reduces the volume of blood you'll lose during a period. Without progesterone, you miss out on its ability to lighten your periods.

Cycles that are shorter than 21 days and longer than 35 days are more likely to be anovulatory than those that are 21 to 35 days long. Prolonged bleeding that lasts more than seven days and/or heavy bleeding can suggest an anovulatory cycle, but your flow can also be lighter than normal or the same as it usually is. The best way to establish whether you're ovulating or not is to track your basal body temperature (BBT), because after ovulation your temperature rises. Tracking your BBT is a great way to establish if and when you're ovulating.

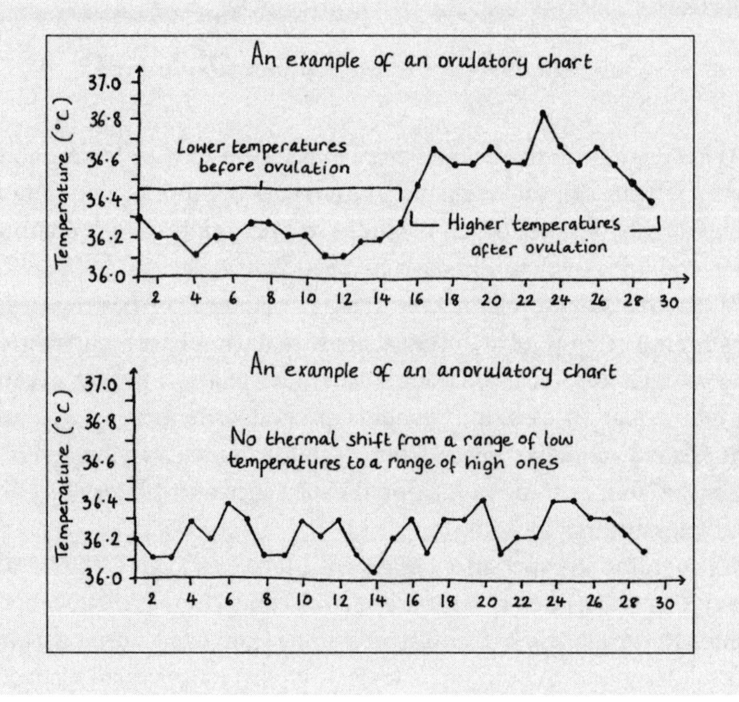

As the dominant follicle continues to grow and ripen, oestrogen levels climb, causing your endometrium to thicken to 10 to 11mm and your cervix to produce fertile-quality mucus. Cervical fluid changes throughout the cycle in response to what oestrogen and progesterone are getting up to. There will be times when you don't produce any and have 'dry days', but once oestrogen is on the scene, you produce mucus that is described as fertile. That's because in its presence, sperm can survive for up to five days. The first type of mucus you might see (might, because we're all different) is what's described as *non-peak mucus*. Non-peak mucus can look white and creamy and is fertile, i.e. if you have unprotected sex during this time, conception is possible. Peak mucus is produced when oestrogen is high in the days before ovulation. It's clear, stretchy, and is thinner and more watery, often resembling egg whites. If you pay attention to how it feels when you wipe yourself after going to the toilet, you might notice that there are times when you wipe and your hand speeds up, and glides past your vulva and perineum. That's due to the presence of mucus that's slippery. As we age, we produce less cervical fluid, which reduces the number of days in each cycle that we're considered to be fertile.

Oestrogen production is maintained at the same level in older women as it is in younger women and can even be higher. A few days before ovulation, oestrogen reaches its peak and a hormonal sequence is triggered, instigating the final growth spurt that your follicle needs in order to release the mature egg it contains. This surge of growth creates a bulge on the surface of the follicle/ovary, which then ruptures, and, just like that, your mature egg is released.

In early perimenopause, raised FSH and normal/high oestrogen means that you ovulate on the early side, which is why cycles often shorten. With time, your sensitivity to oestrogen becomes reduced and messages aren't always received. The LH surge which triggers ovulation becomes erratic, so sometimes you ovulate and sometimes you don't. At the same time, follicles become less sensitive to FSH and LH, and oestrogen levels start to fall, which results in luteal phase defects and more anovulatory cycles.

Luteal Phase: Ovulation to Menstruation

After ovulation, something happens that will always blow my mind. The follicle that released the egg collapses and folds in on itself, turns yellow and is now referred to as the corpus luteum (Latin for 'yellow body'). Now, I don't wanna knock a follicle's ability to change colour, because that's a pretty cool party trick, but there's something else it does that astounds me: it develops its own blood supply, turns into a temporary gland and starts to produce and secrete progesterone – the hormone that supports the second half of the cycle and pregnancy if it were to occur – all in the space of 24 hours. MIND. BLOW. ING.

Progesterone causes cervical fluid to dry up and thicken up. Whereas fertile cervical fluid assists sperm in their journey to the egg and keeps them alive, non-fertile cervical fluid produced after ovulation stops them in their tracks. Due to the warming effect of progesterone, its sudden presence also causes your basal body temperature (BBT) to go up, though in perimenopause this can be slower or less significant than it used to be.

In the second half of the cycle, both oestrogen and progesterone are produced, but for most of our cycling years, progesterone is secreted in far greater amounts. As you get to know your cycle, think about how progesterone might be driving your behaviour in the second half of your cycle. Less interested in going out? That's progesterone trying to keep you safe in case you're housing an embryo. Raiding the fridge? That's progesterone making sure you have enough calories and nutrients to support a pregnancy, especially if you're not eating enough protein. No interest in getting knocked up and wondering if this still applies to you? Your ovaries didn't get that memo.

In the world of hormones, progesterone plays second fiddle to oestrogen. Medical professionals extol the many virtues of oestrogen, but it's rare to see someone showing progesterone some love. Oestrogen loves to sparkle, but progesterone is the supporting actress who carries the film without hogging the limelight.

And progesterone does way more than support pregnancy. It calms and soothes the nervous system, improves sleep, reduces inflammation, stimulates the building of bone tissue and supports breast health. It also keeps oestrogen in check, which is a very good thing. When oestrogen is unopposed by progesterone its ability to make things grow gets a little out of hand. Cysts on your ovaries, breast/chest lumps, the lining of your uterus (the endometrium) and hormone-sensitive tumours are all associated with high levels of oestrogen. But before you start hating on oestrogen, remember that she's awesome too. This isn't about two celebrities being pitted against each other on the cover of a magazine, it's about the relationship between them. They're both essential.

If implantation doesn't happen, the corpus luteum begins to disintegrate 12 to 16 days after it formed and progesterone levels drop. This sends a signal to the endometrium that it's time to break down, initiating menstruation and the return to the follicular phase. The 12- to 16-day lifespan of the corpus luteum is why the luteal phase is relatively fixed in length for most of our cycling years: you can't have a long luteal phase, though it can certainly become shorter once progesterone levels decline during perimenopause.

The Progesterone Drop-off

Progesterone has long been described as having a calming effect on the nervous system, which is why you might find it easier to fall asleep and sleep more deeply around the time progesterone is peaking, which is five to seven days after ovulation or around day 21 in a 28-day cycle. Once your body recognises that conception hasn't taken place, the corpus luteum degenerates and progesterone production stops for the cycle. Oestrogen also declines and the combined effects of this can be felt rapidly. It's where you can go from feeling calm and focussed one day then wake up a teary hot mess the next, or start the day feeling like your usual self and then begin to unravel at some point. I've had many, many clients describe it like their mind and world are falling apart.

Feeling vulnerable, raw, teary, a deep need to be alone, to be surrounded by nature, to abandon daily life in some way or simply feeling slightly out of it are all signs that you're entering this phase. It might occur two days or two hours before you start bleeding, so be aware of yourself in the days before your period is due, because you are being guided to a deep place, one of instinct that you'll potentially miss out on, or dismiss as simply feeling anxious or depressed.

If you're aware of when you ovulate and know how long your luteal phase is, then you can estimate when your period will start and when the progesterone drop-off will hit. If you're tracking your BBT (see page 34) then you might notice that your temperature drops in the days before your period begins. Doing this means that you can at least understand what's going on when it happens and go easy on yourself. But ideally it means you can prepare and compensate for it, so that it isn't as sudden or severe. Here's what clients have found useful:

- Eat regularly. This is not the time to skip meals.
- Have some home-cooked food in the freezer ready to take out, so that you aren't left staring at the dubious contents of your fridge or relying on takeaway.
- Avoid alcohol. This is often when people want to drink, but it will exacerbate how you're feeling. You really don't need a hangover whilst you're in the progesterone drop-off.

- Sit with your feelings and give them space. Cry. And I know that this can be challenging when you're in certain environments, such as your workplace, but if you can give yourself five minutes to allow your feelings to come up, acknowledge and name them, then that puts you in a place where you can move on. If you stuff them down and try to keep the mask on, your feelings will become more intense and it'll take far more energy and effort to go about your day. Feel your feelings.
- Have a comfortable outfit that you feel happy in, cleaned and ready to wear. This is not a time to have all your favourite clothes in the laundry and only have dressy outfits or clothes that don't suit you as well left in your wardrobe.
- No house guests.
- Lie down with a blanket and watch *This is Us*.
- Move your body in a way that feels good and helps you to let go of any pent-up energy and feelings. Channel Taylor Swift and shake it off.

The Cycle Strategy

By the end of this book, you're going to have a chunky toolkit of tips and techniques that you can use throughout your perimenopause and beyond menopause itself too. But I'm going to start with the biggest and most important one: tracking your cycle. Now, I appreciate that if your cycle currently lacks consistency and predictability, then the thought of tracking it may seem pointless, but bear with me.

If you've read my first book, *Period Power*, then you'll already be familiar with the Cycle Strategy – my take on using menstrual cycle awareness to improve your experience of the cycle and to get what you want out of life – but it's worth revisiting it from the perspective of perimenopause as the hormonal variations we experience here can create a very different experience to what you're used to.

If the Cycle Strategy is new to you, then get ready to be fascinated by how your hormones affect your mood, energy and behaviour. Be prepared to feel sad and angry that you didn't have this tool for the past 20 or so years, when you probably could've really done with it. But among those understandable and valid feelings, know that it's not too late to get to know yourself in this way.

In many ways, tracking and working with your cycle during perimenopause is where you can get the most out of it.

After a few months of tracking your cycle (you can download a free guide and charts from my website to help you to do this) you'll get a sense of your personal patterns, powers and pitfalls, and be able to make adjustments here and there to improve your experience of your cycle and make use of each phase.

The goal with this is not to have a perfect experience of your cycle. I don't know anyone who feels amazing throughout all their cycle and I don't expect you to. Life is 50:50 – half the time we feel great and half the time we don't. The menstrual cycle is no different, it's just that the 50:50 split might literally mean that you experience one half of it positively and one half negatively.

If menstrual cycle awareness isn't about having a perfect cycle, then what is the goal? Even if you have a predictable cycle, both in terms of length and experience, it's highly unlikely that you're in a position that allows you to attune daily life to suit your cycle all the time. But menstrual cycle awareness is much the same as knowing the weather in advance. When you know that rain or thunderstorms are due then there may be times where you're able to change your plans and stay indoors, but most of the time you just have to dress appropriately and crack on with your day. And yeah, the weather forecast isn't always accurate, but it does give you a sense of how you can be prepared for sudden downpours in perimenopause.

The Cycle Strategy goes beyond just keeping track of the dates, though that in itself has tremendous value. It is a framework that enables you to deal with the tough days and make the most of the awesome ones, which is essential when your hormones and cycle are liable to go off-piste. One of the biggest gifts of cycle tracking is being able to adjust your diary to suit your cycle, where possible. But I don't know anyone, including myself, who can organise their diary to suit their cycle all the time. And that's especially true during perimenopause, when the cycle can gift you unexpected surprises.

Cycle irregularities along the lines of no period for two months and then two in the space of one month are common during perimenopause, as Vikki, a member of my online membership The Flow Collective told me, 'It's hard to know where you are when your body is not following the script anymore!' Whilst it can seem like there's no point in charting your cycle once all sense of predictability seems to have gone out of the window, there is still tremendous value in the data that you collect. In perimenopause, menstrual cycle awareness can help you to:

- Get to know the range of your cycle's irregularity – are they always shorter, are they becoming more drawn-out or is there a pattern in the occurrence of longer and shorter cycles?
- Identify the emergence of new signs and symptoms.
- Note whether your signs and symptoms are improving or worsening.
- Spot patterns in what aggravates or helps your symptoms.
- Notice how your cycle varies in terms of your experience of it and how your cycle responds to what's going on in your life.
- Pinpoint how your energy, mood and behaviour respond to your hormones.
- Make the most of the times when you feel on top of the world or at least at base camp.

If your life currently feels full, overwhelming and stressful, then you may be reading this and thinking it all sounds great, but it isn't possible for you. You're too busy to bother to keep track. There's no point. Your day-to-day life isn't predictable. You don't have the ability to control your diary. You have kids. You've got all these things going on. And I get it. I told myself all those things too. But that's exactly what they are, they're stories that you're telling yourself. I don't doubt that you are facing challenges that are all-consuming, as is often the case with this phase of life. I don't doubt that you fulfil several roles, all of which require your time, energy and patience, all of which are in short supply. If all this sounds familiar, then congratulations – you've found your why. When it comes to forming a new habit, establishing your motivation for doing it – your why – is essential. And if you're always rushing, knackered and barking at anyone who requests something of you, then you need this because it will change your life.

2

It's getting hot in here

When you're young, you're fertile, you're producing eggs, you're bringing life into the world, right? You're bringing life into the world. And then you get older, no more eggs. You can't bring any more life into the world... so they just set you on fire. What kind of shit is that?

– Wanda Sykes

If you're already experiencing them then you don't need me to tell you that hot flushes are a swift and exaggerated way of dissipating heat. If you aren't experiencing them, then buckle up because you're likely to. Hot flushes are the most well-known menopausal symptom and for good reason – in Western countries, up to 88 per cent of us will experience them. This number does vary and can be as low as 9.5 per cent in Japan, though that particular study was conducted in 1984 and a more recent study found the rate to be 36.9 per cent, which is still lower than that of Western countries.

Their frequency can vary hugely too. Some people will have as few as five per year and others will experience as many as 50 per day, with individuals also experiencing variations in how long they last – the duration of hot flushes has been reported as generally being between one to five minutes, though some can last up to an hour.

As a feature of both perimenopause and postmenopause, hot flushes and night sweats can persist in the years following your last period. In the Study of Women's Health Across the Nation, which studied 3,302 US women undergoing the menopause transition, the average duration was 7.4 years. At the age of 65, 25 per cent of us will still be experiencing them. In one study of women aged 85, around 16 per cent were still experiencing hot flushes and almost 10 per cent of these women were still moderately or very distressed by them.

What each person experiences will vary, but typically hot flushes feature a sudden sensation of heat which is often accompanied by sweating and reddening of the skin. As well as the sense of heat, hot flushes can be accompanied by dry mouth, palpitations, an adrenalin rush, breathlessness, dizziness and nausea. They can occur spontaneously or in response to changes in environmental temperature, stress, emotions such as embarrassment and shame, or drinking caffeine, alcohol and warm drinks. Here's how some of my clients described their flushes:

'Heat that radiates from my chest and tingles. I have to stop whatever I'm doing and take some clothes off or I start to feel sick.'

'It's like molten lava rampaging through you with nowhere to go, followed by having a cold bucket of water chucked over you.'

'The heat swallows me up, like being on fire from the inside out.'

'The combination of heat and panic makes me feel like I'm trapped in a furnace.'

But they can also feel milder, like someone's turned the central heating up a notch or hot prickles on your chest and back:

'You know the sudden flush of heat that you get when you feel embarrassed? It's a bit like that.'

'I feel hot and have to take a layer of clothing off, then five minutes later I have to put it back on again, and that's basically how I spend my day – taking my sweater on and off. I'd rather that than what some of my friends are going through though.'

Hot flushes can have a tremendous impact on the personal and professional lives of those experiencing them, and the consequences of them are often underestimated. Not everyone will view them negatively though. My friend Val swears they're the reason she lost weight during her transition and she told me that her skin looked incredible. Plus, she loved accessorising with beautiful fans and her heating bill plummeted.

Risk factors for developing severe hot flushes include:

- Surgical menopause
- Obesity
- Smoking
- Childhood neglect or abuse (the impact of abuse continues long after it has stopped)
- Prior anxiety or depression
- History of taking the oral contraceptive pill.

Despite their prevalence and impact on quality of life, the underlying mechanism that results in a hot flush remains unknown. Although hot flushes are associated with the lower levels of oestrogen that accompany the later stages of the menopause transition, they can also occur prior to the withdrawal of oestrogen, so the explanation of a low oestrogen state is inadequate.

I hesitate to include a study that's almost as old as I am, but this one is often referenced in more recent research papers because it could find no relationships between the presence of hot flushes and the levels of oestrogens in blood, urine or the vagina – surprising, right? The same study also found no differences in the levels of oestrogen between those who have hot flushes and those who don't. We also know that a drug called clonidine can reduce hot flushes but that it doesn't raise oestrogen levels, which gives further weight to the idea that hot flushes aren't about low oestrogen. What does differ are the levels of activity in a part of the brain known as the central noradrenergic system (CNA) and it's the discovery of these changes that has led to the leading hypothesis of why we get hot flushes.

Your body is skilled at maintaining a core internal temperature of around 37°C, regardless of what the external temperature is up to. Most of the time, you can regulate your internal temperature without much effort. If the room you're in is hot, your body will direct blood flow to your skin in order to get rid of heat and maintain its core temperature, whereas if the room you're in is cool, your blood vessels constrict in order to minimise heat loss (this is why some skin tones will pale in cooler temperatures). When your body maintains its core temperature like this, it's in a thermoneutral zone, i.e. the range of temperatures that you can maintain a normal body temperature at without using energy beyond your basal metabolic rate, which, for simplicity's sake, we'll call what your body can do whilst resting. If more activity is required in order to regulate your temperature, such as shivering when you're cold or sweating when you're hot, then you move beyond your thermoneutral zone.

Changes to this process of thermoregulation are what's thought to result in symptoms such as hot flushes and night sweats. During the menopause transition, the thermoneutral zone narrows and when the upper threshold is crossed, a signal is sent out to get rid of heat. Wanna take a guess at how it accomplishes this? By dilating your blood vessels and increasing blood flow to your skin. And sweating, lots of sweating. In other words, your body has to do more in order to regulate your temperature.

Depressed mood and anxiety are strong predictors of hot flushes during the menopause transition. Those with moderate to high levels of anxiety experienced three to five times greater frequency and severity of hot flushes when compared to those who had lower levels of anxiety. This begs the question, do anxiety, depression and stress trigger hot flushes or is it the other way around? As you might imagine, it's one of those relationships that goes both ways; feeling anxious can precede a hot flush and if you have a hot flush, it can cause you to feel anxious.

How to Play It Cool

So let's run through the options for treating and managing hot flushes and night sweats.

Hormone therapy

When it comes to hot flushes and night sweats that are frequent and/or severe, hormone therapy is the most effective treatment strategy that is also easy to access through your GP (or at least it should be, provided that your GP is following the National Institute of Health and Care Excellence (NICE) guidelines and the supplies of HRT are sorted out). More often than not, oestrogen is the hormone that is focussed on, but during perimenopause oestrogen is often high and erratic, in which case body-identical progesterone can be used to treat hot flushes, night sweats and insomnia. If, however, you're also experiencing symptoms of low oestrogen, such as vaginal dryness and painful joints (see page 54 for a full list), then using oestrogen and progesterone would be more beneficial.

The Problem with HRT

So far I've used the term hormone replacement therapy (HRT) to describe the hormone therapy that is available during the menopause transition, but to be honest, I'm not a fan of HRT – but my dislike of it has nothing to do with how and why it's used. My problem with HRT is its name, because hormone replacement therapy implies that there are missing hormones that need to be replaced and I think we can all agree that all of us experience a decline in hormones during midlife because for some reason, that's what's meant to happen. Now that doesn't mean to say you can't or shouldn't use hormone therapy, but let's ditch the word replacement and call it menopause hormone therapy (MHT) instead, as most research scientists already do.

Tibolone

Tibolone is medication which mimics the activity of oestrogen, progesterone and testosterone. It's a synthetic steroid that's used as an alternative to hormone therapy in those who can't take it, to reduce hot flushes and night sweats, improve genito-urinary symptoms and prevent bone loss. Tibolone is associated with an increased risk of developing breast cancer in those who've previously had breast cancer and who are over the age of 60, but in younger women not affected by breast cancer, no increased risk has been found.

Antidepressant drugs: SSRIs and SNRIs

SSRIs and SNRIs such as venlafaxine, desvenlafaxine, paroxetine, citalopram and escitalopram can be used to reduce the frequency and severity of hot flushes by anywhere from 10 to 64 per cent, depending on the study, though some trials have found that taking a placebo is almost as effective. If you have a history of breast cancer and are taking tamoxifen you should not take SSRIs as they interfere with the action of tamoxifen, but SNRIs such as venlafaxine and desvenlafaxine are safe to take.

Clonidine

Clonidine is a drug that's used to treat high blood pressure and prevent recurrent migraines. It also widens the thermoneutral zone, which means that it can reduce the frequency of hot flushes. Clonidine is licensed for use in perimenopause and postmenopause, but side effects include insomnia, unpleasant dreams, low blood pressure, dry mouth, tiredness and constipation.

Gabapentin

Gabapentin is an anti-seizure medication that's used to treat epilepsy and it can be used to treat neuropathic (nerve) pain, including pain following shingles and trigeminal neuralgia (severe pain in your facial nerves). One trial found that gabapentin is as effective as low-dose oestrogen at improving vasomotor symptoms and it can also improve sleep quality. Side effects include increased appetite, weight gain, dizziness, drowsiness and unsteadiness. Gabapentin can be used in those with hormone-positive breast cancer and, unlike SSRIs, does not interact with tamoxifen.

Pregabalin

Similar to gabapentin, pregabalin is an anti-seizure medication that can be used to treat vasomotor symptoms and, although the same range of side effects applies, they may be less severe.

Paced respiration

Paced respiration refers to slow, deliberate, deep breathing. Instead of the average 15 breaths we take a minute, breathing rate is slowed to six to eight times per minute. Some studies have found that paced respiration reduces the frequency of hot flushes by 50 per cent and there are no known side effects other than feeling calm and grounded. I recommend practising paced respiration in the morning and evening for clients of all ages, as it's a great way to stimulate the vagus nerve (see page 140) and relax your nervous system, and it can be used at the onset of a hot flush too.

CBT

Cognitive behavioural therapy (CBT) is a form of talking therapy that focuses on how your thoughts, beliefs and attitudes affect your feelings and behaviour. Though it doesn't appear to reduce the frequency of hot flushes, CBT is effective at reducing their impact, i.e. how much of a problem they are for the person experiencing them. This is important as we know that our attitude and anxiety about having hot flushes intensifies the severity of them. The North American Menopause Society recommends CBT as a non-hormonal strategy for hot flushes and in the UK the NICE guidelines recommend it for anxiety and/or low mood in relation to menopause.

Acupuncture

As an acupuncturist who has treated a lot of perimenopausal and postmenopausal women, I am of course going to tell you that acupuncture is incredible. I've used it to successfully treat hot flushes, night sweats, palpitations, restlessness in the evening, sleep issues, excessive thirst, anxiety, depression and irritability (not to mention a whole host of gynaecological issues such as menstrual flooding and period pain). Some research has shown that it is effective in treating vasomotor symptoms and some have concluded that it's as effective as a placebo (though trying to conduct an acupuncture trial is tricky, because for the placebo arm of the trial you still have to put needles in someone and that will always do something). Acupuncture isn't accessible to everyone, because only a handful of clinics operate within the NHS. If you're keen to give it a go but affordability is an issue, search for a community acupuncture practice near you or go to a supervised student clinic as these treatments are usually significantly lower in price.

Phytoestrogens

Phytoestrogens are chemicals that resemble oestrogen, which are converted into weak oestrogenic substances in the digestive tract. There are three types of phytoestrogens – isoflavones (the most potent), coumestans and lignans – and they're found in soybeans, hops, flaxseed, fruits, vegetables, whole grains and legumes. Some research has found that supplementing with soy isoflavones for 12 weeks results in a reduction of hot flushes, whereas other trials have found no improvement. Some menopausal herbal remedies such as black cohosh and red clover are phytoestrogens. The types of phytoestrogens and treatment protocols used in these trials have varied greatly and it's possible that the gut microbiome of the participants involved could impact the ability to convert isoflavones into oestrogenic substances. Phytoestrogens can't be taken alongside medication that contains oestrogens, such as the birth control pill and menopause hormone therapy (MHT), and shouldn't be used by anyone with breast cancer.

Black cohosh (*Cimicifuga racemosa*)

Studies have demonstrated that black cohosh – a herb that can be taken as a tincture or capsules – is effective in treating menopausal symptoms such as hot flushes and because it doesn't contain phytoestrogens it can be used safely by those who can't take oestrogens. If you're interested in using herbs during perimenopause then I recommend working with a qualified medical herbalist. If seeing a qualified practitioner privately isn't possible, then look for a student clinic at a university where final-year students see patients under supervised conditions at reduced cost.

Vitamin E

Taking 400 IUs of vitamin E a day for four weeks can reduce hot flushes, and it's an anti-inflammatory and powerful antioxidant, so it can be helpful if you smoke, are exposed to environmental toxins or have high levels of inflammation and/or oxidative stress. It's also great for your skin. When supplementing, pick vitamin E that contains mixed tocopherols and tocotrienols so that the various forms of vitamin E remain in balance with each other.

Pomegranate

Some studies have found that pomegranate seed oil can reduce menopausal symptoms such as hot flushes, sleep issues, depression, exhaustion and vaginal dryness.

Red clover (*Trifolium pratense*)

Red clover is another phytoestrogen and it's said to help with symptoms such as hot flushes and night sweats, though once again the evidence from research is mixed. My personal experience is that a herbal blend that contained red clover stopped my premenstrual night sweats, though it's impossible to say if this was due to the action of red clover or the combination of supportive ingredients.

Sage (*Salvia officinalis*)

Sage has been used for centuries to treat menopausal symptoms, especially hot flushes and night sweats, thanks to its drying effect. Like many herbs, some people swear by it and others find it makes no difference, and the mixed research around its use reflects this. Working with a medical herbalist is a worthwhile investment here, because they'll suggest herbs that suit your particular scenario at an effective dose. Some types of sage contain a chemical called thujone which can cause negative side effects such as rapid heartbeat and vomiting, so be sure to buy 'thujone-free' sage.

Ziziphus (*Ziziphus spinosa*)

Ziziphus is a herb used in traditional Chinese medicine that's derived from red date and it can aid sleep, reduce anxiety and relieve excessive sweating. In Chinese medicine it's said to nourish the heart and calm the spirit, so you can see why it's a popular option for managing menopausal symptoms.

Rhubarb (*Rheum rhaponticum*)

A dried extract from the roots of rhubarb has been commercially available in Germany for several decades and studies have found that it can safely treat menopausal symptoms and reduce the severity of hot flushes thanks to its oestrogenic actions (though because of this, those with oestrogen-dependent cancers should not use it).

CASE STUDY

Simone came to me because she'd been experiencing an interesting array of symptoms and her friend had suggested that they could be hormonal in nature, but it hadn't occurred to Simone that 'hormonal' could mean perimenopausal. Simone was 42, recently single and enjoying the dating scene. On the one hand, she felt full of youth and was excited about her future, but she'd noticed that she didn't have the physical energy to keep up with how she felt mentally. Simone struggled to make it through the day and was reliant on caffeine. She worked as a creative director, which meant she was used to having boozy lunches with clients. And once she was home at night, she liked to unwind with a drink whilst she cooked spicy dinners.

Evenings were when the majority of her symptoms would appear: hot flushes, a feeling of restlessness that bordered on anxiety even when she was feeling relaxed on the sofa, palpitations, trouble falling asleep and then night sweats once she did, and waking up at 4.30am unable to return to sleep. No wonder she was so shattered. But I had to be straight with Simone and I told her that if she wanted to get the most out of her treatments, we'd need to look at her diet and lifestyle, and that meant significantly reducing or cutting out alcohol entirely, and swapping hot spicy food for a more cooling diet.

Simone was keen to negotiate what that looked like, particularly on the alcohol side of things. She decided that she would limit drinking alcohol to two nights a week and that she'd stay clear of client lunches for a couple of weeks (she didn't think she would be able to, in her words, 'stay strong' so she opted to avoid them for the time being). I gave her a list of foods to lean away from – rich meats like lamb, pork and beef, and heating spices like chilli and ginger – as well as a list of foods to lean towards such as seafood, avocado, broccoli, asparagus, cucumber and melon (for a full list of heating and cooling foods from the Chinese medicine perspective, head to www.maisiehill.com/perimenopausepower). We focussed on her eating enough protein throughout the day as she rarely ate a portion until lunch, by which time she was already feeling tired. Once her protein intake was up, she realised that she didn't need as much caffeine and was able to stick with one black coffee in the morning. I suggested she add a teaspoon of powdered cordyceps – a medicinal mushroom (see page 152) – to this for extra energy. Simone started taking a women's multivitamin and magnesium too. We also started with weekly acupuncture. Her symptoms commonly appear together in Chinese medicine and are pretty straightforward to treat, which she was relieved to discover. We discussed the possibility of using micronised body-identical progesterone, and although Simone was glad to know that she could access progesterone through her GP, we agreed that it would be best to assess the effects of everything else we were doing first.

Simone noticed an immediate difference in how she felt after our sessions – the restlessness, palpitations and hot flushes reduced, she started to sleep better and her energy was picking up so that she could actually stay awake when she went out on an evening date. But she was dismayed to discover that drinking alcohol and eating spicy food were massive triggers for her symptoms, and she told me she wanted to reduce her intake of them even more, so we got to work on finding substitutes. We found other ways of adding flavour to her meals and going to restorative yoga classes in the evening helped her wind down instead of reaching for a glass of wine.

Tactics you can employ to improve hot flushes and night sweats include:

- Reduce sources of stress and anxiety that could be causing or exacerbating hot flushes. I know, easier said than done, but I've got some suggestions to help you with this coming up in Chapter 6.
- Avoid spicy food and hot drinks.
- Lower your alcohol intake. The evidence based around whether alcohol worsens vasomotor symptoms is mixed – some studies have concluded that it does, whereas others have concluded that alcohol actually improves them. Most of the clients I've treated have been unwilling to limit their alcohol intake, but once they do, they notice a difference.
- Wearing natural, loose, breathable clothing can make a difference. Linen trousers won't appeal to all of you. Kemi Telford is a great example of stylish clothing for those of you who have no desire to become wallflowers, but who also want to be comfortable.
- If you share a bed with someone, use two single duvets instead of one large one, like the Swedes and Danes do. Doing this can also improve sleep quality and lessen the 'you stole the duvet' disagreements too.
- Keep a bedroom window open at night or use a quiet fan.
- Some people find relief with a cooling gel pad mattress topper and cooling pads can also be inserted inside your pillowcase.
- Use cotton sheets instead of man-made fibres or polycotton blends.
- Make a cooling spritz to use when you feel a hot flush coming on. Using a glass bottle with a spray attachment, add 10 drops of lavender essential oil and 15 drops of peppermint essential oil to 100ml of water. Shake before each use to distribute the oil through the water and spray onto your skin for an instant cooling effect.
- Use electrical or paper fans. Though an investment, I've heard that the Dyson cooling fans are powerful but quiet enough to have running at night without disturbing your sleep.

Be Still, My Beating Heart

Palpitations are common and more often than not harmless. That being said, when your heartbeat becomes more rapid, strong or irregular, it can freak you the fuck out. You might feel palpitations as a flutter or a skipped beat, and you might get them for only a few moments, but that doesn't stop them from being unnerving. Palpitations can happen as a result of:

- Emotions and psychological triggers
- Dehydration
- Caffeine
- Anaemia – have your palpitations started since your periods have become heavy?
- Nutrient deficiencies
- Thyroid dysfunction
- Histamine intolerance
- Medications such as asthma inhalers, high blood pressure medications, antihistamines, antibiotics and antidepressants, such as citalopram and escitalopram
- Recreational drugs
- Low blood sugar and diabetes
- Physical exertion
- Feeling hot(!)
- The hormonal fluctuations of menopause.

Your heart is designed to respond to stress so that it beats faster and can pump blood to the parts of the body needed for a fight-or-flight response, but high levels of these hormones can cause high blood pressure and other heart problems. During our cycling years, oestrogen protects against the toxic effects of these hormones, so when the amount of oestrogen you produce drops in perimenopause and postmenopause, stress hormones have more of an impact on your heart and can lead to palpitations. Palpitations can occur during a hot flush, so that you're not just experiencing the intensity of the heat, but also the feeling of a horse galloping through your chest at the same time. If you get palpitations, here's what you can do:

- Stay hydrated
- Do what you can to reduce anxiety and stress by addressing the causes
- Practise regulating your nervous system with breathing techniques (see page 143)
- Prioritise sleep
- Limit/cut out alcohol and caffeine
- Stop smoking
- Avoid food and drink that triggers a histamine response if you suspect you are intolerant (see page 264)
- Keep your blood sugar balanced by eating regularly
- Address anaemia or any other nutrient deficiencies, such as B vitamins and magnesium
- Consider using body-identical progesterone
- Consider using oestrogen
- Speak to your GP if you suspect medication you're taking could be causing them
- *Speak to your GP if your palpitations last a long time or are getting worse, if you have a history of heart problems, or if you're concerned about them.*

Hot flushes and night sweats during perimenopause and after are associated with changes to blood pressure, cholesterol levels and high body mass index (BMI), though this could be because the risk factors for hot flushes, such as increased weight and smoking, are also risk factors for an unfavourable cardiovascular risk profile. If you're experiencing them then this news is probably going to be concerning to you, but bear in mind that when it comes to serious health issues like heart attacks we often say, 'If only there'd been a warning sign.' It appears that hot flushes *are* an early warning sign, so you can decide to think that reading this is good news and take preventative action by stopping smoking, exercising regularly and eating a healthy diet.

Low, Low, Low

During the early stage of the perimenopause, oestrogen goes wild – the ebb and flow of your cycle turns into a rollercoaster ride with plenty of steep plummets. Symptoms during this phase can be described as excessive: frequent cycles, heavy flow, irritability, rage, breast/chest swelling and tenderness, and bloating, etc. In late perimenopause, though, oestrogen begins to decline and the symptoms switch to those that can be grouped together as signs and symptoms of deficiency. Signs and symptoms of low oestrogen include:

- Absent or irregular periods
- Lethargy
- Depression
- Anxiety
- Feeling fragile emotionally compared to how you used to feel
- Joint pain
- Poor memory
- Vaginal dryness or loss of feeling
- Painful sex
- Low sexual desire
- Night sweats or hot flushes
- Insomnia
- Waking in the middle of the night or far earlier than you'd like to
- A leaky or overactive bladder
- Bladder infections
- Wrinkles
- Dry skin and eyes
- Melasma (sun damage)
- Low bone density
- Loss of hair on the head.

These symptoms are classically associated with menopause, but it's important to know that they can show up at other times too, so experiencing them doesn't necessarily mean that you're menopausal. I've had plenty of clients in their thirties exhibit signs and symptoms of oestrogen deficiency, and only one case was due to premature ovarian insufficiency – a condition in which ovarian function declines prematurely. You can be deficient in oestrogen after coming off hormonal birth control such as the pill, and after having a baby and breastfeeding. High stress levels, over-exercising, disordered eating, low-fat diets, inadequate nutrition, thyroid dysfunction and some medications can also impact on oestrogen production, so you can see why the stage is often set for oestrogen deficiency outside of menopause.

If you start experiencing these symptoms before the age of 45, speak to your GP about having some blood tests done to figure out why. If you're over the age of 45 and experiencing them, then it's safe to assume that you're perimenopausal. If you're over the age of 45, haven't had a period in a year and are experiencing these symptoms, then it's likely that you're postmenopausal.

During your cycling years, the dominant form of oestrogen circulating around your body is oestradiol (E2) and it's produced by your ovaries. It's the kind of oestrogen that we talk about in terms of your menstrual cycle. Once your ovaries stop producing oestradiol in this way, they do still secrete androgens which can be converted into another type of oestrogen called oestrone (E1), and your adrenal glands also supply androgens that can be converted.

In postmenopause it's oestrone (E1) that plays an important role, though it's a far weaker form of oestrogen. E1 is converted from other hormones that are found in your liver, heart, bone, muscles, brain, body fat and skin, and around 5 per cent of it can be converted into oestradiol (E2). Fat tissue is the main source of postmenopausal E2, which is why oestrogen levels can be higher in those with a larger frame. Higher levels of oestrone are associated with the growth of breast and endometrial cancers, whereas lower levels are associated with osteoporosis.

Essentially, what this means is that after menopause, although some oestrogen is produced through the conversion of other hormones, the amount of it is far smaller than was produced throughout your cycling years.

Skin Deep

Your skin is the largest organ in the body and oestrogens assist with hair growth, the colouring of your skin, blood supply, elasticity and its ability to hold water. Your skin actually varies throughout the menstrual cycle as a result of changing oestrogen levels; skin is thinner and drier at the start of the cycle when oestrogen is low and it increases in thickness as oestrogen rises. Once oestrogen starts to decline it has a significant effect on your skin, for example:

- The appearance of fine wrinkles
- Thinning of the epidermis
- Thinning of the dermis, which means that skin bruises easily and hefty bruises appear out of nowhere
- Decreased collagen

- Decreased water
- Dry skin
- Sagging
- Poor wound healing
- Hair loss
- Hirsutism – the appearance of unwanted facial hair – though this can occur for other reasons too (see page 290).

Some Chinese medicine practitioners specialise in using facial acupuncture to stimulate the production of collagen, which can improve the appearance of wrinkles, and gua sha is a technique in which massage tools (often made from jade or rose quartz) are used to scrape the skin in order to reduce tension, smooth away puffy eyes and areas of congestion, and improve circulation. Some of my clients have found that using microcurrent facial devices helps to rejuvenate and tone their skin (the one by NuFACE seems to be a fave), but find a skincare regime that works for you – ideally one using products that aren't laden with hormone-disrupting chemicals and have SPF support. However, as well as taking care of our skin from the outside, we also want to be taking care of it from the inside by eating a nutrient-dense diet that includes sufficient healthy fats (see page 271), avoiding sugar and staying hydrated.

Approximately 30 per cent of the collagen in your skin is lost in the first five years of postmenopausal life, with an average decline of 1 to 2 per cent per year. Researchers also found a relationship between declining skin collagen content and a loss of bone mineral content. A review of 14 studies found that the majority reported a correlation between skin thinness and brittle bones, and concluded that estimating skin changes could prove to be helpful in estimating bone changes – not quite as simple as the more wrinkles you have, the more likely you are to be at risk of postmenopausal osteoporosis, but almost.

All Dried Out

Having less oestrogen doesn't just change your skin, it also causes other parts of your body to dry up, such as your eyes, nose and mouth. As if this weren't enough to deal with, your vulva, vagina and lower urinary tract also undergo changes. This is because the sheets of cells which line them have a high number of oestrogen receptors, so a drop in oestrogen has an effect on all of them. In the joyous world of medical terminology these changes have traditionally been described as vulvovaginal atrophy which – prepare yourself – means they 'waste away'.

Thankfully, in 2014, the International Society for the Study of Women's Sexual Health and the North American Menopause Society recognised the need for a more inclusive and accurate terminology. And one which was less alarming. They came up with the 'genito-urinary syndrome of menopause' (GSM), which describes the menopausal signs and symptoms of the vulva, vagina and lower urinary tract (your bladder, urethra – the tube that takes wee from your bladder to the hole just above your vagina – and the sphincters – which open and close in order to wee or not). GSM encompasses the signs and symptoms associated with the loss of oestrogen at the time of menopause, which can involve:

- Genital symptoms such as burning, dryness and irritation
- Sexual symptoms such as lack of lubrication, discomfort and pain
- Urinary symptoms such as urgency, increased frequency, painful or difficult urination and urinary tract infections (UTIs).

Between 40 and 54 per cent of us will experience some degree of GSM, and both the likelihood and severity of it increases with age. Yet despite the vast number of people affected by it, one study found that only 4 per cent of those experiencing symptoms were able to connect their experience to GSM, which is hardly surprising given the lack of education around menopause. Only 25 per cent of those with GSM will go to a healthcare practitioner to discuss their symptoms. A quarter! Whilst that number is appalling in that such huge numbers of us are suffering in silence, 25 per cent is hardly surprising when you consider how many factors may need to be overcome in order to seek out medical advice.

The most common reasons for not seeking out help with GSM include embarrassment, believing that nothing can be done and believing that it's not appropriate to discuss it with a healthcare professional. Thinking that a healthcare professional is too busy or that they might be embarrassed by the topic, and wishing that someone else would initiate the conversation, can also prevent important conversations about genital, sexual and urinary health from taking place. Please don't let any of the above or anything else prevent you from seeking out help. GSM can damage self-esteem, intimacy in relationships and the ability to enjoy life – even going for a walk can cause pain.

What Can Be Done?

The bad news is that the changes I've outlined in this chapter are likely to happen. The good news is that there are things that can help. Even if you're someone who doesn't mind the idea of less sex, you may still need to explore strategies to take care of your vulva and vagina, because the changes they undergo don't just affect your sex life, they also have consequences for other aspects of your life, such as what menstrual products you use whilst you still have periods, underwear and clothing, activities such as bike riding, walking and even what you can sit on and how long for.

CASE STUDY

Juliana was surprised by what perimenopause did to her. Whilst her friends were complaining of never feeling 'up for it', Juliana's sexual desire had skyrocketed. She smiled as she told me that it was like a fire had emerged in her after years of feeling barely anything, and how much fun and joy it had brought to her relationship. Then she paused and frowned before telling me that penetration was painful. Juliana told me about the frustration of feeling desire again and, now that her son had moved out, finally feeling free to have sex with her husband, whilst at the same time feeling frustrated at her body for what she described as 'not co-operating'. She went on to tell me that the vaginal dryness she was experiencing was also impacting her husband, because he took it to mean that she wasn't turned on.

Juliana and I spoke at great length about how wetness doesn't equal being turned on – you can have cervical fluid literally dripping out of you and not be ready to have sex, and you can feel really turned on and be dry at the same time. We discussed using vaginal moisturiser and the importance of using lube and Juliana slumped in her chair, burst into tears and told me she felt ashamed that she needed them. When I told her that I know twenty-somethings that love to use lube she was astonished and sat up straight again, curious to know more. I also suggested that she speak to her GP about using what's known as a topical or local oestrogen – the kind that's applied to the vulva and vagina directly to help with vaginal dryness and other genito-urinary symptoms.

But Juliana was worried, 'What about cancer?' she asked. 'What about it?' I replied. She looked at me, confused. 'I thought that taking manufactured oestrogen can cause breast cancer.' I went on to explain that the dose of oestrogen in topical preparations is very low and, as such, its use is very low-risk, and that the type of oestrogen in these preparations is body-identical. In other words, it's the same as the oestrogen we make ourselves. Juliana was relieved to know that this was an option and emailed me half an hour after she left to say that she had an appointment with her GP the following day. I asked her to keep me posted and three months later I received an email from her saying that her symptoms had really improved and that she was having lots of fun connecting with her husband.

Lubricants

I'm a fan of lube at any age – it makes such a difference to our experience of pleasure. During your cycling years there will be points in the cycle where its use can feel more necessary, rather than it being a fun add-on, and that's true for the menopause transition too. You can get lubricants that are oil-based or water-based, each producing a different sensation. Water-based ones don't last as long as oil-based ones, but oil-based ones can't be used with condoms. Steer clear of lubricants that contain glycerine and glycols as these are linked to vaginal infections such as thrush. Yes™ has a fantastic range of lubricants and vaginal moisturisers that are pH balanced, hypoallergenic, plant-based and certified organic, and your GP can give you a prescription for them.

Vaginal moisturisers

Unlike lubricants, vaginal moisturisers aren't used for sex, they're used to hydrate your vagina, which can help with itching, soreness and dryness. Some of my clients tell me that they like to use coconut oil to moisturise their vulvas and vaginas, but I recommend being wary of this strategy as coconut oil is antimicrobial, which means it can negatively affect your vulvovaginal microbiome.

Local (topical) oestrogen

Oral and topical oestrogen can improve or reverse many of the symptoms of GSM, improve blood flow and increase production of vaginal fluids. If you're only experiencing symptoms of GSM, but not getting other signs of low oestrogen, then you may just need some local oestrogen that's administered to the vagina as a slow-release tablet, cream or as a hormone-releasing ring that stays in place for three months at a time. Common brand names include Vagifem and Ovestin.

When oestrogen is applied to the vulvovaginal area, it delivers oestrogen to the tissues that need it. Local oestrogen is safe for the majority of people, yet so many resist it and try to do things 'naturally'. As I've said before, you get to decide what's best for you, but please don't let fear of using oestrogen in this way be what informs your decision – a year's supply of local oestrogen only equates to one tablet of the lowest dose of MHT, so it's worth asking yourself if you're making a mountain out of a molehill when considering whether to do this.

If your GP is unwilling to prescribe it or, even worse, if they suggest that you drink a glass of wine to relax, as many of my clients have been told, then please don't accept this and, ideally, provide feedback that this is an inappropriate response and they are not following the NICE guidelines (you can do this through the Patient Advice and Liaison Services (PALS)). If you have active breast cancer or undiagnosed vaginal or uterine bleeding then you can't use a local oestrogen and if you are taking tamoxifen following a previous diagnosis then your doctor will want to speak to your oncologist before prescribing it.

Systemic oestrogen

Systemic oestrogen is worth discussing with your GP when GSM appears alongside other symptoms such as hot flushes, night sweats, disturbed sleep, joint pain and forgetfulness. Although 10 to 15 per cent of those using systemic hormone therapy still experience vulvovaginal dryness, in these cases local oestrogen can be used alongside it. We'll be talking more about this kind of hormone therapy in Chapter 3, so either hold tight or skip ahead.

Vaginal DHEA

As you may remember, DHEA (dehydroepiandrosterone) is what we call a mother hormone because it's the precursor to other hormones like oestrogen, progesterone, testosterone and cortisol. Vaginal DHEA comes in the form of a pessary and, once it's inside you, your body will convert it into oestrogen and testosterone.

Ospemifene

Ospemifene is a selective oestrogen receptor modulator (SERM) that has an oestrogenic effect on the vagina, helping with lubrication and reducing pain from penetrative sex. It's the first non-hormonal treatment for GSM that can be used safely by those who can't use local oestrogen, such as those being treated for active breast cancer, which is helpful as some breast cancer treatments can cause vaginal atrophy and dryness.

Laser therapy

Laser therapy can help to improve blood flow and stimulate the production of collagen, which can help to plump up your labia. This can make a difference when it comes to being able to move and sit comfortably. It can also improve the elasticity and moisture of the vagina, though it isn't available through the NHS and needs to be funded privately.

When It Hurts So Bad

Pain during sex is common in vagina owners of all ages, but can be particularly pronounced when oestrogen becomes low during perimenopause and postmenopause. Pain during sex can impact your identity as well as intimate relationships, and the pain can also exist when you're not having sex – for some, the sensation of menstrual pads, clothing and even simply sitting down can cause excruciating pain. If you experience any of the following then I encourage you to speak to a healthcare professional about what's going on. If they dismiss you, don't accept it – your sexuality is deserving of healthcare, no matter your age or relationship status.

Dyspareunia is the general term for experiencing pain during sex. Unfortunately, too many women are told that it's all in their head. I've lost count of the number of women who've been told by their GP to 'just relax, have a glass of wine' as if that will (magically) take care of everything. If a man went to a GP and described the same experience, I suspect that he would be taken seriously, properly assessed and offered appropriate treatment strategies. Pain during sex can be caused by a number of things – the hormonal changes of menopause, endometriosis, pelvic floor dysfunction, prolapse, adhesions and scarring from surgery, and infection, as well as a history of episiotomy, cancer treatment or pelvic trauma. All can be helped with treatments such as hormone therapy, sex therapy and seeing a pelvic health physiotherapist. Your GP can refer you to a specialist on the NHS and you can also pay to see someone privately.

Vaginismus is a psychosexual condition in which the muscles that make up the pelvic floor that surround the vagina, bladder and uterus involuntarily spasm and tighten when penetration is attempted, making penetrative sex, vaginal examinations and the use of tampons painful or impossible. It's a condition that has implications beyond sexual relationships – those who have it often suffer in silence and feel isolated, and it can impact on mental health and self-confidence too.

Vaginismus can be primary, which basically means it existed prior to any kind of penetration, or secondary, which means it's occurred following a traumatic or painful experience such as birth or sexual trauma, back/hip injuries or repeated thrush infections. After experiencing a negative painful experience where the pelvic floor muscles shorten and tighten, the fear of recurrence then causes the pelvic muscles to brace as they try to protect you from further pain, thus perpetuating and confounding the pain/spasm cycle. Treatment should include seeing a highly specialised pelvic health physiotherapist who can work with you and your comfort level, and might include the use of vaginal dilators, vibrators, sex therapy, relaxation and breathing. It's also worth knowing that even though your GP may not be familiar with vaginismus as a condition, specialist NHS services do exist. The College of Sexual and Relationship Therapists (COSRT) and the Institute of Psychosexual Medicine can steer you in a helpful direction, and the Vaginismus Network do great work when it comes to educating, connecting, supporting and empowering those with vaginismus. I highly recommend joining their community if you suspect or know that you have vaginismus.

Vulvodynia describes pain, burning and discomfort in the vulva, but, in the absence of a particular cause, vulvodynia is a symptom not a condition. The pain might be felt in a specific area – such as the clitoris or entrance to the vagina – or it can be generalised and felt across the whole vulva. It can be continuous (which is described as unprovoked vulvodynia) or it may occur as a result of touch (this type is described as provoked vulvodynia), though those with vulvodynia may experience an overlap of the two types. For some, the pain will extend to around the anus, inner thighs and upper legs, and the hypersensitivity can be triggered during sex, using tampons or menstrual cups, wiping after going to the toilet, and during a vaginal exam or cervical screening, but for some any form of touch, clothing or simply sitting down will result in pain. When symptoms are limited to the entrance to the vagina, it's known as vestibulodynia.

Ointments and gels that contain a local anaesthetic and tricylic antidepressants may be prescribed, but a multidisciplinary approach is usually needed. This may include: working with a highly skilled pelvic health physiotherapist who can develop a treatment plan that's specific to your particular experience (people with vulvodynia often have a hypertonic pelvic floor, which means that the muscles are too tight); acupuncture; using hormone therapy to improve lubrication; calming the nervous system and improving sleep (hormones can help with this too); reducing emotional stress; reducing the intake of inflammatory foods; following an elimination diet to identify any dietary triggers; improving gut function and nutritional deficiencies; and working through issues such as exhaustion, abuse and birth/sexual trauma.

Atrophic vulvovaginitis is when the tissue of the entrance to the vagina and the vagina itself thins ('atrophies') and becomes inflamed as a result of low levels of oestrogen. It can therefore develop after having a baby, during breastfeeding, whilst taking oestrogen-decreasing medication prescribed in order to manage uterine fibroids and endometriosis, following the surgical removal of the ovaries (which instigates instantaneous menopause) and after natural menopause. Treatment involves the local application of oestrogen in the form of a vaginal cream, tablet (sometimes referred to as a pessary) or vaginal ring (see pages 117–118) that's similar to the contraceptive ring. This lowers the pH of the vagina, stimulates the maturation of the cells lining the vagina and urethra, decreases the frequency of UTIs and reverses atrophy.

Interstitial cystitis (IC), also known as painful bladder syndrome, is different to 'regular' cystitis because it's not caused by an infection. The actual cause of it is unknown and the symptoms vary from person to person, and they can also change with time, and come and go. Interstitial cystitis is a chronic condition that causes painful urinary symptoms such as abdominal or pelvic pain; persistent, unpleasant sensations in the bladder; discomfort with bladder filling and only partial relief upon emptying; bladder pressure; frequent urination; and urgent and frequent urination at night. In people with IC, 75 per cent experience pain with intercourse and 90 per cent of women with it report low sexual desire, difficulty with arousal, bladder pain during sex and an urge to urinate during sex. One study found that 87 per cent of participants with IC had pelvic floor dysfunction – the inability to use the muscles of the pelvic floor to control bladder and bowel movements – so, yet again, this is a condition that can be improved by working with a specialist pelvic health physio.

Hold On

Your bladder has two jobs: to store urine and to let it out. Simple, right? All it has to do is fill up and then release at the appropriate time. This makes the bladder sound like a really basic organ when compared to the majestical and all-important heart, for example. But your ability to store urine and release it at the appropriate time requires complex co-ordination of the brain, nervous system, bladder, sphincters and pelvic floor. In other words, there are plenty of ways that things can go wrong.

Your pelvic floor muscles lie across the base of your pelvis and provide support to your bladder, uterus and bowel, helping to keep them where they ought to be. The pelvic floor undergoes changes as a result of hormonal changes, pregnancy and life events. It impacts how you wee, poo and have sex. Considering how essential it is, it's odd that not much thought is given to it until it struggles to do its job. And by that point, it becomes very clear how important a functioning pelvic floor is.

Up to a third of us will experience a problem with our pelvic floor muscles at some point, and this can manifest as leaking urine and pelvic organ prolapse, which is when it feels like something has dropped down into your vagina. Like the other muscles in your body, the muscles which make up your pelvic floor can become weak, too tight, overstretched, torn and slow to work. Common causes of pelvic floor problems include:

- Pregnancy and childbirth, especially if you've had an assisted (instrumental) birth, an episiotomy or a significant tear, a very large baby or a protracted pushing stage.
- Being very overweight as this can increase the pressure on the pelvic floor muscles.
- Chronic constipation – straining isn't good for any muscle.
- Chronic coughing as a result of smoking or conditions like asthma.
- High-impact exercises and vigorous gym activities can create strain, as can heavy lifting. Now, I appreciate that for some of you exercise with a pelvic floor issue will bring its challenges, but it's not a reason to avoid it. You just need to work with a trainer who is mindful of the pelvic floor and creates exercise plans which target the pelvic floor.
- And, of course, menopause.

When there's less oestrogen reaching the hormone receptors in your bladder, urinary tract and pelvic floor, this results in changes to both the actual anatomy of the bladder (its physical structure) and its function. The effects of oestrogen deficiency include loss of collagen and adipose tissue. This causes thinning, which can make it difficult or painful to wee and causes an increase in the frequency that you need to wee, as well as urinary incontinence.

Many of these changes can be reversed with the use of oestrogen therapy. Urge urinary incontinence, an overactive bladder and recurrent UTIs are particularly improved with oestrogen, but there is much debate on how useful it is in treating stress incontinence. Although the loss of oestrogen causes a decline in collagen production and strength, which can weaken bladder support and therefore increase the risk of stress incontinence, the use of oestrogen therapy to treat pure stress incontinence is not recommended. It's been suggested that reduced oestrogen levels can affect the tissues surrounding the urethra, contributing towards a loosening effect and subsequent incontinence.

Pelvic Floor Dysfunction

Pelvic floor dysfunction is an umbrella term which includes a range of issues caused by the muscles of the pelvic floor being either too weak (hypotonicity) or too tight (hypertonicity). Pelvic floor dysfunction affects how able you are to control your bladder and bowel, causing you to leak, need to go urgently or break wind without warning, and it can also change the position of your uterus, resulting in a bearing down sensation whilst exercising, during your period or when you have sex. When it comes to incontinence, there are also more specific terms:

Urinary incontinence refers to the involuntary loss of urine. In other words, you wee when you don't want to.

Stress urinary incontinence is when 'stress' placed on the bladder through activities such as sneezing, coughing, tripping, lifting or trampolining, results in leakage. This type is often about small leaks.

Urge incontinence is when you have a sudden urge to wee and leak shortly thereafter. It's unpredictable and usually results in a large loss of urine. It's associated with overactive bladder syndrome.

Overactive bladder (OAB) syndrome is when your bladder squeezes (contracts) without warning, day or night, giving you an urgent need to wee and not much time to get to a toilet, resulting in urge incontinence. People with OAB often need to wee more frequently than usual and in small volumes. A diagnosis of overactive bladder syndrome is made when these symptoms occur in the absence of an infection or other obvious cause.

Mixed urinary incontinence is when you have some stress incontinence and some urge incontinence.

Overflow incontinence occurs when the bladder doesn't empty normally and becomes very full as a result.

Nocturia describes the need to urinate at night.

Anal incontinence (AI) refers to leaking of stools (solid or liquid) and wind. The highest risk factor for developing AI is in those who've had obstetric anal sphincter injury (OASI) as a result of tears and episiotomies from giving birth, though most won't develop AI until hormone levels reduce and/or there's loss of pelvic floor function.

Although pelvic floor dysfunction can occur at any stage of life – particularly after pregnancy and childbirth – it becomes more common with age. Between 40 and 59 years of age a quarter of us will experience it, and between 60 and 79 this goes up to a third. By 80 half of us will have pelvic floor issues. But less than 40 per cent of women report seeking treatment for urinary incontinence, often because of the belief that it's a normal part of ageing and that nothing can be done. This misconception, which healthcare practitioners may hold too, can have devastating consequences on quality of life. Whether it's occurred as a result of pregnancy, vaginal or caesarean birth, menopause, illness or surgery, incontinence is never something that you should accept or put up with.

Despite urinary incontinence costing the NHS £353.6 million a year(!), pelvic floor education is low on the healthcare agenda and if you ever receive instruction from a doctor (or, more likely, a magazine), it'll be along the lines of 'Do your Kegels to strengthen your pelvic floor.' Although well-intended, this can sometimes *cause* pelvic floor dysfunction as the emphasis on squeezing and tightening can cause hypertonicity – excessive tone, tension or activity of the pelvic floor. Your pelvic floor does need to be strong to do its job, but it shouldn't be tense. A hypertonic pelvic floor can cause bladder and bowel issues, such as urgency and leakage, and other conditions, such as dyspareunia (pain during sex), vaginismus, vulvodynia and pudendal neuralgia. By the way, if there's a man in your life who suffers from chronic prostatitis, a hypertonic pelvic floor could be the reason why.

You already know that we should all be taking care of our pelvic floors, but the pelvic floor is a bit like the kid in the class who does what they're supposed to do and doesn't cause any issues, so they don't get the attention that the ones who are struggling and being louder do. With time, lack of attention starts to cause issues, but at this point they can be nipped in the bud. Left untended, however, the issues become more severe and that's what we see with the pelvic floor. A bit of leakage when you sneeze now is distressing, but you might dismiss it, hoping that it'll get better. This is unlikely to happen, particularly once oestrogen starts to decline in perimenopause. There is no better time to address your pelvic floor than now – and that includes those of you who don't have any issues. Not giving your pelvic floor the TLC it needs means you're more likely to have it impact your day-to-day life. I don't imagine you spend a lot of time trampolining, but what if you go on a date or meet up with friends and can't enjoy yourself because you're on guard in case you suddenly need to go? How about if that night out involves a train journey to get there, so you decline the invitation because you can't trust your bladder? You might not be able to do the kinds of exercise you love or worry about being in a group class or gym environment in case others notice your pad or that you've leaked.

And then there's the irritation that leaking can cause. The pH of normal healthy skin is around 5.5, but with exposure to urine it can jump up to 8.0 and this creates opportunities for infection, as well as a more challenging environment for your outer layer of skin to heal itself. Add to that the inflammation that can be caused by rubbing pads and a cycle of damage results in incontinence-associated dermatitis, all at a time when your vulva is possibly in a sensitised situation too.

What's the Remedy?

- Clearly, pelvic floor training and bladder training can't be underestimated. Ask your GP to refer you to a pelvic health physiotherapist or pay to see someone privately – compared to the amount you could end up spending on incontinence pads over the next three to four decades, it's a small investment. #pantsnotpads is the way to go.

- Download (and use!) Squeezy, an NHS-approved, physiotherapy-led, pelvic floor muscle exercise app. At the time of writing it costs £2.99, which is less than the cost of a small pack of incontinence pads.
- Stay hydrated. You might think that drinking less will be helpful. It won't. It'll leave you feeling like crap and your urine will be pungent, which can irritate your bladder as well as your vulva.
- Only go when you actually need to. Don't get in the habit of going 'just in case' – this includes the last tinkle before bed.
- Don't hold on till you're ready to burst. You wouldn't force a small child to do this so please treat your own bladder with the same respect.
- There's no award for pissing the quickest, so take your time and don't squeeze it out.
- Constipation and straining can cause and exacerbate pelvic floor dysfunction. You need enough water to float the boat so stay hydrated, eat plenty of fibre (see page 274), move your body and go when you have the urge to – don't miss your chance. You can also put something in front of the toilet like a small stool that you can place your feet on, so your knees are slightly above your hips. That way you can lean forward and adopt the position that humans are designed to poo in – squatting.
- Limit caffeine, alcohol and fizzy drinks.

Strength Training and Bladder Training

I spoke to women's health coach and pelvic floor guru Baz Moffat about how strength training classes rarely consider pelvic floor function and why they really should. Here's what Baz told me:

> There's a lot of attention given to how important strength and impact training is for women, especially those over 35. The main reason for this focus is primarily the positive evidence base supporting these forms of exercise when it comes to maintaining, and even building, bone health and muscle strength. Impact training also helps with cardiac health, which should be a key focus of any exercise programme in midlife women.
>
> This is all brilliant stuff and much-needed. We need to get our bodies ahead of the inevitable curve, when oestrogen leaves our system – it's good to build muscle, have strong bones and a healthy heart. It helps

us to have a better quality of life as we age and protects us against many chronic diseases.

The piece missing from most of these discussions, however, is the pelvic floor – nobody, or very few, even mention it. In my opinion this is because the model to which the fitness industry subscribes to is one based on men and there are very few over-30 women in the fitness industry. So most trainers are young and most are male, which means that women's health is rarely on the agenda, outside of pre/post-natal. Midlife women don't seem to be catered for outside of pilates classes, which is important for many reasons, but does not tick all the boxes.

So, in my opinion, yes, strength training is fundamental to all midlife women. I'd go so far as to say it's a non-negotiable, but under the umbrella of a fully functioning pelvic floor. Our continence is our independence, and we must acknowledge and respect this part of our body, and work with it. We can all learn how to exhale as we lift and work with the core, so not only do we get to work out hard, but we also don't do ourselves any harm. I believe that more and more women and coaches are getting really interested in this, and change will come, but in the meantime my advice is to do your own research and not just do whatever you're told if it doesn't feel right. No woman should be leaking whilst working out or be in pain or have feelings of heaviness. There is so much that you can do without being anywhere near this place, both in terms of the types of exercise that you do and what you do within an exercise session. When most people think of exercise, what springs to mind will be aerobics and running, but there are lots of other options – dancing, paddle-boarding and functional movement to name a few. During an exercise session, most women will already be aware of the types of movement that will be an issue for them – jumping, skipping and star jumps are usually top of the list of no-goes, but it's important to know that these movements can be swapped for lower-impact options that you can benefit from without issue.

Feeling the Burn

Your urethra, the tube which takes urine from your bladder to the outside of your body, is shorter than it is in males. That means that it's easier for bacteria from around your anus to reach your bladder. That's why we're taught to wipe ourselves from front to back – to avoid causing a urinary tract infection (UTI). UTIs aren't pleasant at any age and the risk factors for developing one include a new sexual partner, frequent sexual intercourse, using a spermicide and … menopause. Structural changes which take place as a result of menopause and ageing, such as the thinning and weakening of the urethra, make recurrent UTIs more likely in postmenopause. Pelvic floor dysfunction can result in reduced flow and residual urine being left in the bladder after urination which both increase the likelihood of recurrent UTIs. It doesn't help that your vagina also becomes less acidic, which alters the vaginal microbiome, leaving you with less friendly bacteria and more of the troublesome varieties. Symptoms of a UTI can include:

- Peeing more frequently during the day and/or night-time
- Pain, stinging or burning whilst peeing, though possibly only passing a small amount of urine
- Pain or pressure in your lower abdomen or lower back
- Urgency
- Strong-smelling urine
- Cloudy urine
- Blood in the urine
- Nausea and/or vomiting
- Feeling tired or under the weather
- Shaking and fever.

Your doctor will do a dipstick test to analyse your urine and may arrange for further testing, particularly if you don't respond to the standard treatment of antibiotics or have two or more episodes within three months. Other measures you can take include:

- Drinking enough water. I appreciate that it's hard to do when it hurts when you wee, but it's really important.
- Always wiping from front to back to prevent bacteria from your anus reaching your urethra and vagina.
- Supporting the health of your vaginal microbiome – no douching, scented soaps, bath bombs, bubble baths or 'feminine cleansers' (FYI, you're not dirty and your vagina never needs to be cleaned, it takes care of that all by itself).
- Avoid spermicide. Nasty stuff.
- Use condoms that are vagina-friendly (see page 119).

- Use lube during sex to prevent friction (and pain!), which can lead to inflammation and infection.
- Address pelvic floor dysfunction.
- Keep some barley in your kitchen cupboards to make lemon barley water when you get the first telltale signs of a UTI. Drinking homemade lemon barley water drastically reduces symptoms within 24 hours and resolves them entirely soon after. You can make it by taking 150g of pearl barley and rinsing it until the water runs clear. Place it in a saucepan along with the zest of two lemons, 1 tablespoon of grated ginger and 2.5 pints of water. Bring it all to the boil and then turn it down to a gentle simmer for 10 minutes. Remove from the heat, strain and save the liquid, then add the juice of the two lemons (and 2 tablespoons of honey if you'd like). Set aside to cool and drink at room temperature throughout your day.
- D-mannose, the active ingredient in cranberries, can be taken as a supplement and is a much better option than store-bought cranberry juice, which contains a lot of sugar that aggravates UTIs.
- Topical oestrogen – the kind of hormone therapy that's applied locally to the vagina – can help to reduce and prevent the occurrence of UTIs.
- Believe me, antibiotics absolutely have their place when it comes to UTIs, but using them is also a risk factor for developing thrush and also for getting a subsequent UTI, so we want to do all we can to prevent them in the first place.
- If you get recurrent UTIs, evaluate the health of your microbiome. Your bladder has its own community of microorganisms, but it's important to address your gut microbiome too as it's the command central for all the other microbiomes around your body.

Prolapse

Prolapse is when an organ falls out of its usual position and drops down into the vagina. According to the Royal College of Obstetricians and Gynaecologists, half of womb-owners over the age of 50 will experience symptoms of pelvic organ prolapse and by the age of 80 one in 10 will have had surgery to treat the prolapse. There are several types of prolapse:

- Urethrocele happens when the urethra (the tube urine travels in from the bladder to the outside) prolapses into the vagina.
- Cystocele is where the bladder prolapses into the front wall of the vagina.

Types of Prolapse

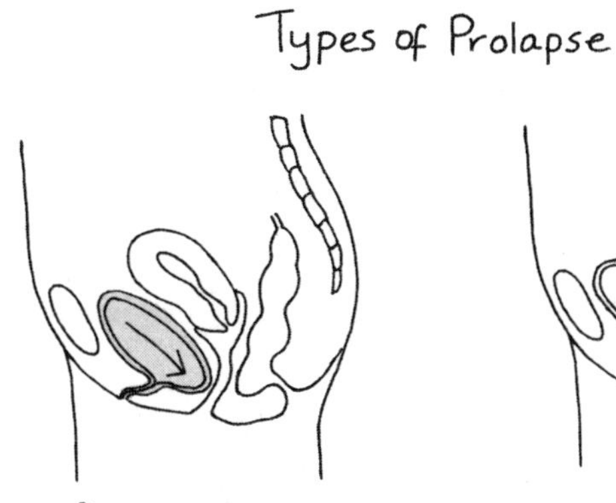

Cystourethrocele

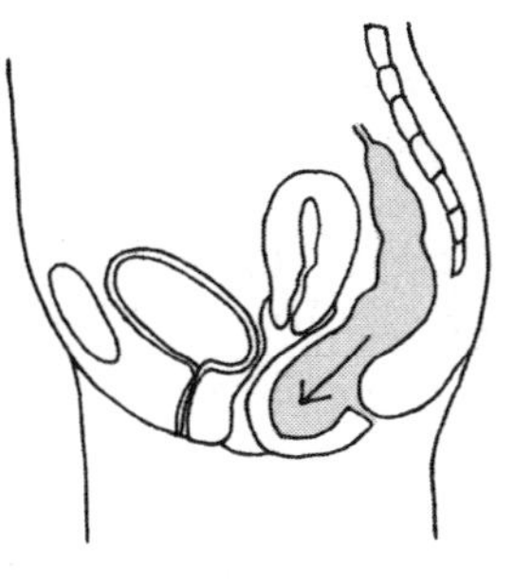

Rectocele

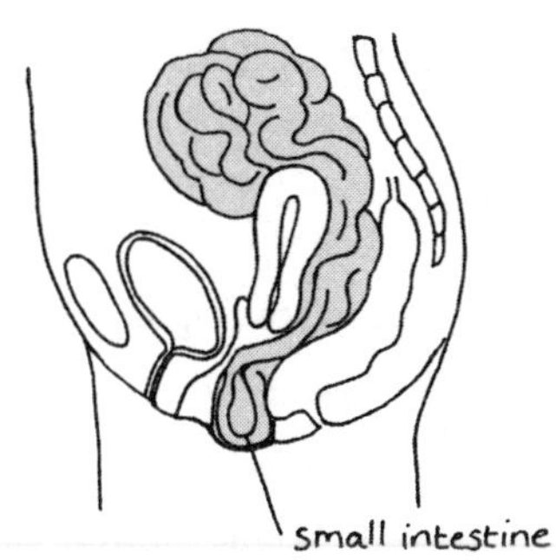

Enterocele

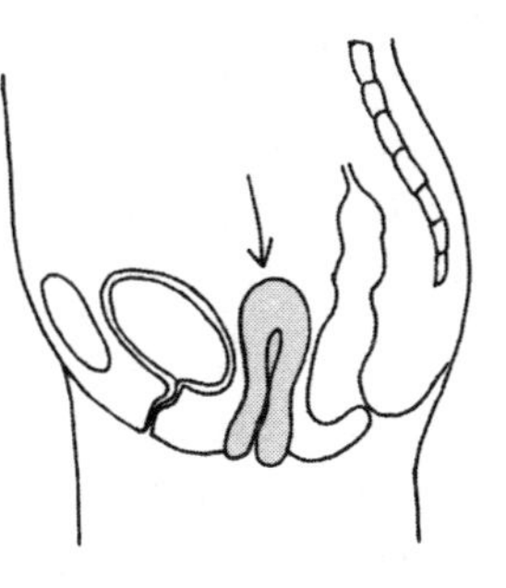

Uterine prolapse

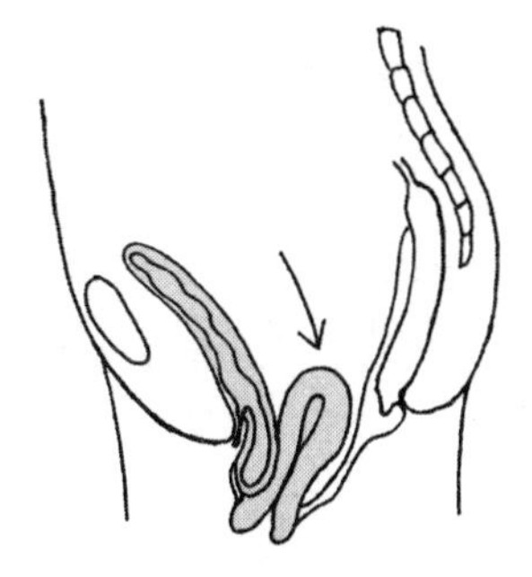

Procidentia

- When both the bladder and the urethra prolapse, it's called a cystourethrocele.
- Rectocele is where the rectum prolapses into the back wall of the vagina.
- Uterine prolapse is when the uterus hangs down into the vagina. This type of prolapse is often described as being first, second or third degree, which refers to the pelvic organ prolapse quantification system:
    - Stage 0 – no prolapse
    - Stage 1 – the cervix has descended into the vagina, but is more than 1cm above the hymen
    - Stage 2 – descent has reached within 1cm of the hymen to protruding 1cm
    - Stage 3 – descent has reached beyond 1cm of the hymen, but not more than 2cm
    - Stage 4 – the uterus protrudes outside the body (procidentia).

Symptoms of pelvic organ prolapse include:

- A sensation of dragging, discomfort or a lump coming down, which may intensify after standing or sitting for a long time or towards the end of the day. This feeling may also improve after lying down.
- Needing to wee frequently.
- Struggling to wee.
- An awareness that your bladder isn't emptying properly.
- Leaking when sneezing, coughing, laughing or lifting heavy objects (like kids).
- Frequent UTIs.
- Lower back pain, constipation and incomplete bowel movements (two-parters) can occur when the bowel is involved.
- You might be able to feel or see a bulge around the entrance to your vagina or inside it.

Or you might not have any symptoms at all and only find out you have a prolapse after attending a cervical screening appointment or other gynaecological investigation. None of these symptoms are pleasant, yet so many people stay silent and suffer. Please don't. Make an appointment to speak to your GP so that they can assess you.

Prolapse is diagnosed by vaginal examination. A speculum is used to separate the walls of the vagina so that your doctor or pelvic health physio can see which organ(s) are prolapsing. My former boss, pelvic health physiotherapist Christien Bird, told me about the importance of carrying out examinations whilst standing, as some prolapses are less problematic or disappear when lying down and can therefore be missed by inexperienced practitioners. Once a prolapse has been diagnosed you'll hopefully be referred for pelvic muscle training and you may receive advice relating to other factors that can contribute to prolapse, such as constipation and straining, heavy lifting and weight loss if your BMI is high. If prolapse occurs alongside signs of genito-urinary syndrome (GSM), then you may be prescribed a vaginal oestrogen cream or an oestrogen-releasing ring, which is inserted into the vagina and worn for three months at a time. Vaginal pessaries are soft, removable devices that are made of silicone or plastic, that can be inserted into your vagina to hold a prolapsed uterus or vaginal wall in place. They can be used prior to surgery or long term if surgery isn't wanted or is contraindicated. Vaginal pessaries may require a bit of trial and error to get the right fit, and they can have an effect on penetrative sex. They need to be replaced every six months and potential complications from their use include bleeding, discharge, difficulty removing them and expulsion.

If these treatment strategies don't work, or don't work well enough, then surgery may be suggested. Surgery may involve the use of a mesh, but this is controversial. When mesh implants arrived on the scene, they appeared to be a fantastic solution to incontinence and prolapse. The mesh was flexible and allowed body tissue to go through it so that the body's tissue could help to hold it in place, and it only took an hour to implant via keyhole surgery, which is why it became the standard treatment. But the use of vaginal mesh implants has triggered class action law suits in the UK, US and Australia, due to complications arising from the mesh eroding and poking through the vaginal wall or cutting through internal tissue, creating issues such as vaginal scarring, pain during sex, and pelvic, back and leg pain. It's been labelled a 'high-risk device' by the U.S. Food and Drug Administration and the NHS has suspended its use in the treatment of stress incontinence. If you've had mesh implanted then I recommend joining Sling the Mesh, a Facebook group set up by journalist Kath Sansom, who had a mesh inserted and then removed seven months later.

When it comes to incontinence and our reproductive organs remaining in place, it may feel like an uphill battle. You might be struggling already, particularly if pregnancy and birth left their mark on you, but I hope that in reading this chapter, you can see that there is a lot that can be done to improve pelvic floor function, and that starts with speaking to your GP and/or a specialist pelvic health physiotherapist. And the sooner you do that, the better.

3

HRT: devil or saviour?

I imagine that you've reached this chapter, or possibly skipped ahead to this chapter(!), in the hope that I'm going to tell you whether you should take HRT or not. I get it. Newspaper headlines about hormone replacement therapy are usually scary and sometimes contradictory, and you're possibly thinking that it would be nice to find someone whose opinion you can trust (which may or may not be me).

Before we delve into the details, I want to be very clear that I cannot tell you whether you should take hormones or not (and whilst we're on the topic, I can't do that via social media or email either). It's not in my professional remit. That is a discussion for you to have with your medical team. What I will do is give you its history and what I aim to be a balanced overview of the research that's available. And, yes, I'm aware that we all have our biases and so what I consider to be 'balanced' is likely to be judged differently by others.

Like most areas of reproductive health, discussion around HRT is polarised into love it or loathe it camps. Some will say that menopause is natural and a positive transition to go through, others that it's awful and a design flaw that hormones can counteract. My take on it is that menopause can be both a positive transition *and* a situation where the use of hormones, along with other lifestyle measures, can be hugely helpful.

The menopause transition is a stage of life, not a disease. For some reason, our hormones are meant to decline in midlife, which is why I'm not a fan of the term hormone *replacement* therapy (HRT), because it implies that we should have hormones. Now, that doesn't mean that you or I won't choose to use hormones, but we're not replacing them, because they shouldn't be there in the first place. This is why I prefer the terms hormone therapy and menopausal hormone therapy (MHT).

Many women have told me that the discussions they've had with their GPs have been inadequate, either because of time constraints, feeling that they weren't being heard or that their symptoms were being dismissed, that the only option presented to them was MHT when they hoped for something else, *or* that they weren't prescribed MHT when the evidence base and current guidelines state that they should have been offered it. I've also had clients who've had marvellous GPs who were clearly invested in understanding and supporting their patients through menopause.

When it comes to hormone therapy, I don't claim to have all the answers and that is not my aim. I want to help you to make sense of the history of their use and the claims that have been made about hormone therapy, so that you are informed and ready to speak to medical professionals about what options are appropriate for you. Some might call it a cop out; I call it staying in my lane.

The History

Hormones have been given to patients since the 1940s, though they've come on a lot in the intervening decades. Back then, a vast amount of raw material was needed: the corpora lutea of 50,000 pigs were needed to produce a few milligrams of progesterone; 4,000 gallons of urine provided less than one hundredth of an ounce of testosterone; one scientist processed nearly a ton of bulls' testicles and another the ovaries of more than 80,000 sows to get 12 thousandth of a gram of oestradiol. At the time, progesterone cost $200 per gram. In 1941, Premarin, an oestrogen made from pregnant mares' urine, was licensed for use in Canada and in 1942 the US followed suit.

Fast-forward to the 1960s and hormone therapy was widely used and accepted, in part due to the publication of *Feminine Forever*, a bestselling book written by Dr Robert Wilson in which he claimed that, 'Menopause is a hormone deficiency disease, curable and totally preventable, just take estrogen.' Given the appalling title, you can gather that Wilson presented HRT as a way of preserving femininity. In the 1970s, it was found that taking oestrogen without progesterone to counterbalance it was associated with an increase in endometrial cancer, which is what led to smaller doses of oestrogen and the addition of progestins (a synthetic form of progesterone), known as combined HRT, to protect the endometrium (coming up, we'll be looking at progestin, progestogens and progesterone, so for an explanation of the differences, see page 101).

In 1993, the largest piece of clinical research into women's health began – the Women's Health Initiative (WHI). The 1-billion-dollar US study would analyse the risks and benefits of a variety of healthcare strategies that were used to improve the health of postmenopausal women, part of which, of course, involved observing the effects of hormone therapy. It's still largely this piece of research that the public, patients and medical professionals use to form their views around the safety of hormone therapy, so let's get to grips with what the researchers found – or thought they found. In the section of the trial which looked at the use of hormone therapy, 16,608 women with uteruses were allocated to receive a combination of Premarin (the older type of oestrogen made from pregnant mares' urine) and Provera (a synthetic form of progesterone), or a placebo. A second arm of the trial looked at 10,739 women who'd had hysterectomies and these women either received Premarin (oestrogen) on its own or a placebo.

The first article to discuss the findings on the use of Premarin and Provera with regards to the long-term health of women was published by the *Journal of the American Medical Association* in July 2002, but a week before its publication, a bizarre decision to share the results with a group of health journalists was made. What followed was a series of frightening front-page headlines stating that HRT causes a 26 per cent increase in breast cancer, a 29 per cent increase in heart attacks and a 41 per cent increase in stroke among women using Premarin and Provera. The WHI study was subsequently called off, because to continue in the face of these findings would have been unsafe and unethical.

As you can imagine, this had a tremendous impact on public perceptions of menopause hormone therapy (MHT) and, arguably, on public health too. The concern that hormone therapy can cause or increase the risk of breast cancer caused many of those happily taking it to stop using it and some physicians to stop prescribing it. By the time the paper was actually published a week later and the data could be analysed by others, the damage had been done. The prescription rate for MHT fell by 65–70 per cent in 2002, the year the WHI was published. In California, the Kaiser Permanente health organisation carried out a six and a half-year study which evaluated the impact of MHT cessation following the publication of the WHI study on the incidence of hip fracture. This was a large study of 80,955 postmenopausal women and it found that those who stopped taking MHT had a significantly increased risk of hip fracture compared with those who continued – they were at 55 per cent greater risk!

Twenty years later, the impact of the WHI study continues; some doctors and members of the public still associate the use of HRT with breast cancer and heart attacks. Are they right to?

Flaws and All

The WHI report itself stated that, 'The 26 per cent increase in breast cancer incidence among the HRT group compared with the placebo group almost reached nominal significance,' but as Dr Avrum Bluming and Dr Carol Tavris, authors of *Oestrogen Matters*, a 2018 book that analysed the WHI study in forensic detail, point out, '*Almost* means it did *not* reach statistical significance, and that means it could be a spurious association.' Updated findings on this group of women were published in 2006 and there was no increased risk of breast cancer, but that helpful piece of information wasn't juicy enough to make headlines, and it seems that the papers and news channels forgot to tell us.

Later, in 2010, the WHI authors reported that there were more deaths from breast cancer in those who had been taking MHT than those who had taken a placebo, but this was 2.6 versus 1.3 deaths per 10,000 women, so we're not talking numbers that are enough to be statistically significant either.

The WHI study, which is where the majority of unfounded scary headlines stem from, was fundamentally flawed in its design and reported irresponsibly. Yet it has had, and continues to have, an enormous – arguably harmful – effect on the health of those who are peri- and postmenopausal.

Breast Cancer

If you're interested in the data surrounding breast cancer and the use of MHT, I recommend you read an amazing review that was published in the journal *Climacteric* by Hodis and Sarrel in 2018, but in case you're not up for that I'll summarise their points in relation to breast cancer.

In the oestrogen-only (Premarin) arm of the study:

- Among those who actually took their oestrogen-only pills at least 80 per cent of the time, there was a statistically significant reduction in the breast cancer rate of 32 per cent when compared to those taking the placebo.
- Regardless of how much participants adhered to their treatment protocol there was a statistically significant reduction of 29 per cent in rate of ductal carcinoma – the most common type of breast cancer.
- Among the deaths of the participants in the WHI during the 18 years of ongoing follow-up, the group taking oestrogen showed a statistically significant decrease in the rate of dying from breast cancer (by the way, that's low anyway).
- Of the 7,489 deaths from all causes, no increased risk of death from cardiovascular disease or cancer was found in those who took hormone therapy.

The Premarin and Provera group was made up of women with an average age of 63 years old who had experienced menopause 12 years prior to the start of the trial. And as Bluming and Tavris point out in *Oestrogen Matters*, '35 percent of the women were considerably overweight, and another 34 percent were obese; nearly 36 percent were being treated for high blood pressure; nearly half were either current or past cigarette smokers.' Only 10 per cent of those who were randomised to take hormone therapy were aged between 50 and 54. The combination of increased age and time since menopause, and inclusion of women who were overweight or obese, should really have meant that these women were excluded from participating in the trial as obesity by itself is associated with an increase in cancer and cardiovascular disease. Yes, it's really shocking, isn't it? But what the hell, let's plough on and use the flawed data anyway.

In the oestrogen (Premarin) and progestogen (Provera) group:

- A grand total of eight additional cases of breast cancer were detected per 10,000 women per year of use – that's an increase, but not much of one.

In the group of women taking a placebo instead of oestrogen and progestogen, there was a decreased incidence of breast cancer. It's one of those situations where something happened randomly during the trial that couldn't initially be explained – there was just an unusually low incidence of breast cancer. But it meant that when the two groups were compared, it gave the false impression that there was a higher incidence in those taking hormone therapy, resulting in the data being considered as statistically significant. The increased risk of breast cancer in those taking oestrogen and progestogen was not due to an increase in breast cancer rates among those taking hormones, it was because those in the placebo arm of the trial *who had previously used hormone therapy* had a decreased risk.

As you can see, there were many, many issues with this trial. Yet it is the one that still most informs physicians, patients and the press. But the WHI wasn't the only large study to report a negative association between hormone therapy and the long-term health of women. In 2003, yet another stop-the-press moment happened when the senior author of the Million Women Study (MWS) stated that 20,000 new cases of breast cancer in the UK were attributable to the use of HRT. But, similarly to the WHI, once the data were analysed, this incidence was found to be a 0.3 per cent increase per 1,000 women per year, which nullified the apparent risks.

In 2019, the media stated that, 'Breast cancer risk from using HRT is "twice what was thought,"' once again striking fear among the public. The headlines made it seem like a recent scientific trail had found this association, but the study being referred to was in fact a review which analysed data from 58 studies which took place between 1992 and 2018. Many of these studies were observational, which means that study participants were not randomly selected to take a particular MHT regimen or a placebo, and often what the participants took was down to personal choice. Some of the studies used older types of MHT that are no longer used, so this research is not representative of current prescribing guidelines. A significant amount of data used in this analysis also came from the WHI trial and the MWS. Now that I've given you the take-what-I'm-about-to-say-with-a-pinch-of-salt chat, let's talk about what they actually found.

They concluded that the relative risk of developing breast cancer was higher among those taking oestrogen and progestogen every day than in those taking progestogen intermittently (by this they mean cyclic hormone therapy, where you take progestogen for 10 to 14 days a month or every three months) and in those taking oestrogen alone. They also found an association between being obese and developing breast cancer in those taking MHT *as well as those who had never used it*, but the newspapers didn't run with that important public health message.

We should absolutely consider the risks of using hormone therapy, which will, of course, vary from person to person. We should also consider that there is a stronger association between drinking more than two units of alcohol a week and breast cancer than there is for using MHT. But nobody is up in arms about radically changing drinking behaviour. Whilst it is always a good idea to assess how safe a form of treatment is, including the use of medication, imagine what eating a nutrient–dense diet, not smoking and not drinking would do to reduce your risk of breast cancer. And for that matter, every other form of cancer and type of disease. But it's more convenient to blame mass-prescribed medication than a glass of cabernet. One third of the deaths attributed to breast cancer are from diet, environment and lifestyle factors. It's estimated that a whopping 50 per cent of cases could be prevented by avoiding risk factors and improving lifestyle choices.

Risk factors for developing breast cancer that you can't do anything about include:

- A family history of breast cancer
- Getting your period before the age of 12
- Menopause after the age of 55
- Inheriting gene mutations.

Ready for the risk factors that you CAN do something about?

- Smoking
- Moderate to heavy alcohol use
- Being overweight
- Radiation exposure
- Xenoestrogen exposure (that's things like BPA which mimic oestrogen – see page 277 for more info)
- Antibiotic exposure
- Stress
- Nutrient depletion
- Breastfeeding less than 12 months
- Type 2 diabetes
- Low omega-3:omega-6 ratio
- Consumption of polycyclic aromatic hydrocarbons (see box overleaf).

WTF are Polycyclic Aromatic Hydrocarbons?

Well, let's just start off by abbreviating them to PAHs, shall we? PAHs are a group of over 100 chemicals that are classified as persistent organic pollutants. They occur naturally in coal, crude oil and gasoline. They can also get into food from the environment or as a result of food processing, and they're a problem because they're known to damage DNA and cause cancer. Elevated levels of PAH have been found in smoked fish and meat, dried fruit and vegetable oils, and barbecuing, smoking or charring food over a fire can increase the levels of PAHs in food.

You can support breast health by:

- Checking. Your. Breasts. I cannot emphasise this enough. Checking your breasts and chest on the regular is essential, because it means you can get to know your normal (no two boobs are the same, even your own) and spot any changes so that you can get them checked out, pronto. It's not just your breasts that need to be checked. You need to feel in and around your armpits, and all the way up to your collarbone.
- Attending screening appointments. If you're in the UK then you'll be invited to attend a mammogram screening appointment every three years between the ages of 50 and 70. Early detection of breast cancer can save lives, although the NHS also points out that around three in every 200 screenings picks up a cancer that wouldn't have otherwise been picked up or become life-threatening: 'This adds up to about 4,000 women each year in the UK who are offered treatment that they did not need. Overall, for every one woman who has her life saved from breast cancer, about three women are diagnosed with a cancer that would never have become life-threatening.' Indeed, Dr Margaret McCartney, a GP who writes about evidence-based medicine, points out that 'Overdiagnosis – picking up "diseases" that were never going to cause any problem – is a major problem in most screening programmes.'

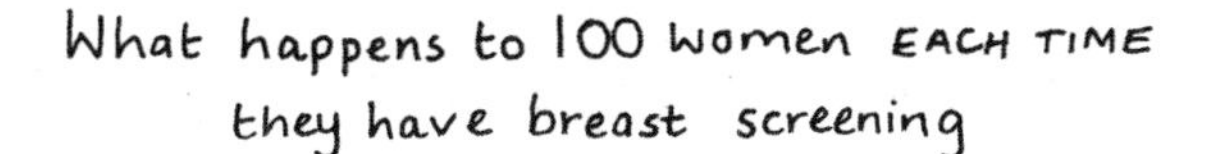

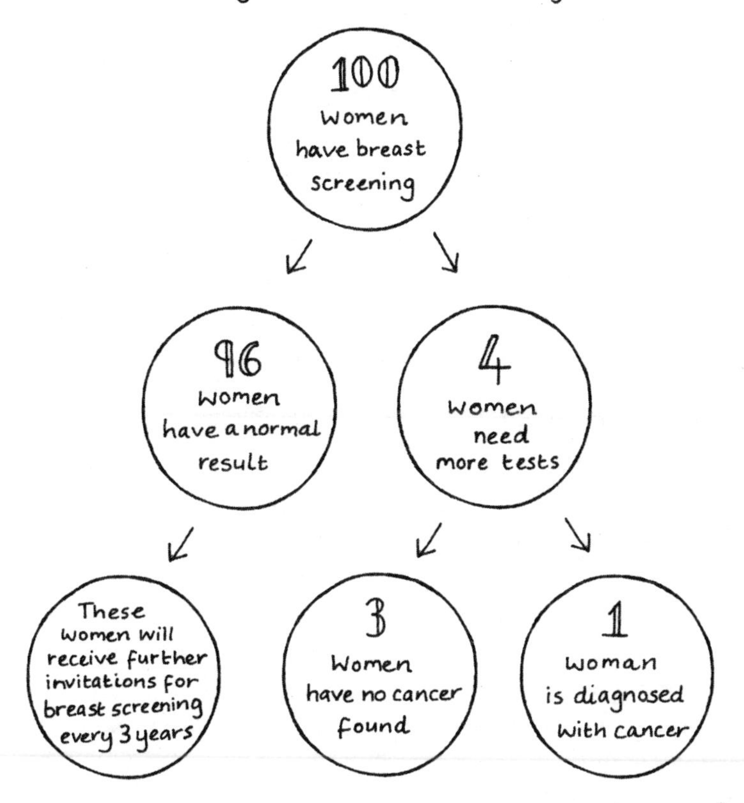

Source: NHS Breast Screening Helping You Decide (online pdf)

- Dry skin brushing and lymphatic massage.
- Avoid endocrine disruptors – chemicals present in personal care products, food and the environment which interrupt your natural hormones (see pages 276–280).
- Support oestrogen detoxification through diet and lifestyle measures (see pages 253–257).
- Preventing or improving insulin resistance.
- Getting enough sleep. Melatonin, your sleepy hormone, is a powerful antioxidant, so do all you can to support its production (see pages 247–251). Breast cancer rates are higher among shift and night workers.

Breast Screening

Mammograms are a type of X-ray that detects masses and areas of calcification, even ones as tiny as 1mm that would be too small to feel. The sensitivity of mammograms does go down if you have breast tissue that's very dense.

Thermograms use infrared to pick up areas that are cool or heated by your blood vessels. It doesn't pick up masses or calcification. Cancerous lumps develop their own blood supply and the idea with using thermography is to detect changes to your blood flow – 'hot spots' – before a lump becomes large. However, thermograms only detect changes in surface blood flow, so if cancer has developed at a deeper level then it is unlikely to be picked up by thermography unless it's recruited a blood supply significant enough to disrupt skin flow, which is why thermograms are not available through the NHS. They can be used in addition to mammography.

Ultrasound does not use radiation and it can pick up things like cysts, but it's not good enough when it comes to detecting breast cancers. If you find a lump in your breast tissue, then you may be offered an ultrasound followed by a mammogram.

Thermography and ultrasound can both incorrectly identify non-cancerous features as breast tumours more frequently than mammograms.

Heart of Glass

When my clients and friends talk about the serious illnesses they worry about getting, the focus is always cancer. And whilst considering cancer risks and how to reduce them is undoubtedly important, the main cause of death in females, particularly in those over 70 years old, is cardiovascular events such as heart attacks and stroke. Even if you were to be diagnosed with breast cancer (which I very much hope you won't be), you are still more likely to ultimately die from cardiovascular disease. And I know you're probably thinking that 70 is ages away, that you have time, but one third of non-fatal cardiovascular events occur in women below the age of 60.

Prior to menopause, cardiovascular disease (CVD) is less common in women than in the postmenopausal years. This is widely accepted as being due to the presence of oestrogen during our reproductive years, which is thought to offer protection from heart disease. Oestrogen improves the health of your blood vessels, dilating them and helping them to retain flexibility. It also exerts an anti-inflammatory effect on them. In the 1970s, data from observational studies were collected that showed the use of oestrogen therapy was associated with a decreased risk of developing cardiovascular disease, and that you were less likely to die from CVD too. These findings led to clinical trials which explored whether the use of oestrogen really did protect against CVD, by comparing women who were randomly assigned to either take oestrogen or a placebo.

Initially, a few studies that had enrolled women who had already experienced a heart attack or stroke concluded that MHT did not offer cardiovascular protection and that its use may have a negative outcome. Then came the Women's Health Initiative (WHI), the large-scale study which was stopped prematurely in 2002 (see pages 79–80), due to concerns over safety and what was *thought to be* a high risk of breast cancer and cardiovascular disease among the women taking combined HRT. In 2004, a separate arm of the trail which looked at oestrogen-only HRT was also halted due to a *perceived* increased risk of stroke in those taking oestrogen.

The data collected in the WHI study was independently reanalysed by Leon Speroff, who, at the time was professor of obstetrics and gynaecology and director of the Women's Health Research Unit of the School of Medicine at Oregon Health Sciences University (in other words, he knew what he was talking about). Speroff noted that the increased risk of cardiovascular events such as heart attack and stroke were *only* seen in the women who had been postmenopausal for 20 or more years at the time they were enrolled into the study. In other words, by the time these women began taking HRT, they likely already had physical manifestations of cardiovascular disease, such as atherosclerosis (see box overleaf). Particularly when you consider that 70 per cent of them were very overweight or obese, 50 per cent either smoked or used to smoke, and over 35 per cent had already been treated for high blood pressure, it is ludicrous that these women were enrolled in the study, let alone described as being 'healthy'. As the authors of *Oestrogen Matters*, Dr Avrum Bluming and Carol Tavris, point out, women with these well-established risk factors for cardiovascular disease should have been excluded.

Although oestrogen can help to maintain healthy arterial walls, there ain't much it can do if they're already covered in plaques. In 2006 Shelley Salpeter led a large meta-analysis, where researchers group together all the data from several trials in which similar participants are randomly put into groups to test a drug or intervention. In this case, the data from 23 randomised controlled trials (RCTs) with a total of 39,049 participants, including those from the flawed WHI, were reviewed and it was found that using MHT significantly *reduced* coronary heart disease in younger women, but not in older women.

What is Atherosclerosis?

Atherosclerosis is a disease in which plaques formed of cholesterol, fatty deposits and cellular debris build up on the inside of your arteries. These plaques block the flow of blood and reduce the supply of oxygen and nutrients, and they also tighten the walls of your arteries. They can cause coronary heart disease and angina, and if a plaque becomes loose, it can travel until it gets stuck somewhere. If it gets stuck in an artery that supplies the heart, it causes a heart attack. If it gets stuck in one that supplies blood to the brain, a stroke occurs. It's a slow, progressive disease that can become more of a problem once oestrogen does a runner. As we age, the walls of our arteries become damaged and lose some of their function, which includes the loss of oestrogen receptors found in them. Once circulating oestrogen begins to fall, the oestrogen receptors that populate the artery walls start to disappear, which is why supplementing with oestrogen might be useful when it comes to preserving oestrogen receptors and their function during the postmenopausal years.

The Danish Osteoporosis Prevention Study (DOPS) provided what's regarded as 'good' evidence on the use of HRT and cardiovascular risk. In this, 1,006 healthy women aged between 45 and 58 who had recently become postmenopausal were randomly selected to either take combined HRT, oestrogen-only (if they'd had a hysterectomy) or nothing. They were followed for 10 years and the data collected showed that starting HRT soon after menopause significantly reduced the risk of heart failure, heart attack and the risk of dying from cardiovascular disease. And no increase in risk of cancer, blood clots or stroke was detected. This trial was planned to follow participants for 20 years, but sadly it was called off 10 years prematurely due to the alarming publication of the WHI study.

The International Menopause Society states that according to the clinical evidence available, taking a standard dose of oestrogen-only MHT may decrease the risk of heart attacks in women under the age of 60. The current NICE guidance is as follows:

- HRT does not increase the risk of cardiovascular disease when it's started before the age of 60.
- HRT does not increase the risk of dying from cardiovascular disease.
- Using combined HRT is associated with little or no increase in the risk of developing coronary heart disease (this is estimated as being an additional five women per 1,000) or in having a stroke (six more per 1,000).
- The risk of developing a blood clot in your vein (venous thromboembolism) is increased when using oral HRT, but the risk is smaller when using a transdermal preparation like a patch or gel. In fact, using HRT this way brings the risk down to the baseline population risk.
- For those who are at an increased risk of blood clots, such as those with a high BMI, using gels or patches is recommended instead of an oral tablet, and many GPs will favour these routes for most people anyway.

Mighty Mitochondria

Think back to your biology classes in school. Do you remember being told that mitochondria are the 'energy powerhouses' of a cell? Don't worry, I'm not about to spring a test on you, but we do have to talk about the importance of your mitochondria because their health relates to ageing and chronic diseases such as cardiovascular disease, diabetes, metabolic syndrome, Alzheimer's, Parkinson's, chronic fatigue syndrome, gastro-intestinal diseases, autoimmune conditions such as multiple sclerosis (MS), and neurobehavioural disorders such as autism spectrum disorders, schizophrenia and bipolar disorder. With a list like that, I hope it's clear that we should all have a vested interest in keeping our mitochondria happy.

When mitochondria are struggling to do their job, one of the most significant ways we feel it is fatigue, because they create our main source of energy. As we age, mitochondrial function is impaired as a result of oxidative damage, which basically means the harm caused to DNA and cells as a result of the presence of free radicals. To save you from a chemistry lesson, let's just say that free radicals are unstable molecules that run around your body stealing electrons from atoms in your body, and oxidative stress is when your body can't keep up with repairing the damage done. This is particularly relevant to menopause, because research suggests that oestrogen reduces the quantity of free radicals generated by mitochondria, helping to keep our brains and hearts healthy. Once oestrogen drops off, mitochondrial function declines, leaving us open to the impact of oxidative stress, which includes the development and progression of neurological and cardiovascular diseases.

Other common sources of oxidative stress include:

- Rancid vegetable oils – the industrial process of making vegetable oils such as canola, soybean and safflower means these oils are subject to heat, metals and other chemicals, which damage their fatty acids. They're usually then stored in clear plastic, which doesn't do them any favours because they're subject to heat and light. And finally, they're used in cooking, which damages them even further.
- Insufficient levels of antioxidants – not eating enough colourful fruit and veggies.
- A disrupted circadian rhythm – not getting enough sleep, exposure to blue light in the evenings and whatever else is interrupting your beauty sleep.
- Smoking.
- Stress.
- Environmental toxins such as air pollution, mould, pesticides and endocrine disruptors (see pages 276–280).
- Infections.
- A sedentary lifestyle.
- Overeating.
- Long-term stress.
- Mould – it's present environmentally in damp areas of homes and businesses, and messes with mitochondrial function.

- Mycotoxins – these are toxins present in food and they're produced by mould in the growing, cooking and fermentation processes. Organic veggies and wild-caught fish bind to mycotoxins, giving them a way out of your body, so eat more of them.
- Heavy metals and pesticides such as glyphosate, the active ingredient that's commonly used in weed killers, reduce how much energy your mitochondria are able to produce (glyphosate has also been linked to tens of thousands of cancer cases). You can minimise exposure to it by buying organic food (particularly the Dirty Dozen – see page 270), and washing fruit and vegetables before eating them. Staying hydrated, sweating through exercise and using saunas will help to excrete toxic chemicals. Hanging out in a sauna isn't going to be your plan of action if you're experiencing temperature regulation issues, but it's a great option if you're not.

So if you want to reduce oxidative stress and support your mitochondria, you can:

- Avoid rancid vegetable oils
- Don't overeat
- Get enough sleep, and go to bed and wake up around the same time
- Eat lots of colourful fruit and vegetables
- Stop smoking
- Limit exposure to environmental toxins
- Move your body
- Deal with stress
- Increase your intake of nutrients such as coenzyme Q10, L-carnitine, magnesium, alpha-lipoic acid (ALA), creatine, B vitamins and iron to support the health of your mitochondria.

Making a Decision

As each of us progresses through peri- and postmenopause, the risks of using MHT versus the benefits will change, so I encourage you, as with most things to do with this stage of life, to keep a degree of flexibility in your approach. Your views about what is the best path for you to take may well alter as your experience unfolds. It is okay to change your mind and opt for something that you previously dissed. You are not weak. You haven't given up. You are doing your best to take care of yourself with the help that's available to you. You can also blend strategies as long as it's safe to do so.

Different Types of Hormone Therapy

Combined hormone therapy is a menopausal hormone therapy that combines an oestrogen and a progestogen. If you have a uterus then you must take a progestogen alongside oestrogen to prevent the lining of your uterus from thickening up and causing endometrial hyperplasia. The progestogen may be synthetic, such as the type that's in pills and in the Mirena® coil or, more commonly, it may be natural progesterone, which is described as body-identical.

Cyclical hormone therapy is appropriate if you have regular periods. You take oestrogen every day, but only take the progestogen component towards the end of your cycle. Once your periods become irregular, you take the progestogen component for a set number of days once every three months.

Continuous hormone therapy is appropriate once your periods have stopped. You take oestrogen and progestogen every day, rather than following a cyclical pattern.

Systemic hormone therapy is a form of menopausal hormone therapy that affects you system-wide. This is the type of hormone therapy used to treat symptoms such as hot flushes, sleep issues, cognitive function and joint pain. It can be used in addition to topical (vaginal) oestrogen.

Topical hormone therapy is a form of menopausal hormone therapy which is applied to the vulva and vagina to produce a localised effect. This can help with the genito-urinary syndrome of menopause (GSM), but won't have a system-wide effect.

Please don't wait until your menopausal symptoms are severe before you see your GP or consider hormone therapy. If this is you, then stop and think for a moment. A major plus of the menopause transition is that you can decide what's best for you and starting hormone therapy later can mean missing out on the window in which its use appears to protect against Alzheimer's disease and cardiovascular disease. For those of you who do decide to use MHT, I encourage you to see it as part of a strategy, not the sole component. Alcohol consumption, exercise, mental health, nutrition, weight and giving up smoking are all crucial to your experience of menopause and the years that follow.

When Menopause Hits Earlier Than Expected

Just to be clear on the terms, early menopause describes the temporary or permanent loss of ovarian function before the age of 45. It can occur temporarily if, for example, you are prescribed a medication to manage fibroids prior to surgery and prevent them from growing further. Whereas premature ovarian insufficiency (POI) – often referred to as premature ovarian failure, a phrase which conjures up all sorts of terrifying imagery – is when someone under the age of 40 has had no periods for four months or more, in addition to at least two measurements of follicle stimulating hormone (FSH) in the menopausal range (> 40mIU/ml) which have been obtained more than a month apart, in addition to low oestrogen levels.

There are several reasons why periods can go AWOL (we refer to this as amenorrhoea) and if yours have stopped it doesn't mean you have POI, but absent periods should *always* be investigated to determine the cause and decide upon an appropriate treatment strategy. One rather dated study found that for around 25 per cent of those eventually diagnosed with POI, the time to diagnosis can take longer than five years, which is frustrating given how straightforward the diagnostic tests are. Hopefully this figure has reduced since the paper was published in 2002. It's important that you find out what's happening so that you can be proactive in supporting your health and hormones, and make decisions around fertility and trying to conceive (see box on pages 95–96).

Early menopause is the term used when you go through menopause between the ages of 40 and 45, and although they share similar symptoms, it's not the same as POI. Menopause is irreversible and permanent, whereas although POI involves a halt in ovarian function, it may not always be permanent. Around 50 per cent of people with POI retain some ovarian function, and research suggests that 5 to 10 per cent of those diagnosed with POI will conceive and have a baby post-diagnosis. You can see why premature ovarian insufficiency is a more helpful term than premature ovarian failure, which implies that your ovaries have shut up shop for good.

Surgical menopause is when surgery, rather than the natural ageing process, instigates menopause. If you have both your ovaries removed (oophorectomy – see page 95) then this will cause immediate menopause due to the sudden loss of the hormones that are produced in the ovaries: oestrogen, progesterone and testosterone. Whilst oestrogen and testosterone can be produced in small amounts elsewhere in the body, it's the abrupt shift from having these hormones prior to surgery, to not having them afterwards, that comes as a shock. Oestrogen is involved in a vast number of bodily functions, including mood, energy, memory and verbal recall. When oestrogen plummets after oophorectomy you may not feel like yourself at all. Recovering from surgery is one thing. Recovering from it with menopausal symptoms is another, so it's crucial that you prepare for it and speak to your doctor about whether MHT is appropriate for you to take.

In those with, or who have had, oestrogen-receptor cancer, the use of hormone therapy and tibolone are generally not recommended to treat menopausal symptoms such as hot flushes, night sweats and genito-urinary syndrome of menopause. That being said, some patients with a history of hormone-dependent cancers will make the informed decision, in conjunction with their doctor (usually a menopause specialist), to use MHT when other treatments haven't provided adequate relief. In those with a history of breast cancer, topical application of oestrogen can usually still be used to improve symptoms such as vaginal dryness.

If you've had a risk-reducing salpingo-oophorectomy (RRSO) in which healthy ovaries and uterine tubes are removed in order to reduce the risk of ovarian cancer, then you're at increased risk of developing osteoporosis and coronary heart disease. MHT can decrease these risks though you might be wondering if it's a good idea to take it if you carry a BRCA mutation and have an increased risk of breast cancer. If you have no personal history of breast cancer, have a BRCA1 or BRCA2 mutation and have your ovaries removed before the age of natural menopause, the current NICE guidelines recommend the use of hormone therapy up until the time you would have expected menopause. Short-term use of HRT following risk-reducing surgery is not associated with an increased risk of breast cancer and in one small study it decreased the risk.

More on POI

Due to the varying levels of ovarian function in POI, 'menopausal' symptoms may be milder than in regular menopause, which means that there can be a delay in seeking out medical help and receiving an accurate diagnosis. It's a condition that affects at least 1 per cent of those under the age of 40, 0.1 per cent of those under the age of 30 and 0.01 per cent of those under 20.

The underlying causes of POI are not fully understood and, in most cases (around 80 per cent), no underlying cause will be identified. Approximately 10 per cent of cases are due to genetic causes and these are more common in people with a family history of POI. Genetic causes of POI can be chromosomal and involve the X-chromosome or be a result of a single gene mutation. Of the 10 per cent of cases that have genetic causes, the most common abnormality is Turner syndrome. Other conditions such as Fragile X syndrome and galactosaemia can also result in POI, and tend to run in families.

Autoimmune is a term used to describe situations where the body's immune system mistakenly attacks the body and there is a connection between POI and other autoimmune conditions such as Hashimoto's autoimmune thyroiditis, type 1 diabetes and Addison's disease – in fact, 5 per cent of cases are autoimmune in origin. Due to the line between POI and autoimmune conditions, it is recommended that blood tests to check for thyroid and adrenal antibodies should be carried out following diagnosis of POI and, if present, further testing needs to be carried out.

POI can also be caused by medical treatment such as the surgical removal of an ovary (oophorectomy) and/or uterus (hysterectomy), because even if an ovary, or both of them remain, there is an increased risk of ovarian function diminishing following surgery. Radiotherapy and chemotherapy can also affect your ovaries, though techniques to preserve fertility, such as shielding reproductive organs from X-rays and egg-freezing, are usually employed.

If you're wondering what signs and symptoms might alert you to the possibility of being someone who develops POI, I'm afraid that there are no early warning signs. Most people with POI have a normal menstrual history and a common scenario is that their periods don't return following pregnancy or when they come off the contraceptive pill. It's worth pointing out here that it is normal and common for it to take a while for your periods to return post-childbirth. It can also take a while for periods to return post-pill.

The use of MHT is widely accepted as an essential treatment strategy for those with POI as the premature loss of oestrogen has major consequences in terms of health and quality of life. Regardless of the cause of premature oestrogen deficiency, it increases the rate of cardiovascular disease, stroke, bone density loss, osteoporosis and fractures. Add to this the presence of symptoms such as hot flushes and night sweats, sleep issues, mood changes, vaginal dryness and bladder dysfunction, and you can see why the use of MHT for those with POI is recommended by both the British Menopause Society and the International Menopause Society until *at least* the average age of natural menopause – 51 years old. Given alarming newspaper headlines about the use of hormone therapy, it is understandable that those with POI are cautious about using MHT, but even if we were to accept the research methods of the Women's Health Initiative study – the piece of research behind the headlines – as rigorous (they weren't), it's important to know that the findings did not apply to those using MHT in the case of premature menopause. Not using MHT increases your risk of cardiovascular disease, fractures and osteoporosis. Not to mention the vaginal dryness, urinary tract infections and painful sex that's associated with genito-urinary syndrome of menopause. In all honesty, when I speak to women with POI who aren't taking MHT, my body clenches with worry for them.

Although ovulation and therefore conception is possible for those with POI, it is not predictable. The most reliable fertility treatment is IVF through the use of donor eggs and the male partner's (or donor) sperm.

Choices, Choices

There over 50 different combinations of MHT. This might feel overwhelming, but it's actually fantastic news, because it means you have options. We don't want our varying needs to be lumped together as one option and there is no 'one size fits all' with hormone therapy; all our needs will be different. Plus, what is most appropriate for you may change according to the symptoms you experience and any other health issues that develop, particularly ones that would increase your risk of using MHT. There are different types of hormones and ways of taking them, and brands and dosages vary too. If you want to know more about MHT (you do, don't you?), then I highly recommend heading to menopause expert Dr Louise Newson's website, www.menopausedoctor.co.uk. Dr Newson is committed to dispelling the myths around MHT and improving access to it, and she has some great resources to help you prepare for, and get the most out of, your GP appointments.

Most MHT involves oestrogens, but during early perimenopause, when oestrogen levels are often initially high, you can question whether that's a good idea. I certainly would if I were you. Given that perimenopause can be a time when oestrogen is high and progesterone is low, I'm going to start off examining what hormonal options are available to you by talking about the hormone you might want to consider using first: progesterone.

Progesterone Therapy

Progesterone is the hormone that's made as a result of ovulation. As we age, progesterone production ain't what it used to be (we looked at the signs and symptoms of low progesterone earlier – see pages 26–27). Progesterone keeps oestrogen in check, so less of it means that oestrogen gets to party, and the signs and symptoms associated with high oestrogen levels will then emerge, such as:

- Heavy menstrual bleeding
- Breast tenderness
- Cysts
- PMS
- Painful periods
- Endometriosis
- Fibroids

- Menstrual migraines
- Mood swings and irritability
- Moodiness and meltdowns
- Depression
- Weepiness
- Mid-cycle pain
- Brain fog
- Weight gain around the middle
- Bloating, puffiness, or water retention
- Abnormal smear tests.

Oestrogen imbalance can be caused by:

- Anovulatory cycles (common during teen years and perimenopause)
- Declining levels of progesterone
- Impaired oestrogen detoxification
- Poor diet
- Histamine intolerance
- Gut issues like constipation
- High levels of cortisol competing for and blocking progesterone receptors
- Environmental toxins such as BPA and phthalates that are commonly found in plastics which mimic oestrogen and interfere with its action in the body
- Alcohol consumption
- Weight gain and obesity (because fat cells produce oestrogen)
- Diabetes
- Some autoimmune conditions.

In this situation – one where there is an absence of symptoms caused by low oestrogen – supplementing with oestrogen would add fuel to the fire, whereas supplementing with progesterone would help to dampen it. Progesterone can also improve hot flushes, bone density, breast cysts and anxiety, and it supports sleep, so much so that it must be taken at bedtime.

Other ways you can improve symptoms of oestrogen imbalance include:

- Supporting liver detoxification and improving gut function.
- Increasing your intake of dietary fibre to support oestrogen detoxification via your colon (and poo).

- Increasing your water intake to support oestrogen detoxification via your wee.
- Supporting sleep. Before you roll yours eyes at me, I get that during this stage of life, there's probably nothing you'd love more than to be able to sleep but your brain and body won't comply. I get it and I've got some solutions for you, including the use of progesterone.
- Reducing alcohol intake.
- Exercising, particularly types which are high intensity and make you sweat.
- Losing excess weight.
- Eating broccoli sprouts. You can sprout them at home in three days which makes them a very affordable way of supporting your health. They contain the highest concentrations of glucoraphanin and sulforaphane which encourage oestrogen metabolites that are going down the unhealthy quinone 4OH to head back to the start of the pathway so that it has a chance of going down a better route. Sulforaphane also has antioxidant, antimicrobial, anticancer, anti-inflammatory, and anti-diabetic properties, and can help to protect against cardiovascular and neurodegenerative diseases – bring on the broccoli sprouts!
- Using supplements such as calcium D-glucarate, iodine (which makes oestrogen receptors less sensitive), vitamin D, N-acetyl cysteine (NAC), and resveratrol.

Bio-identical Hormones

Bio-identical hormones are, quite literally, exactly the same as the hormones made by your ovaries: oestrogen, progesterone and testosterone. Except they're made in a lab using plant sources such as yams (a tropical fruit) and formulated into oral micronised tablets, patches and gels, which your GP can easily prescribe. These are different to the older types of MHT, which are made from the oestrogens that are present in the urine of pregnant mares (such as Premarin, which is not identical to the oestrogen we produce) and synthetic forms of progesterone, and they can cause unwanted side effects such as impaired glucose metabolism, acne, water retention and weight gain.

Regulated bio-identical hormone replacement therapy (rBHRT) products have been developed in the conventional way and, as the name of them may have tipped you off to, they're regulated. On the other hand, you may also come across compounded bio-identical hormone replacement therapy (cBHRT) products. These are marketed as bespoke hormone treatments, 'compounded' or created for individuals, in specific doses, based on blood and saliva tests. Compounded bio-identical hormone replacement therapy products are available as creams, lozenges and vaginal preparations, but crucially they aren't tested or regulated in the same way that conventional pharmaceutical products are. The British Menopause Society does not recommend the use of compounded bio-identical hormones, and to avoid confusion that's why it distinguishes between cBHRT and rBHRT, referring to the regulated hormones as *body*-identical rather than *bio*-identical.

Taking Progesterone

Oral micronised progesterone (Utrogestan in the UK, Prometrium elsewhere) is a body-identical progesterone that's taken in tablet form and can be easily prescribed by your GP. Body-identical means it's a precise duplicate of the hormone progesterone that the ovaries produce and it's considered to be safer than older types of progestogens (synthetic progesterone) – even though, as you've seen, the data from that research is highly questionable. Micronised just means that it's been made into a very fine powder. As progesterone soothes the nervous system and aids sleep, you'll need to take it before bedtime and how frequently you take it will depend on what type of MHT regimen you're on. Cyclical MHT, also known as sequential MHT, is usually recommended if you have menopausal symptoms, but still have periods. It can be taken in two ways:

1) With monthly MHT you take oestrogen every day and take progestogen for the last 14 days of the cycle. This is what's recommended if you have regular-ish periods.
2) With three-monthly MHT you take oestrogen every day and progestogen alongside it for around 14 days every three months. This is usually recommended if your periods have become less frequent.

Some people using cyclical MHT will bleed at the end of the progestogen phase, but there may be cycles that don't feature any bleeding and, in some cases, you won't experience any bleeding. It's important to know that if you don't bleed that doesn't mean you're not benefitting from the endometrial protection aspect of this kind of MHT.

Continuous combined MHT is what's recommended once your periods stop and you're postmenopausal. With continuous combined MHT you'll take oestrogen and progestogen every day without a break.

When it comes to body-identical micronised progesterone, it's use isn't associated with an increase in breast cancer rates; four separate studies have found no risk or a lower risk of breast cancer with the use of micronised progesterone. Micronised progesterone can be used in addition to oestrogen-only patches and gels, so once oestrogen levels decline around the time your periods stop, they can be added in.

Progestogen can also be administered by an intrauterine system (IUS) such as the Mirena® coil, which means that it doubles as a form of contraception. This form of progestogen – levonorgestrel – is older and synthetic so doesn't carry the benefits that micronised body-identical progesterone does, such as supporting sleep, improving hot flushes, and supporting breast and bone health.

It's important to remember that progesterone/progestogen decreases the risk of endometrial cancer and that, although progesterone will soothe the nervous system and improve mood in most people, one in 10 of us will experience lower mood whilst taking it, which may be due to progesterone/progestogen intolerance (see pages 133–136).

Progesterone, Progestogens, Progestin – What's in a Name?

Progesterone refers to the hormone progesterone that's manufactured by the ovaries as a result of ovulation.

Progestogens are medications which include body-identical progesterone as well as progestins. This is the type that you're likely to be prescribed by your GP.

Progestins is a term used to describe synthetic progestogens. This refers to a group of synthetic hormones that share a similar molecular structure to progesterone, enough for them to bind to progesterone receptors and activate them. Common progestins include medroxyprogesterone (MPA) and norethisterone. They're found in some types of hormonal birth control, but they are not the same and therefore do not act in the same way as progesterone.

The North American Menopause Society recommends that progestogen be used to describe progesterone and synthetic progestogens, and that progestin is used solely to describe synthetic progestogens. Hopefully that's cleared that up then.

Oestrogen Therapy

Oestrogens are used to improve vasomotor symptoms such as hot flushes and night sweats, genito-urinary symptoms such as vaginal dryness and UTIs, mood changes and sleep disturbances. They also have a positive impact on bone and heart health, skin, and your cholesterol and triglyceride levels.

Oestradiol is a body-identical oestrogen that comes as a patch or gel. It's usually preferred over older, synthetic oestrogens such as Premarin, which is taken as an oral tablet and can slightly increase your risk of blood clots. Patches are changed once or twice a week, and if you use the gel, your doctor will advise how much and how frequently you should apply it. The gel and patch can even be used together in order to create an ideal dose.

It can also be supplied as a topical oestrogen such as a pessary, cream or ring, each of which can be used on their own to improve vaginal dryness, though these won't have a system-wide effect and therefore won't improve other symptoms such as hot flushes. Because the risks of vaginal oestrogen are so low – a year's worth of vaginal oestrogen equates to one oral dose of oestrogen – you can take it without a progestogen. It can also be taken in addition to any systemic oestrogen that comes in the form of gels, tablets and patches if it's needed. Oestrogen is only prescribed on its own if you've had a hysterectomy.

Combined HRT

If you have a uterus then you'll be prescribed oestrogen in combination with a progestogen, either as body-identical micronised progesterone or as a synthetic form of progesterone – this is what's known as combined MHT.

Taking oestrogen on its own causes the lining of your uterus to build up, increasing your risk of endometrial hyperplasia, a condition in which the lining of your endometrium becomes abnormally thick, which can lead to uterine cancer (see page 135). Using a progestogen minimises these risks, because whereas oestrogen tells the lining of your uterus to grow, progestogens cause changes to the endometrium that stop it from thickening up too much.

Once your periods stop and you go through menopause, you'll move to continuous combined MHT, whereby you'll take oestrogen and progesterone/progestogen every day.

Androgens

Testosterone can be prescribed to support sexual function when other forms of hormone therapy have not succeeded in improving sexual desire and function. This does not mean that testosterone will definitely improve things, but it's an option and will make a difference to levels of sexual desire in some cases. It can also help with mood, concentration and motivation. Using testosterone in this way is described as 'off-label', meaning that it's being used in a way that it's not licensed for (lots of medications are used in this way, but you might need to see a doctor who specialises in menopause in order to have it prescribed – none of my clients have been able to get it without seeing a menopause specialist). It seems that those who have POI (premature ovarian insufficiency – see page 291) or who've gone through early menopause benefit the most from taking testosterone, but they're not the only ones who can benefit from it – a low dose of testosterone can sometimes help to improve energy, mood and concentration, and in some people it can improve sexual desire too. I do wonder if the main reason it's so hard for women to access testosterone is because the medical establishment frown and shake their heads at the idea of older women being sexual.

Testosterone is usually supplied as a cream or gel that you apply to your skin, usually your lower abdomen or inner thigh, so that it can be absorbed into your bloodstream. Occasionally it can stimulate hair growth in the area where it's applied, which is why it's recommended that you change the area that you rub the cream or gel into. It can also be given as an implant.

DHEA (see page 27) can be prescribed as an androgen therapy, but the evidence base from clinical trials doesn't support its use for improving sexual function, mood and cognition.

Key Points Regarding the Use of MHT

- The Women's Health Initiative study that has resulted in most of you being worried about using hormones was hugely flawed, much of the data was analysed incorrectly and the forms of hormones used in that trial aren't typically used these days anyway.
- Taking oestrogen as MHT does not cause breast cancer.
- Taking oestrogen as MHT does not increase cardiovascular risk, it decreases it.
- Unopposed oestrogen increases the risk of developing endometrial hyperplasia and endometrial cancer, whether that's the oestrogen your body produces on its own, or oestrogen taken as MHT. This is why, if you have a uterus, you will also be prescribed a progestogen (but there are other benefits to taking a progestogen too).
- You may need progesterone before you need oestrogen. Remember, oestrogen can vary but is often high in early perimenopause. Progesterone can help with hot flushes, sleep, anxiety and bone mineral density.
- Oestrogen MHT can help with hot flushes and night sweats, genito-urinary syndrome of menopause (GSM), cardiovascular health and bone mineral density.
- Testosterone isn't licensed for use in MHT but it can be prescribed 'off-label'.
- MHT may also help with cognitive function.
- MHT tablets (not patches and gels) are associated with a higher risk of developing a blood clot, so if you have a history of clots or have other risk factors of developing them you will be recommended to use patches or gels instead; most people are given MHT in these forms anyway).
- If you experience premature ovarian insufficiency (POI) or premature menopause, you should take MHT until *at least* the age of 51.
- In the absence of any risk factors developing, you can take MHT for as long as you want to – you don't need to stop after five years.
- You can use vaginal oestrogen in addition to oestrogen that you take for other symptoms.
- The sooner you start taking it, the more benefits there are in terms of protecting against cardiovascular disease and osteoporosis.
- You can be of the opinion that menopause is not a disease *and* use MHT.

What Are You Waiting For?

Deciding to take MHT is very much an individual choice and something you'll need to weigh up the benefits and risks of in conjunction with your doctor. Just remember that the risks are possibly far fewer than possibly you and/or your GP realise. In fact, don't assume that your GP has received any training in menopause management; in 2017, Louise Newson and Rob Mair ran a menopause survey to assess the level of menopause education and training among GPs, and they found that 48 per cent of participants had not. I do not wish to slate GPs, the breadth of what they know and do astounds me, particularly on such limited resources, and some of my clients have had fantastic experiences with their GPs. Unfortunately, that isn't the case for everyone. Take my client Rosie. Rosie suspected that she was perimenopausal so she asked her local GP surgery if there was a menopause clinic that she could attend. They were thrilled to tell her that yes, the menopause specialist saw patients on Tuesdays, but they went on to explain that because her assigned GP worked on that day, she would only be able to attend the clinic if her GP was ill because it was the surgery's policy that if your doctor is working on the day of your appointment, you can't have an appointment with another doctor. If you're shaking your head or swearing out loud already, then prepare yourself for what came next. Rosie's GP refused to prescribe her MHT, not because Rosie has a risk factor, no, her GP wouldn't prescribe hormones because … she still has periods therefore she cannot be menopausal!!! Instead, Rosie was prescribed citalopram, which did improve her mood but left her with brain fog and her libido plummeted too. When she raised this with her GP, he shrugged his shoulders and said, 'Well that's what citalopram does'. After three years of being on citalopram, which included times where she felt suicidal, Rosie decided to come off it. During this transitionary period of coming off citalopram, she was on holiday with her partner in Spain and he read up about using oestrogen, and they managed to get some from a chemist. Within a week, Rosie felt a lot better. Her mood had improved, her body felt better and the brain fog had cleared. On returning to the UK, Rosie met with her GP, placed the oestrogen on his desk and said, 'I want that one please'. She got it, but why did she have to go through six years of hell to get something that the NICE guidelines recommend?

When it comes to speaking to your GP, I recommend keeping a symptom diary (you can download the one I give to my clients from www.maisiehill.com/perimenopausepower) and reading through the NICE guidance beforehand (see Resources) – you could also take a printed copy with you. If you're not happy with your experience, it's important that you speak up. I know that can be hard if you're in a dark place, which is why you might want to ask a loved one to come with you for support.

You might decide to take MHT for a few years or use it for longer, in which case please know that as long as your risk for taking it doesn't go up, there is no limit at which you should stop using hormone therapy. MHT is safe for the vast majority of us when we start taking it prior to the age of 60. But it appears to do more harm than good if started after 60. And starting it too late can mean missing out on the window of opportunity, where it can protect against cardiovascular disease, oesteoporosis and Alzheimer's disease.

Often, women wait until their menopause symptoms are severe before they're willing to consider MHT. If this is you, then what are you waiting for? Seriously, stop and think where waiting is getting you. Is there a part of you that thinks that taking it means giving in, so you have to wait until you absolutely cannot bear it before you relent? As I've said, this is not some test with awards for those who endure the most. The great reward of the menopause transition is in deciding not to put up with things anymore and to care for yourself at last. You are deserving of a life without suffering. We all are.

4

Let's talk about sex

In perimenopause and postmenopause, the impact of less oestrogen on sex is significant. Your vulva and vagina change, there's less lubrication, reduced sensitivity or increased sensitivity, which may be painful, and changes in blood flow and nerve transmission, as well as whatever your pelvic floor is up to. All of which means that even when your brain is saying yes, your body may feel like it's saying no.

Add to that interrupted sleep, hot flushes, fatigue, sore joints that may make certain positions hard and it's no wonder that so many will experience a lower level of sexual desire and activity. Medications that treat depression, anxiety, mood disorders, blood pressure, epilepsy and multiple sclerosis (MS) can all impact on desire and orgasm, as can menstrual cycle changes, alcohol, hypothyroidism, the pile of laundry seen only by you, emptiness from years of having sex to try and conceive, the grief of losses along the way and strain in your relationship.

Reading this might feel depressing, but if you want to have a fulfilling sex life, whatever that looks like to you, it's important to be aware of the reasons that could get in the way of having one. That way you can be empowered to make changes where you're able to. And it's good to bear in mind that not everyone will experience a drop in desire. For some it will heighten, even surge. Without concerns about pregnancy, sex following menopause can be liberating and highly enjoyable. Other factors such as improved communication in your relationship, regaining privacy once the kids move out or entering a new sexual relationship can all have a libido-boosting effect, and as progesterone and oestrogen lower, testosterone can also be relatively high, which is another reason why you might suddenly have an insatiable appetite for sexual pleasure.

Sex Doesn't Stop at 50

When I was 17, I used to volunteer at an HIV/AIDS centre, and I remember being told during my training that sex doesn't stop at 50. At the time I was mortified at the idea that my mum could be having sex – particularly as she was doing the same training as me and we were sat next to each other – and so that fact has always stayed with me, but some medical professionals do have an ageist attitude to sex and either don't even think to consider the sex lives of those over 50 or they do but are unwilling to go there. Worryingly, this means that STIs can be missed – yes, even people over 50 can have casual sex. Sexual health and wellbeing are therefore yet another neglected area of menopause and that needs to change, because 60 to 75 per cent of older women say that their sexuality is important to their wellbeing and lives.

At this stage of life, you might feel desire, but not feel physically able to have sex due to pain and other symptoms. You may feel fine physically, but have low or non-existent desire. Your desire might be sky-high, for your partner or someone else. Or perhaps not much has changed for you, but your partner's sexual desire and function is changing. You might feel quite glad about not having sex or it could upset you deeply. What matters is whether you're happy with where you're at and, if you're not, that you get appropriate help. Exploring other ways of connecting and being intimate in your relationship, hormonal support, sex therapy, relationship therapy, vibrators, other sex toys and masturbation are all great ways of adapting to your changing sexual needs.

Many women in heterosexual relationships have expressed concern to me that not wanting to, or not being able to, have penetrative sex in the way they used to leaves them feeling 'bad' for their male partner. And whilst some of my clients have expressed *their* desire to feel connection and pleasure through penetration, this worry is more frequently based in wanting to please men. Now, there's nothing wrong with wanting your lover or partner to experience pleasure, but how many male partners have you had who've expressed this level of concern about your right to experience sexual pleasure and orgasm? All that's happening here is that men are now in the position that we have been in for most of our lives; the sexual activity most associated with orgasm – penetration for them, clitoral stimulation for us – is denied them.

If it's included in a sexual act at all, clitoral stimulation is considered as foreplay – a term I cannot stand because it implies that everything that comes before penetration is only a precursor to the main event and it prioritises vaginal penetration as being the ultimate place to get to, with male orgasm signalling the end of sex. In her excellent book *Mind the Gap: The Truth about Desire and how to Futureproof Your Sex Life*, clinical psychologist and psychosexologist Dr Karen Gurney asks us to consider the following:

- Ninety-five per cent of men and women can orgasm from masturbation (in other words, there isn't a difference in orgasm rates between the sexes).
- The clitoris is the source of sexual pleasure in women.
- Penetrative vaginal sex is the type of sex least likely to result in orgasm.
- Less than 5 per cent of women use penetration by itself to masturbate.
- When straight couples have sex, men orgasm at the same rate as they do when they masturbate, but for women this drops to 65 per cent, or as low as 18 per cent during casual sex.
- When women have sex with other women, the orgasm rate only drops to 85 per cent.

With all of the above in mind, it's clear that most women in heterosexual relationships have sex lives that are rooted in male pleasure (and penetration). Gurney cautions against framing orgasm as the goal of sex and states that:

> Heterosexual women are often having the types of sex that are not the ultimate fit for their anatomy, then feeling shame and guilt for not experiencing the 'right amount' of pleasure or orgasms from these experiences, or experiencing a knock-on effect on their desire for sex with their partner, without even realising these limiting and dissatisfying scripts are to blame... the type of sex which equates to 'real sex' is vaginal penetration (suiting men's anatomy and their most reliable route to orgasm, not women's).

Use It or Lose It

Scientific papers on the genito-urinary syndrome of menopause (GSM) frequently report that increased sexual activity helps to maintain a 'robust vaginal muscle condition' and by sexual activity they of course mean vaginal penetration. This, at the point in life where *if* you are attracted to men you may also find them irritating and unbearable, science says that you need their penis if you are to maintain vaginal elasticity and pliability. And not just their penis, you need their semen too! Semen contains sexual steroids, prostaglandins and essential fatty acids, all of which are apparently *essential* to the health of your vagina. And for those of you who *aren't* partnered up, masturbation and sex devices are 'options'. Heaven forbid that those be options when you've got a penis – I mean, man – lying around the house.

First of all, let's set aside that heterosexuality is assumed, as is a preference for vaginal penetration, and that they also seem to think that when we masturbate we focus on penetration. Now that we're past all of those incorrect assumptions, let's talk about the evidence base for using penetration to keep your vagina in tip-top shape.

The belief that penetration can help with GSM comes from one small outdated study which didn't involve microscopic examination of vaginal tissue. A more recent study that did look for cellular differences in the vaginal tissue of postmenopausal women having penetrative sex and those who weren't found no differences whatsoever. There are some instances where the use of dilators and vibrators can help, such as for vaginismus, but that appears to be about it.

Basically, if you're experiencing GSM, your vulva and vagina are likely to be feeling dry and delicate. Do you really want to force yourself into penetration when there's no evidence suggesting that it will help? Penis-in-vagina sex is upheld as the societal norm and menopause is a great time to do away with that if you want to.

So, you think you're sponge-worthy?
–Elaine (Julia Louis-Dreyfus) in 'The Sponge', *Seinfeld*

The unplanned pregnancy rate in those over 40 is 40 per cent, so assume that if you're having penetrative sex and there's a penis involved, then there's a chance of pregnancy. Once in the 45 to 50 age bracket, during which menstrual cycle frequency becomes more irregular and anovulatory cycles become more common, the likelihood of conceiving declines further, but is still estimated to be around 10 per cent chance per year for those not using contraception. Don't assume that longer cycles mean you're in the clear; 25 per cent of cycles longer than 50 days are ones where ovulation takes place.

If you're wondering when you can do away with contraception, the current guidance is that contraception should be used for at least two years following your last period. So by the age of 55, most of us won't need it.

At this point your ovaries still contain some remaining follicles, but whilst they can undergo a degree of hormonal activity, for the majority of the time it's not enough to result in ovulation.

Taking hormonal contraception can mask the signs and symptoms of perimenopause and menopause itself. If you're on the combined pill then you might be thinking that because you're still having periods you haven't reached menopause, but the episodes of bleeding whilst on the pill aren't actually periods, they're withdrawal bleeds. If you'd like to find out where you're at, you can ask your doctor to check your FSH levels as they can indicate if you're peri- or postmenopausal. FSH can be checked whilst taking the progestogen-only pill or an IUS like the Mirena®, but if you're taking the combined pill or injections then you need to come off them before being tested.

When it comes to conceiving, if you're in the not-on-your-nelly camp, you need to decide on how you'll prevent it from happening. You get to decide what form of contraception is most appropriate for you. Consider all your options and discuss them with your partner (if you have one) and your doctor (if appropriate), but know that you are the only person who can truly decide whether the risks outweigh the benefits of each choice. So, when it comes to contraception, what are your choices?

Male sterilisation

I'm shocked but not surprised at how many research papers discuss contraception, but do not mention vasectomy, which is why I'm starting with it. Vasectomy is a minor surgical procedure in which the tubes which carry sperm from the testes to the penis – the vas deferens – are cut or sealed. The procedure is carried out under local anaesthetic and takes around 15 minutes. After a vasectomy, sperm are still produced, but they're soaked up by the body, and semen is still produced, but sperm aren't present in it. However, it's important to know that sperm already in the pipes will be present until they've all been ejaculated, so another method of contraception needs to be used until a sperm test confirms that there aren't any present in your partner's semen, which is usually tested 12 to 16 weeks following the procedure.

I've had several clients discuss their options with their partners and they've decided to go ahead with a vasectomy, but upon going to their GP for a referral, they've been sent home with a leaflet about the pill to give to their wife. One man had to switch GP surgery in order to get a vasectomy! Another client asked her GP about what contraception she could use during the three-month period following her boyfriend's vasectomy, whilst they waited for the sperm already present in his tubes to be ejaculated, and she was astonished to hear them suggest the coil – which remains in place for three years.

Female sterilisation

You can also have your tubes tied. During this surgical procedure, which is usually carried out as a laparoscopy under general anaesthetic, two small cuts are made in your abdomen, one which allows the surgeon to see what they're doing with a telescope and one in which the instrument used to block your tubes is inserted. Clips or rings are applied to the uterine (fallopian) tubes, which create a block and prevent eggs and sperm from getting together. Around two to five women in every 1,000 will become pregnant following laparoscopic sterilisation and these pregnancies are more likely to be ectopic, where the pregnancy develops outside of the uterus. According to the NHS, male steriliasation is 'a simpler, safer and more reliable option than female sterilisation'. So why isn't it recommended more often?

The Essure Coil

The Essure device is a set of nickel-titanium coils which, until recently, were inserted into the fallopian tubes as a method of permanent contraception. Because the implantation of Essure could be done via a hysteroscopy and didn't require surgery, it was a favoured method of female sterilisation. But from 2002, when Essure was approved for use, until the end of 2019, the Federal Drug Administration (FDA) in America received 47,856 medical device reports related to Essure. The most frequently reported problems were abdominal pain, heavier periods, painful periods, irregular periods, headaches, painful intercourse and *device fragmentation in patients.* It turns out that those titanium coils are prone to turning into shrapnel and can pierce internal tissue and migrate into the abdomen. Being allergic to the nickel used in the coils can also cause pain and further problems. Eight adult deaths have been linked to Essure and thousands have undergone keyhole surgery or hysterectomies to remove the coils. If you had, or have, the Essure device, then I recommend joining the Life After Essure UK and Ireland support group on Facebook.

Hormonal contraception

Hormonal contraception is used for all sorts of reasons. Sometimes it's used for what it was intended for – contraception. Other times it's prescribed to try and manage period problems. Fifty-eight per cent of people using the combined pill take it for non-contraceptive reasons, such as to 'regulate' their periods. This is highly problematic because it cannot achieve this. Regulating periods means supporting ovulation, not suppressing it as the pill does. When you're on the pill you don't get periods, you have what's known as withdrawal bleeds. Having a menstrual cycle is good for your heart, bone and breast health, and has many other benefits too, so unless there is a clear reason to stop having one, I suggest making the most out of it whilst you can.

Perimenopause is a time when new period problems can emerge and existing ones can worsen. Hormonal contraception is often prescribed to 'treat' period pain, heavy periods, PMS, PMDD (premenstrual dysphoric disorder – see pages 127–131), PCOS (polycystic ovarian syndrome – see page 291), endometriosis and adenomyosis (a condition in which the lining of the uterus breaks through to the muscular wall, causing cramps and heavy bleeding). There are plenty of people with periods who suffer from these debilitating hormonal and reproductive conditions who will experience significant or total relief from hormonal birth control, so that they can actually live their lives, but whilst the pill can reduce some symptoms, it doesn't actually treat any of these conditions. It simply acts as a band-aid, which in some cases can unfortunately cause further problems.

Long-acting reversible contraception (LARC) such as the coil, implant and injection offer a high rate of preventing pregnancy.

The injection

The injection contains the hormone progestogen, which is released into your blood to prevent pregnancy, with each injection lasting for between eight and 13 weeks. With perfect use, it's 99 per cent effective. With typical use, such as getting an injection later than instructed, it's 94 per cent and it's common for periods to stop altogether. Whilst to some of you (I'm looking at you, heavy bleeders), this may sound fantastic, it can also cause breakthrough bleeding, breast tenderness, weight gain, depression, diminished sexual desire, hypertension and temporary bone loss. Not what you need at this stage of life when the odds of developing all those health issues are already stacked up. It can also increase your risk of cervical dysplasia and of developing breast cancer.

The implant

The implant is a small plastic tube that's around 4cm long, which is inserted under the skin of your upper arm. It also releases progestogen, which works by thinning the lining of your uterus and altering cervical fluid, preventing sperm from getting to an egg and making the endometrium unsuitable for implantation, but it can also prevent ovulation from taking place. The implant can remain in situ for up to three years, with a 99 per cent effectiveness, but its use is associated with weight gain and erratic bleeding.

Intrauterine devices and systems (IUD and IUS aka the coil)

The coil is a T-shaped plastic or copper device that's placed inside your uterus and can provide contraception for three to 10 years. The IUS and IUD both have a 99 per cent perfect use rate and the typical use is the same. It's insertion shouldn't take any longer than five minutes and the process is similar to a cervical screening appointment in that a speculum is inserted into your vagina to separate the vaginal walls and access the cervix. Once it's placed inside the uterus, a couple of thin plastic strings hang down through the cervix and can be felt high up inside your vagina. In the first year of use 6 to 8 per cent of coils can come out, with this figure reducing to 2.5 per cent in the second year and coming down year after year thereafter. This is why your doctor will ask you to check and feel for the strings, as either feeling that they've lengthened or not being able to feel them at all is a sign that it's come out. Other signs of expulsion include cramping and spotting. In case it's not obvious, if your coil has come out then you need to use another method of contraception. Getting an appointment to have a coil inserted always seems to be quick and easy. Sadly, my clients frequently report that if they request its removal, they're told there is a six-month waiting period. This is unacceptable, particularly as the procedure to remove it is usually quick and straightforward. If this happens to you, complain.

Mirena® or Skyla® intrauterine systems (IUS)

The hormonal coil, which you may know as the Mirena® or Skyla®, is what's known as an intrauterine system. It can remain in place for three to five years. It releases progestogen and, although it works primarily by thickening your cervical fluid so that sperm can't penetrate it and reach an egg, and by thinning the lining of your uterus so that a fertilised egg can't implant, it can also suppress ovulation in up to 85 per cent of cycles in the first year of use, with this figure reducing to around 15 per cent of cycles thereafter. It is often used to manage the heavy periods that are a common feature of perimenopause and it can also be used to treat endometrial hyperplasia (see pages 226–227).

Copper intrauterine device (IUD)

The non-hormonal or copper coil is an intrauterine device that releases copper and prevents pregnancy by stopping sperm and eggs from surviving once they're inside the uterus. If it's inserted after the age of 40 then it can remain in place until after menopause and, because it doesn't contain hormones, you'll still experience a menstrual cycle until your periods stop. It can also be used as emergency contraception. You might experience an increase in flow and/or period pain and, because heavy periods can cause anaemia and anaemia can cause heavy periods, it's worth getting your iron levels checked and addressing any deficiencies through diet and supplementation, as well as looking at any other reasons that could be contributing towards heavy periods, such as low progesterone. There is a small but serious risk of pelvic inflammatory disease (1 per cent in the first month following insertion and 0.1 per cent following that), though this is not due to the device itself and usually a consequence of an existing infection such as chlamydia or gonorrhoea, which really just gives you another reason to be up on STI tests. There is some concern that continued exposure to copper can upset the delicate balance between zinc and copper in the body. This is more likely to happen if you're already deficient in zinc, which can be the case if you've been on the pill or don't get enough through your diet.

The combined pill

The combined pill contains oestrogen and progestin, and is 99 per cent effective with perfect use, dropping to 91 per cent with typical use. It's not recommended if you're over the age of 35 and you smoke and/or are overweight because of the risk of developing blood clots. It's also not recommended if you are 35 or older and experience migraines.

The combined pill can be prescribed to manage menopausal symptoms if you're under the age of 50. There are times when taking the pill might be suggested to you, but I would argue that there are better ways of improving menopausal symptoms, including the use of body-identical hormones (see page 99).

The pill increases your risk of breast, cervical and liver cancers, and shouldn't be taken if there is a history of breast cancer in your family or if you smoke, because of the increased risk of blood clots. It also lowers production of cortisol, testosterone and DHEA, hormones which all impact your experience of perimenopause.

The pill increases production of thyroid hormone binding globulin (THBG), which binds to your thyroid hormones and inhibits their actions in the body, preventing them from helping you to feel energised, maintain a healthy weight and have a full head of hair. As you will read in Chapter 7, being born a female and getting older puts us all at greater risk for thyroid dysfunction. Our thyroid hormones are trying their best during perimenopause without us causing more issues through pill use.

It also increases production of sex hormone binding globulin (SHBG) – the protein that takes care of any excess hormones that are circulating. This is a perfect response to pill use, because it's how your body protects itself. The problem is that it also binds up the small amount of testosterone that you do have circulating whilst on the pill, so that testosterone can't be used, which lowers sexual desire. Dr Claudia Panzer, an endocrinologist and researcher, found that, even after four months of not taking the pill, levels of SHBG still remained high when compared to participants who had never taken the pill and she recommended that long-term research should be carried out to evaluate whether this change could be permanent. Panzer states that, 'It is important for physicians prescribing oral contraceptives to point out to their patients potential sexual side effects, such as decreased desire, arousal, decreased lubrication and increased sexual pain.'

SHGB also binds up oestrogen, which can unfortunately have a shrivelling effect on genital tissue, as well as causing a decrease in lubrication. Again, this is a feature of late perimenopause, so do you want to potentially instigate it sooner? One study of 22 healthy women found that after three months of being on the pill that:

- The labia minora decreased in thickness.
- The size of the entrance to the vagina decreased.
- Frequency of intercourse decreased.
- Frequency of orgasm decreased.
- Pain during sex increased.

I admit a study of 22 women is a small one and I'd love it if we had more data to discuss, but I've met so many women over the years whose experiences echoed the findings of this study and we do need to talk about side effects such as these. Another small study found that clitoral volume decreases too. A history of pill use is also associated with vulvodynia – the chronic pain condition that affects the vulva. All this makes me wonder, is our focus on suppressing reproductive function at the expense of healthy and enjoyable sexual function? Again, it may not reflect your experience, but if it does, speak to your doctor. Your sexuality matters.

The progestogen-only pill (POP)

This type of pill is also known as the 'mini-pill' or 'progesterone-only pill' and it's also 91 per cent effective with typical use. Although it suppresses ovulation 60 per cent of the time, it mainly works by thickening your cervical fluid, so it's not sperm-friendly, and thinning your uterine lining, so it's not suitable for implantation. Your periods may become irregular, light or stop altogether. You may also experience acne, breast/chest tenderness and ovarian cysts. It's also not effective if it isn't taken at the same time every day.

A large Danish study of more than 1 million women aged 15 to 34 found that women taking hormonal contraception were more likely to be diagnosed with depression and, among the teenage participants, this risk was increased in those taking the progestogen-only pill.

The patch and the ring

The contraceptive patch (Evra) and vaginal ring (NuvaRing) also contain oestrogen and progestogen. Its perfect use rate is 99 per cent, and typical use is 91 per cent. Like the combined pill, they should be avoided if you're over the age of 35 and if you're a smoker or if you're over 40 and have cardiovascular disease or a history of migraines. When compared with the pill, the patch and the ring come with a higher risk of developing a blood clot. This is because when you take the pill orally, it goes through your digestive system and via the liver, where it can be processed. When you use the patch or the ring, the synthetic hormones don't pass through the liver. Instead, they go straight into your bloodstream.

MHT and contraception

The progestogen-only pill, injection and implant can all be used whilst taking MHT, though given their significant risk factors and the fact that the symptoms they're often prescribed to manage can be dealt with in other, less damaging ways, I'm not sure why you'd want to if you have a choice.

MHT can't be used as a method of contraception, but if you have an IUS like the Mirena®, then this can provide the progestogen component of MHT that you need to take whilst taking oestrogen.

The combined pill can also be used 'off label' to manage menopausal symptoms such as hot flushes and night sweats, but shouldn't be used if you're over the age of 40 and have cardiovascular disease or a history of blood clots or migraines. Given all the health risks of using the pill, again, I'm not sure why you'd opt for it if body-identical hormones are an option for you.

Emergency hormonal contraception

Depending on the type you take, the morning after pill can be used three to five days after unprotected sex. It works by preventing ovulation, which means that you need to take it before you ovulate. This is a 'you can't put the toothpaste back in the tube' situation, so if you want to use it, get it and take it as soon as you're able to. Because of the unpredictability of perimenopausal cycles, some of my clients like to have some on standby for emergency use.

In contrast, the copper coil can be used as emergency contraception up to five days after unprotected sex and can be used after ovulation has taken place.

Male condoms

Condoms are the only contraceptive method that protects against pregnancy and sexually transmitted infections. With perfect use, they're 98 per cent effective. With typical use this goes down to 82 per cent. Condoms are made of very thin latex (rubber), polyurethane (plastic) or polyisoprene (synthetic latex). They need to be applied prior to genital-to-genital contact and your partner's penis needs to be withdrawn carefully straight after ejaculation before their penis goes soft, so that no semen leaks.

Condoms may slip off or split if they're the wrong size or shape, so it's worth experimenting with different brands and types to find what feels good to you and your partner. Stay away from condoms that have spermicide, colours and flavourings as not only do they smell and taste rank, but they disrupt the vaginal microbiome and can cause bladder infections too. My favourite brands include Hanx, which are made of rubber and certified vegan, and Hex™, which are latex and made in a hexagonal web which is designed to stretch and securely fit a wide range of sizes.

Lubricants – which I heartily recommend at any life stage – should be water-based if you're using latex condoms as oil-based ones weaken latex and can break them. Oil-based lube can be used with polyurethane condoms.

Female condoms

Female condoms are 95 per cent effective if used correctly every time. With typical use they're around 79 per cent effective. They're sheaths made of soft polyurethane that have a flexible ring at each end. One covers your vulva and one sits inside your vagina so that the tube connecting the two rings loosely lines your vagina. They can be inserted hours before you have penetrative sex, you just need to ensure that your partner's penis is inside the condom and not between the condom and your vagina. As is the case with male condoms, you need to use a new condom each time and additional spermicide isn't needed or recommended. Oil-based lube can be used with female condoms.

Cervical cap

A cervical cap is a little cup made of silicone that's shaped like a sailor's hat. You place it inside your vagina so that it covers your cervix, blocking sperm from entering it. Its perfect use rate is between 92 and 96 per cent, with typical use dropping to 71 to 88 per cent. It needs to be left in place for six hours, but can be left inside for up to two days. It's removed by breaking the suction and pulling it down and out and, as with the diaphragm, should be washed with soap and water only, left to air-dry and stored appropriately. Cervical caps such as FemCap™ can be ordered online and the FemCap comes in three different sizes.

Diaphragm

A diaphragm is a shallow, bendable cup that's shaped like a small saucer. It's made from soft latex or silicone, and you bend it in half and insert it into your vagina so that it covers your cervix. With perfect use, it's 94 per cent effective at preventing pregnancy and its typical use is 88 per cent. It can be placed inside up to two hours prior to having sex and needs to be left in for at least six hours after the last time you had sex, so that when you remove it sperm cells are no longer active. (It shouldn't be left in for more than 24 hours.) After each use, you take it out by hooking your finger around the rim of it in order to break the suction, much as you'd do to remove a menstrual cup. You then wash it with soap and water, leave it to air-dry, and store it in a clean place away from direct sunlight and extreme heat. The Caya® is a one-size-fits-most diaphragm that can be ordered online. It can be used for two years and oil-based lubricants should be avoided with it.

Withdrawal method (pull out)

It may surprise you that, if practised properly, the withdrawal method has a perfect use rate of 96 per cent (though its lowest typical use rate is 78 per cent). It's a method that's scoffed at, despite its enduring popularity, largely because of the belief that pre-ejaculatory fluid contains sperm. Unsurprisingly, research comparing pre-ejaculatory fluid with ejaculatory fluid is lacking, but one small study of five men didn't find a single sperm in the collections of pre-ejaculatory fluid. However, a later study of 27 men found that sperm were present in 11 participants' samples. Clearly, this is a method that relies upon trust, communication and skill, as well as a roll of the dice.

Fertility awareness method (FAM)

The sympto-thermal method is a highly effective contraceptive method when practised properly. With perfect use and training by qualified instructors, it's 99.4 per cent effective at preventing pregnancy. With typical use this falls to 76 to 98.2 per cent and this wide range is attributed to variations in the fertility awareness methods used in the study, what level of instruction participants received and whether they stuck to the rules of the method.

FAM relies upon being knowledgeable and consistent in charting your cycle and following the rules. When followed, it's a highly effective contraceptive method. It involves taking your basal body temperature (BBT) first thing in the morning as well as monitoring your cervical fluid in order to identify when you're fertile and need to abstain from penetrative sex or use a barrier method of contraception, or if you're safe to crack on and have unprotected sex. Yes, I really do mean that there are points in the cycle where you can have unprotected sex and you can't conceive. The irregularities in cycle length that happen during perimenopause do not reduce how effective the sympto-thermal method is as long as you follow the rules. One study of 160 couples where the women were 40 to 55 years old found that over a 12-month period the unintended pregnancy rate was 1.5 per cent with perfect use of the method followed and 6 per cent with typical use.

If you're interested in using FAM as a contraceptive method you need to chart for several cycles before taking the plunge. Ideally, you'd work with a practitioner as well to help interpret your charts. At the very least, you need to read a dedicated book and educate yourself. I don't recommend relying on apps to tell you when it's safe to proceed without another method of contraception or, for that matter, when you're in your fertile window and should be trying to conceive.

Beyond preventing pregnancy, charting your cycle like this helps you to get a sense of what your cycles and hormones are up to, and that in itself enables you to own your experience rather than be a victim to it. It can suggest hormonal imbalances such as low progesterone and poor thyroid function and can help you to develop a positive relationship with your body. See Resources for my favourite FAM books, thermometers and apps.

5

Moody bitches

Anger is only one letter short of danger
– Eleanor Roosevelt

Perimenopause changes how your brain works. Hormone receptors are found in your brain so it makes sense that when hormone levels fluctuate, and then eventually decline, this is going to have an impact on your mental health and cognitive function. In early perimenopause, you might have an intensified experience of the premenstrual phase of your cycle. As progesterone levels fall, you could find yourself feeling anxious, depressed, irritable and angry in the second half of your cycle thanks to the imbalance of progesterone and oestrogen. Oh so angry. Then, once oestrogen levels start to fall in late perimenopause, depression, anxiety, memory loss and an inability to focus might creep in. The brain changes that take place in our forties and fifties even impact on dementia and Alzheimer's disease. Life events and stressors in this stage of life are numerous and undoubtedly have an impact on mental health, but we can't ignore that many of these symptoms occur as a result of what your hormones are up to, which is why the standard medical approach of treating with antidepressants is unlikely to cut the mustard.

All Fired Up

If there's one thing that unifies the experience of perimenopause it's the ability to instantly switch from feeling calm to being filled with rage. Hot, burning anger that builds up like a volcano, the lava pouring out onto whoever or whatever is closest. All within a split-second. What my clients find most disturbing about this is the lack of control, going from zero to 60 without realising that your foot is on the accelerator until it's too late; the words already out of your mouth, the damage done. Angela, a member of The Flow Collective, describes her experience:

> It's like I can see the words that are about to come out of my mouth and my brain is going, 'Don't say that, don't say that,' and it just comes out anyway and I feel horrible. I feel really, really bad about myself. It just makes me feel a failure in that regard, because I've been working my whole life, trying to be more caring in how I express myself, but then there are these moments where it's like there's no link between the brain and the mouth, and it just comes straight out.

Whilst irritability and mood disturbances can be driven by fluctuating hormone levels and/or sensitivity to hormones, anger and rage are common during perimenopause thanks to the toll of the increased mental load, emotional labour and unpaid work that are typical features of being a forty-something. Perimenopause highlights the gross imbalances of life and wakes us up to the need for change, in our homes, our workplaces and on a global level. Anger can be an ally. It is there to instruct us and we can use it in powerful ways without our relationships being razed to the ground. Rage can actually be very reasonable, bringing with it a level of clarity and directness that may not have been available to us previously. Britta, another member of The Flow Collective, is finding that her perimenopause has brought mood changes and anger:

> I don't really feel like apologizing for myself. I'm just angry, you know. I've had enough. That's it. It's often my husband who gets it, but I've just had enough, you know. You come to this age and just when it's the same thing, every time it's because of patriarchy. I just get angry and I feel like I've got the right to be angry, rather than apologizing for it.

Being born female means that we're expected to be gentle, passive and caring. It's our nature, according to archaic nonsense. It's natural for men to be angry, though. It's expected and justified. They are admired, respected and rewarded for their anger. But we are punished for daring to step out of the role that patriarchy has deemed acceptable for us: passive victims, sad, teary and grief-stricken. It's not acceptable for us to be burning with rage and when we are, we're unreasonable. Hormonal. We are punished for feeling angry. We're bitches. So we just keep swallowing all that rage until it destroys us from the inside out, because the world doesn't want us to be angry. The world wants us to be nice and polite and always fucking smiling.

I Hate You So Much Right Now

There are times when we're angry, pure and simple. And there are other times when there's something else going on. Once someone has had a chance to express their anger properly, other emotions often emerge. The Gottman Institute describes this as the 'anger iceberg': anger is the emotion that's visible, but beneath the surface are other emotions such as embarrassment, feeling scared, shame, humiliation, insecurity, guilt, and feeling attacked and trapped. In this sense, anger can be seen as an emotion that protects us from other emotions. Knowing this is enough to change your relationship with it.

When you feel anger, pause and allow yourself to actually feel it. Usually, when we feel anger we try to get rid of it by yelling and clanging pots and pans around, or by drinking alcohol, which, of course, never works. However, allowing your anger, and, in turn, allowing others to feel and express their anger, is something that allows you to respond instead of reacting. It helps you to come out of fight or flight and get back into your prefrontal cortex, which means that you decide what you want to do and you're able to take in what's going on around you. You can do this by taking slow, deep breaths and reminding yourself that you're safe, your body is just trying to protect you. Then, drop into the anger, feel it in your body and describe it to yourself. Have a conversation with your anger and see what lies beneath. Ask what your anger is really about. Is it that you're fed up with the rubbish not being taken out (hello Paul, if you're reading this!), or is it that you interpret a full rubbish bag as meaning that they don't love you? You're also gonna want to mentally calculate when you last ate some protein, because it may be that you're more hangry than angry.

My clients who are in straight relationships often tell me about the anger they feel towards their boyfriends and husbands for their ability to take care of themselves. Amy, a perimenopausal member of The Flow Collective, described a common situation that she finds herself in:

> The one thing my husband is really good at is giving himself time and it's always been what I get angry about. Every day he runs for 10–15 miles and it's part of what he does to regulate himself. On days when I've been at home with the kids, or I've been at work and get home to everyone asking 'What's for dinner?' and I say to myself, 'Why am I always the one that has to have the answer?', he says, 'I'm just going out for a run' and he just gets to go.

How often do you find yourself getting mad at those around you for doing something that you yourself would love to do? My favourite way to deal with this was taught to me by my mentor, Brooke Castillo. Brooke teaches the importance of looking at a situation for what it actually is by describing it in a way that we could all agree on. As in, the grass is green, the sky is blue. When you reduce a situation down to something that's completely neutral like this, it takes the oomph out of it, and prevents your thoughts and feelings from escalating. For example, let's use a thought that used to run through my head on a regular basis and resulted in me feeling angry: 'I can't stand it when he doesn't take the rubbish out. Why do I have to do everything in this house?' Now in this situation, the completely neutral description of what's going on is that there's rubbish in the bin. That's all. But I used to have a whole load of thoughts about there being rubbish in the bin and it's those thoughts that would make me feel angry. Establishing a practice of separating out fact from fiction, i.e. what we could all agree to be true versus the stories we tell ourselves, will change your life. It's a way for you to see what's going on and notice what you're making it mean.

Observe the sentences you say in your head and out loud, and be on the lookout for words such as 'always', 'never' and 'everything', because they're often a sign that you're throwing around inaccurate generalisations that make a situation more extreme than it actually is. Try to catch yourself out when you do this – spotting 'always', 'never' and 'everything' is a game you can play with yourself that will give you pause when your brain is getting carried away. It adds an element of light-heartedness to a charged situation and that in itself can soften your reaction, allowing you to move from reacting to responding. These days a full bin is just a full bin. I can ask him to take it out or do it myself without putting myself through some kind of mental anguish over it.

Last on the List

Whilst changing hormone levels do impact on mood, we can't ignore that this stage of life is full of stressors that increase the risk of psychological distress. Strained relationships, divorce, parental illness, kids who need you, the stress of infertility, moving home, employment changes, financial responsibilities, extended family members who need you, friends who are struggling, interrupted sleep and other perimenopausal symptoms you're going through, plus whatever else is on your list of stressors – they all add up. It's no wonder once we're in our forties that so many of us are pissed off, knackered and depressed.

A significant part of my work involves helping my clients to prioritise themselves. It sounds unbelievably simple, but for most of them it's intensely uncomfortable to do so. Their brains throw up all sorts of obstacles as to why they can't go to Pilates once a week or not cook dinner for their family occasionally. We're not talking about anything radical here by any stretch of the imagination, yet after decades of living to serve others, daring to do things differently is revolutionary. But to get to that point we have to get past the layers of people-pleasing, guilt, fear of judgement and self-criticism, and underneath all that we often uncover a feeling of unworthiness that's been sat there for far too long. Stacey described a situation that many of my clients find themselves in:

> I tell myself that I have to get up. I have to get the kids ready for school. I have to get to work. I have to come home. I have to get the dinner ready or make the dinner before I leave to go to work so there's something for everybody to eat if I'm not back in time. I've felt tied to a pen. These are things that I thought I must do in order to be a good person, but they were making me a horrible person, especially with my kids. Now I realise that taking care of myself is a necessity for me and that I'm worth it.

The premenstrual, or Autumn, phase of the cycle acts as a proving ground for self-awareness and self-development, and perimenopause is one epic, continual Autumn – the kind that can break you and make you. Just as the premenstrual phase of your cycle is when the cracks in your life that can usually be glossed over with a bit of oestrogen become crevices, so it is the case with this phase of life. It's time to take stock of your life so far, decide what's important to you, and then simplify and streamline so that you're not stressed out beyond belief.

Raging PMS

It's 100 per cent normal to experience physical, emotional and behavioural variations throughout the menstrual cycle, and I certainly view these changes as beneficial, as long as you know how to work with the shifts that come about as a result of hormonal changes. But I also know, from my personal and professional experience, that these shifts can be intensely challenging. They can turn the smallest task into a mountain that feels impossible to scale. In some instances, an underlying hormonal imbalance will be at the route of the issue, but it can also be due to the relationship between hormones and your particular sensitivity to them. Some people are hugely affected by the sudden drop off of hormones just after ovulation and just before a period starts, others will be impacted by hormones peaking just before ovulation and a week or so before their period starts. And then we have the hormonal shifts during perimenopause, which can feel gargantuan. However, when it comes to the mood changes experienced by some people, I suspect that our hormones are simply revealing something that's going on all the time, but which oestrogen glosses over in the first half of the cycle. The shifting hormonal landscape of perimenopause can leave you vulnerable to premenstrual syndrome (PMS) – a term we use to describe the emergence of a collection of physical and emotional symptoms in the second half of the cycle – and a far more severe disorder called premenstrual dysphoric disorder (PMDD).

Premenstrual Dysphoric Disorder (PMDD)

If you've always had a particularly challenging experience of your luteal phase, such as intense premenstrual mood disturbances, or you've noticed that things have intensified since having children and/or entering perimenopause, then you might have premenstrual dysphoric disorder (PMDD).

PMDD is often described as an extreme form of PMS and its symptoms can include mood disturbances, depression, sadness and despair, bouts of crying, extreme irritability, anxiety, intrusive thoughts, self-harm, feeling overwhelmed and panic attacks. It's estimated that 3 to 8 per cent of people with periods suffer from PMDD, and it can be mild, moderate or severe. It can start during the 'hormonal events' of our reproductive lifespan, such as when someone first starts having periods, or it can be triggered or aggravated following a pregnancy, miscarriage and during perimenopause. It's associated with an increased risk of postnatal depression and suicide, and because of the on/off feeling great then feeling fucking awful cyclical nature of these symptoms, PMDD is commonly misdiagnosed as rapid-cycling bipolar disorder (also, because medicine is viewed through the male lens).

PMDD is a recognised disorder. In 2013 the Diagnostic and Statistical Manual of Mental Disorders (DSM-5) included PMDD as an official diagnosis – the first and only diagnosis related to the menstrual cycle. It's diagnosed by taking a detailed menstrual and reproductive history, so tracking how your mood, energy and behaviour shifts through the menstrual cycle is essential when it comes to recognising your experience, and sharing this information with your doctor. You can use the Get Cracking with Cycle Tracking guide on my website to help you with this (see Resources) and the Me v PMDD app is purpose-built to support those with PMDD in getting a diagnosis and monitoring their symptoms.

To receive a diagnosis of PMDD, you must experience at least five of the following 11 signs and symptoms (and one of the first four must be present):

1) Marked changes in mood swings or increased sensitivity.
2) Marked irritability or anger or increased personal conflicts.
3) Marked depressed mood, feelings of hopelessness or self-deprecating thoughts.
4) Marked anxiety and tension – feeling on edge.
5) Decreased interest in usual activities and relationships.
6) Difficulty concentrating.
7) Lethargy and marked lack of energy.
8) Marked change in appetite – for example, overeating or specific food cravings.
9) Excessive sleepiness and/or insomnia.
10) Feeling overwhelmed or out of control.
11) Physical symptoms – for example, breast tenderness or swelling, joint or muscle pain, or a sensation of 'bloating' and weight gain.

The symptoms must occur specifically in the week before your period starts, improve once it begins and become minimal or resolve entirely in the week after your period, have featured in most of your menstrual cycles for the past year and be severe enough to affect your work, education, social activities or relationships with others.

People with PMDD often describe themselves as living a Jekyll and Hyde life; their extreme symptoms appear premenstrually, sometimes immediately after ovulation, and respite from them finally comes around the time their period starts. They can then feel pretty good up to ovulation, but if you add in a sprinkle of period problems such as heavy or painful periods, then those days might be a write-off. Then there's the 'PMDD hangover' where you're trying to feel human again and get your life back on track, which often involves repairing everything that was undone premenstrually. All of which means you're left with a handful of days where you feel like yourself. Even those days are hard to embrace because of the awareness of what will happen after ovulation.

Levels of sex hormones don't differ between those with PMDD and those who don't have it, which is why a diagnosis of PMDD cannot be made by measuring hormone levels through a blood test. I'm continually disappointed to hear from people who clearly meet the diagnostic criteria for PMDD and who tell me that they're convinced they have PMDD, but whose doctor has told them that their hormone levels are normal, so they don't have it. It must be appreciated how hard it is to rock up to a GP when you're already in a vulnerable position and try to talk about a disorder that most members of the public and the medical profession aren't aware of. When I voiced my concerns to my male GP, I was told to come back and speak to a female nurse. It had taken a Herculean effort to get to the GP practice and allow those words to come out of my mouth, and at the time I didn't have it in me to go through it again. Between my professional knowledge, and the support of loved ones and colleagues, I was able to figure things out and my symptoms improved. But how many of those with PMDD fall through the cracks in the system? The denial and dismissal of their experience is damaging and dangerous. Those with PMDD experience severe mood changes, intrusive thoughts and suicide ideation, and 30 per cent of those with PMDD will attempt suicide. It is a grave mistake for any doctor to minimise what's reported to them, as it is for them to exclude a diagnosis of PMDD based on hormone tests.

My client Holly has always experienced severe mood changes related to her cycle and these became more of an issue once she entered perimenopause. Immediately after ovulation her mood would plummet and her energy would crash too. Between crushing anxiety, panic attacks, intrusive thoughts and brain fog, she was unable to function. Within a day or two of her period starting, she'd start to feel better, but she would still be recovering from the trial of the previous two weeks and she'd often feel swamped with shame, so it was only really the week in the run-up to ovulation that she felt like herself. That meant that for 75 per cent of each cycle, and throughout her cycling years, she was drowning in hormone-related mental health challenges. Holly had been tracking her cycle for some time and knew that her experience was tied into the hormonal shifts of her cycle, so she took this information to her GP. Her attentive and kind GP referred her for some blood tests to check her hormone levels, which came back as normal, and she was told that she doesn't have PMDD. The impact of this was significant, because not only did being told this leave her thinking that she had imagined the whole thing, but it also prevented her from getting appropriate help in that instance.

PMDD is believed to be a genetic disorder and studies have demonstrated that individuals with PMDD have an altered brain response to normal levels of hormones. When you have PMDD, genetic differences mean you process sex hormones differently. In simple terms, you're more sensitive to them. In science terms, variations in the oestrogen receptor alpha (OSR1) gene and an over-expression of ESC/E(Z) genes have been shown to affect how your cells respond to the hormones of the menstrual cycle. This is important – it's not all in your head. You likely have a genetic predisposition that means your body is wired to respond differently to hormones and your body will flag this up to you during the main hormonal events of life: the beginning of your cycle years, when your cycle returns after having a baby and during perimenopause. Dr David Goldman, Chief of the Laboratory of Neurogenetics at the National Institutes of Health (NIH), stated that his team's research into PMDD 'establishes that women with PMDD have an intrinsic difference in their molecular apparatus for response to sex hormones – *not just emotional behaviours they should be able to voluntarily control*' (emphasis mine). Genetic testing such as this is carried out as part of medical research studies, so you won't be tested for it in order to receive a diagnosis.

Remember how progesterone calms and soothes the nervous system? That's down to a neurosteroid called allopregnanolone (ALLO). ALLO generally makes people feel calmer by calming GABA receptors in the brain, especially when ALLO is at its highest in the cycle, which is when progesterone is peaking. But in those with PMDD it has a different effect, causing anxiety, agitation, irritability and depressed mood.

PMDD can also occur alongside other mental health conditions such as depression, anxiety and bipolar disorder, exacerbating them premenstrually. This is referred to as premenstrual exacerbation/magnification and can also affect other physical conditions such as digestive disorders. Those of us who are neurodivergent (autism spectrum, ADHD, sensory processing disorder, etc.) may also notice that the particular way your brain functions is emphasised premenstrually. In fact, perimenopause itself may be what helps you to realise that you are neurodivergent! Lots of parents I know are discovering that they have autism and ADHD in midlife, because their children have been assessed and 'diagnosed', which has led to the realisation that they too are neurodivergent. But in addition to this, the hormone fluctuations during perimenopause mean that it's no longer possible to mask autism struggles such as sensory sensitivities, difficulty socialising with others, planning and adjusting to change. There is only one study which looks at autism and menopause – a pilot investigation conducted in 2020 that involved an online discussion with seven autistic women.

Meet Your Neurotransmitters

Neurotransmitters are chemical messengers that your nerve cells use to communicate.

Glutamate is the most abundant neurotransmitter in the brain. It activates or excites cells in the brain that are important for brain development, cognitive function, memory and learning. I think of it as get-things-going-glutamate and like most aspects of human physiology it's great and important, but too much of it is a problem; when glutamate is high it kills your brain cells.

GABA is a neurotransmitter that dials things down by inhibiting nerve transmission in the brain. It helps you to feel calm, improves sleep and induces a general feeling of tranquillity and wellbeing. Caffeine inhibits GABA, resulting in more nerve transmissions, which is why you feel pumped up after drinking too much coffee. Anxiety disorders, addiction and Parkinson's syndrome are all linked to low GABA activity. GABA is affected by hormonal fluctuations, i.e. when oestrogen is high, low or swinging between the two, and low progesterone levels also result in less GABA stimulation, which is why anxiety and insomnia can suddenly appear in perimenopause. GABA is produced from another neurotransmitter (glutamate) and it needs vitamin B6 in order to do this. Feeling anxious? B6 could be your new best mate (though taking high doses of more than 200mg can cause tingling and nerve damage).

ALLO or, to give it its full name, allopregnanolone, is a neurosteroid. Remember how progesterone can calm and soothe the nervous system? Well, that's down to ALLO, which is made from progesterone in the brain, adrenal glands and ovaries, and from cholesterol in the brain. Levels of ALLO fluctuate through the menstrual cycle, with its highest concentration occurring when progesterone is high in the second half of the cycle. Low ALLO levels are associated with the onset of depression and anxiety during perimenopause. MHT can increase ALLO and reduce these mood changes.

Here Comes the Rain Again

My first experience of depression began when I was 14, the same age that I started menstruating. Throughout my teens and twenties I experienced on-off depression that would alternate with amazing highs, leading me to wonder if I had bipolar disorder. I wish I'd been tracking my cycle, because, with hindsight, I'm convinced this was tied into the hormone changes of my cycle. At the age of 16, I went on the pill for five years, but instead of on-off low mood, I felt depressed most of the time. With time, therapy and menstrual cycle awareness I was able to find ways of managing and then improving how I felt in my luteal phase. Fast-forward to pregnancy, where I half-expected to feel depressed, but actually felt incredible. Knowing that a history of depression meant that I was at risk of developing postnatal depression (PND), I waited for it to hit. But it didn't. Then my cycle returned, and I found that my mood would plummet after ovulation and my irritability was sky-high. I told myself it was the stress of having a toddler whilst writing a book and even whilst writing about PMDD in *Period Power*, when I realised that I met the criteria, I was still in denial that I might have PMDD. Now that I've thoroughly researched reproductive depression for this book, I've realised that breastfeeding protected me from developing PND, because it suppressed my cycles until my son was almost two. It was only when my cycle returned that the extreme mood changes in my luteal phase hit.

If my story sounds familiar to yours, if you're prone to mood changes and depression that's related to the ebb and flow of hormones during the cycle or during hormonal points in life, then you could be experiencing *reproductive depression*. Reproductive depression includes PMDD, PND and what scientists refer to as climacteric depression. Climacteric refers to the period of time when fertility and sexual activity decline in menopause > eye roll < and this type of depression is often more severe in the two to three years before periods cease than in the years after. What these forms of depression have in common is that they're related to the production of ovarian hormones. People who have experienced PMDD and/or PND often experience great relief during pregnancy and that was certainly my experience.

If you've experienced some form of reproductive depression in the past, then you're more likely to experience it during perimenopause. That may have got the wind up you, but just remember that to be forewarned is to be forearmed and this is crucial information to have when it comes to seeking out appropriate treatment during perimenopause, as it will influence your options for using menopausal hormone therapy. As consultant gynaecologist and expert in reproductive depression Professor John Studd points out, 'Premenstrual depression, postnatal depression and climacteric depression are related to changes in ovarian hormone levels and can be effectively treated by hormones. It is unfortunate that psychiatrists have not accepted this form of treatment.' Studd recommends the use of oestrogens that can be applied to the skin, such as patches and gels, to suppress ovulation and improve mood, and states that testosterone can also be used to enhance mood, energy and libido.

The use of progestogen, which for menopause hormone therapy must be used alongside oestrogen for a minimum of 12 days to prevent the endometrium from becoming too thick, can be problematic in some people as those who experience reproductive depression are often *progestogen/progesterone-intolerant*, which basically means that instead of progestogen/

progesterone making us feel good, it makes us feel like crap. Some people are intolerant of the progesterone that they themselves produce during the luteal phase of the cycle, others of body-identical micronised progesterone such as Utrogestan, and some will 'just' be intolerant of the synthetic progesterone found in some forms of HRT and the pill. And of course there are the lucky buggers who are intolerant to all forms.

Progestogen intolerance produces symptoms such as:

- Anxiety
- Irritability
- Aggression
- Restlessness
- Panic attacks
- Depressed mood
- Poor concentration
- Forgetfulness
- Lethargy
- Emotional lability
- Increased insulin resistance
- Acne
- Greasy skin
- Abdominal cramps
- Bloating
- Fluid retention
- Weakness
- Headaches
- Dizziness
- Breast tenderness.

Symptoms often appear upon taking progestogens and continue for a few days after you stop taking them, and similar symptoms may appear in response to your body's own progesterone being produced during the luteal phase.

Doctors often prescribe the combined pill to treat PMDD, the theory being that by preventing ovulation and the subsequent hormonal changes, the cyclical symptoms will stop. The dilemma with this is that because people with reproductive depression are often progesterone/progestogen-intolerant, taking the pill often results in depression and means you miss out on the part of the cycle where you feel normal again.

If you suspect that you could be progesterone and/or progestogen-intolerant, then this is important to bear in mind when it comes to the use of hormone therapy in perimenopause and postmenopause. The use of progestogens in MHT is important because they prevent the lining of your uterus from building up too much, which is what would happen if you were to take oestrogen on its own. When the lining of your uterus thickens like this, it can cause a condition called endometrial hyperplasia, which is a risk factor for developing uterine cancer. But, for those who are intolerant, this can be a precarious position to be in, because of the need to balance out what's good for your uterus and what's good for your mental health. In fact, a significant number of women discontinue hormone therapy because of the way it affects them. In these cases, some practitioners recommend using the lowest dose and for the shortest duration possible (seven to 10 days instead of the usual 14). If you take a smaller dose or if you take it for a shorter duration then it's recommended that you have regular scans to check on the thickness of your endometrium, as taking body-identical progesterone for less than 12 days is associated with an increased risk of endometrial hyperplasia, because it's not enough to counterbalance the action of oestrogen. Some doctors may suggest that you have a Mirena® IUS or the contraceptive injection. Although the Mirena® is touted as having a localised effect that's limited to the reproductive system, substantial systemic absorption of progestogen does happen – blood tests have found levels of progestogens that equate to taking two 'mini-pills' on a continual daily basis. When it comes to the injection, well, you tell me. Do you think having a problematic hormone injected into someone who is possibly intolerant to it is a good idea when the effects of it last for three to four months?

Progesterone Intolerance vs. Progesterone Drop-off

Progesterone and progestogen intolerance differ from the progesterone drop-off that occurs at the end of the menstrual cycle, in the day or two before your period begins. Those who are intolerant find that their symptoms emerge after ovulation or around the time progesterone peaks (five to seven days after ovulation) with this being sustained until progesterone levels drop off just before menstruation. Many of the people I speak to tell me how they feel like their world falls apart in the final one to three days of their cycle, and this is down to falling levels of oestrogen and progesterone. Some people who are progesterone-intolerant will feel better once this happens, but some will get hit by the hormonal drop-off.

There are ways to improve PMDD and many of my clients and readers of *Period Power* have experienced partial, even total, relief of their symptoms without needing to suppress their cycle. I've also had clients for whom it was entirely appropriate and necessary to use hormone therapy, and I'm currently working with someone who is contemplating having a full hysterectomy. As you'll read in Chapter 9, I'm a big fan of holding onto your ovaries and uterus unless there is a clear medical need to remove them. Unrelenting PMDD that hasn't responded to other treatment strategies is a clear medical need. A hysterectomy can be a hugely positive decision that can be life-changing and life-saving.

Everybody Hurts

In women, the lifetime prevalence of experiencing major depression is 20 per cent and the rate of experiencing depressive episodes is roughly the same. A 2001 study of 10,374 women aged between 40 and 55 found that, during premenopause, rates of psychological distress were 20.9 per cent, with this increasing to 28.9 per cent in early perimenopause, 25.6 per cent in late menopause and 22 per cent in those who were postmenopausal. Unsurprisingly, this study also found a strong link between sleep problems, night sweats, hot flushes and psychological distress; 39.7 per cent of women with sleep issues reported distress compared to 15.4 per cent in those not experiencing difficulty sleeping. Similar rates were found among those with vasomotor symptoms (36.6 per cent vs. 18 per cent). Depressed mood alongside other symptoms of perimenopause will often improve under hormone therapy and many women experiencing reproductive depression have commented to me that body-identical hormones have quickly restored their mood.

Depression in midlife can't always be blamed on falling oestrogen levels, though. If you're experiencing financial strain and your marriage is on the rocks, taking oestrogen might help you to feel more resilient in the face of these challenges, but it can't magic away the discomfort of life. Study after study has found that the high prevalence of depressive symptoms is more likely to be related to demographic factors and health habits (such as smoking and lack of physical activity) than hormone levels. Upsetting life events such as divorce or the death of a loved one make you two and a half to five times as likely to experience depressive symptoms.

Major depressive disorder (MDD), which is also known as clinical depression, is characterised by persistent feelings of sadness, low mood or a sense of despair, all of which may prevent someone from taking part in, and enjoying, activities that they usually find enjoyable. The symptoms of major depression are defined as lasting longer than two weeks, though it can continue for months or years. The risk of developing MDD is one and a half to three times higher in women than men, and there's an increased vulnerability to it during perimenopause and in the first few years following menopause. The age range where rates of suicide peak in women is between 50 and 54, which is yet another reason why it's imperative that healthcare providers receive adequate training in menopause.

The NICE guidelines are that when it comes to low mood and anxiety that arise as a result of perimenopause, hormone therapy and CBT should be considered (you'll find some of my favourite ways to support mental health later on in this chapter). Essentially, even though you're feeling depressed, your depression may be a symptom of perimenopause rather than classical depression itself. The NICE guidelines state that, 'There is no clear evidence for SSRIs or SNRIs [selective serotonin reuptake inhibitors and serotonin-norepinephrine reuptake inhibitors – both antidepressants] to ease low mood in menopausal women who have not been diagnosed with depression.'

Women I speak to often say that they are okay with taking antidepressants, but are scared of taking MHT because they believe – thanks to inaccurate newspaper headlines – that going on MHT increases your risk of breast cancer (see pages 79–80 on why this isn't the case). The lasting impact of the Women's Health Initiative study continues, sometimes with both patient and doctor being fearful of prescribing MHT. Given the potential side effects of taking antidepressants, the questionable effectiveness of taking them, and all the benefits of taking body-identical hormone therapy (see page 288), I know what I'd rather be taking.

Anxiety

If you've started to experience crippling anxiety, this could also be down to perimenopause. You might feel like you're losing your mind, particularly if anxiety is a new experience for you, but you're not losing your mind, you're losing your hormones. Anxiety can appear in a variety of ways, including:

- Worrying about anything and everything
- Social anxiety
- Health anxiety
- Confusion
- Feeling overwhelmed by the smallest of things – you never used to be like this
- Feeling fearful
- Feeling unable to cope
- Panic attacks.

It's often exacerbated by lack of sleep, fatigue and blood sugar dysregulation. Anxiety can also trigger a hot flush and if you feel anxious because of a hot flush, then that can intensify it. Data from the Penn Ovarian Aging Study demonstrates a strong association between anxiety and hot flushes, with the most anxious study participants experiencing the most frequent hot flushes.

Endless worrying about things that never used to bother you can feel terrifying, both because of the physical sensation of anxiety, and because of the ensuing thoughts that only deepen the gnawing pit of doom and leave you feeling very aware of your heartbeat. This affects your appetite in that you might lose it or you might find yourself eating more in an attempt to dampen down what you're feeling. A mind that does a fantastic job of imagining the worst will suck you into a whirlpool of worry that screws with your sleep, and sleep deprivation causes anxiety, making this another vicious cycle to get out of as soon as you can.

There are all sorts of ways of managing and improving anxiety, with the standard medical approach being to prescribe SSRIs, a type of antidepressant. The trouble with this is that those who are perimenopausal (and bear in mind that they may not realise that they are) will be prescribed an SSRI for their anxiety and/or depression (and possibly for hot flushes too), painkillers for their painful joints and something to help them sleep at night, when what they really need is hormone therapy.

When I feel myself moving into fight, flight or freeze, I notice the feeling in my body; what it is and what it feels like. For me (and your experience may be different), I feel a tightness in my chest that's hot and centralises between my boobs and around my bra line. My heart rate picks up and at the same time I notice that I'm hyper-aware of what's going on in my periphery. This is my body doing an excellent job of trying to protect me and were there to be a true threat, this kind of response would serve me well, because I'd be aware of my surroundings and be able to respond swiftly. But I'm not currently under threat. I'm just wondering if I have enough time to write this section before picking up my son from preschool and it's that thought that has created a general feeling of unease and panic in me. I could let the anxiety run wild and, were I to do so, I would absolutely not finish this section. Instead, I'd get carried away with my thoughts, come up with even more thoughts that would create a feeling of anxiety in my body, and go check out what's happening in my fridge. Then I'd panic about lost time and not achieving what I needed to, and end up running a highlight reel of everything that could go wrong with my day and life along the lines of, 'Why can't I get anything done? I'm useless, my book won't be done in time, my publishers are going to hate me, nobody is going to buy my book, the world is going to end.' Okay, now my heart is really beating, but you get the point: anxiety quickly spirals when we allow it to. But I'm practised at handling this, so I notice my body's response, pause, smile and thank it for trying to keep me safe because that's exactly what it's trying to do. That gives me enough space to figure out why I'm feeling anxious. Sometimes there's a physical reason for it, such as drinking caffeine or eating something that triggers my histamine intolerance, but most of the time it's because I have an incredibly inventive imagination that likes to create scenarios that my body thinks it needs to respond to. Telling my body that it can stand down is an incredibly kind and loving way to deal with this. Then I can focus on breathing deeply, which stimulates my vagus nerve, which, in turn, regulates my heart rate.

Your Wandering Nerve

There are two halves of your nervous system. One half – the sympathetic – brings you into the stress response of fight, flight or freeze and the other half – the parasympathetic – is where you're relaxed and in what's described as rest and digest, which in case you were wondering is where most of your time should be spent.

The vagus nerve is a major part of the rest and digest half of your nervous system, and it's the longest pathway of nerves in the body, so much so that it wanders (*vagus* means 'wandering' in Latin) throughout the body. When the vagus nerve is stimulated, your heart rate slows and you move out of fight, flight or freeze, and the more you give your vagus nerve some TLC, the more time you'll spend feeling relaxed and able to connect to yourself and others. Practices which improve vagal tone – the quality of the vagus nerve – include:

- Deep, slow breathing (six breaths a minute)
- Laughing
- Humming
- Singing
- Splashing your face with cold water
- Showering with cold water
- Acupuncture
- Yoga.

The thing is though, if your brain has come up with a question it needs an answer. It'll keep asking it until it does and if you try to ignore it (which you won't be able to do anyway), your anxiety will spiral. The solution is to do what it's asking for and give it an answer. Write the questions it's coming up with down and write the answers down too. They're most likely to be 'what if…' questions, so start by noticing when the what if brigade shows up. Give your brain the answer it's in search of and, in the process, you'll not only come up with a plan for if the source of imaginary impending doom actually happens, but you'll also be able to see things for what they are. The key is to get them down on paper so that you can separate yourself from them and see them, and to do so without judgement. Allowing them to run around in circles inside your head isn't helpful, but neither is bringing out the self-flagellation whip. My favourite ways to support mental health include:

Feeling Your Feelings

It is unhelpful and unreasonable to expect to feel happy all the time. Life isn't just sweet-smelling roses and, if you're on a quest to be in a constant state of positivity, you're going to fail, because there are always two sides of the coin. Life is fraught with testing times, disappointments, losses and shitstorms, and perimenopause is no different. So how comfortable are you with getting uncomfortable? Are you able to sit with your emotions and experience them fully or do you distract yourself with mindless scrolling on social media, a packet of biscuits (my favourite way to comfort-eat) or a bottle of wine? Were you raised to know that it's okay to feel sadness, grief and anger or were these emotions that were frowned upon? Are you able to allow yourself to let emotion run its course?

Squashing feelings down and trying to avoid them never works. It's like trying to push a beach ball filled with air under water – it's hard to get it under in the first place and once you do it pops up again with even more force, causing water to splash all around. When we do this with an uncomfortable feeling, the same happens. Running away from the discomfort of emotions such as anger, sadness, grief and shame, we cause more harm to ourselves and our relationships. Truly inhabiting our bodies, allowing feelings, and leaning into the discomfort and pain is a tremendous gift to give yourself. If you're having trouble getting your head around this, think about the last time you were upset or angry and you shared how you felt with someone, but they dismissed or minimised what you told them, or they just ignored what you said altogether. How did that feel to you? Not great, right? But we do this to ourselves all the time. When it comes to experiencing emotional pain, most of us are highly adept at eating a treat, having a scroll or sinking a glass of wine in order to try and solve the problem. But being a human who feels emotions isn't a problem. Telling yourself that you shouldn't have these feelings is.

Whilst experiencing 'negative' emotion can be intensely uncomfortable, it is part of being human. When we bottle things up, sweep them under the rug and rush to move on, it might feel like you've won the battle with your brain, but the reality is that you've suppressed it and saved it for later. Denying ourselves opportunities to feel angry, anxious, depressed, frustrated, grief-stricken and sad means that we miss out on letting our nervous system calibrate and reach a place of resolution. Instead you've squashed it down and, depending on the situation and your personal tendencies, you might have lashed out at a stranger or loved one/demolished a pack of biscuits/had too much to drink. Of course, much of this will be dependent on the circumstances in which you find yourself – experiencing emotion is likely to be very different if you're in the privacy of your own home versus your workplace, but there are always ways to allow emotion instead of resisting it. Attempting to suppress your feelings with alcohol, food, drugs, Instagram, Netflix, work and keeping busy isn't going to improve your experience of perimenopause.

Get Help

Speak to your GP about the symptoms you're experiencing. If you're in early perimenopause, ask about using body-identical progesterone. Remember, progesterone increases GABA function, helping you to feel calm and serene, and it also helps you sleep. If you're experiencing longer gaps between periods along with mood changes, forgetfulness and cognitive changes, then speak to them about using oestrogen (and progesterone). They can also refer you for cognitive behavioural therapy (CBT), which can help with mood changes and symptoms such as hot flushes too.

A naturopath or functional medicine practitioner can identify any underlying hormone and health imbalances, and refer you for any relevant tests, as well as come up with an individualised treatment strategy. Functional medicine practitioners – some of whom are medical doctors – have undergone specific training so that they can assess and address the root causes of your symptoms. Seeing a functional medicine practitioner is a very different experience to seeing a GP, though some of the testing they refer you for can be accessed via your GP. Working with a professional is ideal, particularly if you have other health issues, are taking medication or considering coming off SSRIs (which, by the way, should be done slowly and carefully, and with the support of a naturopath or functional medicine doctor). Don't just grab a load of supplements and hope for the best. Depression and other mood changes often occur alongside other health issues, such as chronic pain and metabolic syndrome. When there are several components, which there often are, working with someone who can piece it all together saves you time and money in the end. Not to mention your sanity.

Talking therapies are always useful and I wish every human could access them, and life coaches will help you look at everything from negative self-talk to mindset, boundaries and people-pleasing.

The importance of being part of a community that gets you cannot be emphasised enough. Since opening the doors to my online membership, The Flow Collective, I'm continually blown away by the impact of having a dedicated community where we can share our experiences of the menstrual cycle and life cycle. Feeling connected and having a place to truly be yourself is so freeing and nourishing, and having a high level of social support protects against developing depression by as much as 20 per cent.

Focus on Your Body

As well as focussing on what's going on with your mind, look at how you can support your body such as reducing the inflammation that can be involved in depression (see pages 181–182). Give yourself a schedule and stick to it. Wake up and go to bed around the same time, and eat at set mealtimes.

Massage and touch stimulate the flow of oxytocin, the love hormone, so I teach my clients a fabulous self-care massage to put in their perimenopause toolbelt and if you have a willing partner then they can do it to you. Go to www.maisiehill.com/perimenopausepower for my video on how to do this.

Weighted blankets can help to regulate your nervous system, reduce anxiety and improve sleep. Turning your Wi-Fi off overnight and when not in use, and packing your phone away for significant periods of time, can also make a difference. Don't try and tell me that all those alerts aren't having an impact on your nervous system.

Avoid stimulants such as tea and coffee. Even green tea, which does have caffeine in it, can be too much for some people. Alcohol and fags are also stimulants, by the way.

Breathing techniques are a simple and quick way to regulate your heart rate and nervous system. The NHS website, for example, has some very straightforward, easy-to-follow exercises.

Get Out

Leaving the house can feel so hard when your mood and energy are low, but in my personal and professional experience, spending time outside gives us energy, and makes a huge difference to recovering from anxiety and depression. Exposure to daylight, especially in colder darker months, can make a big difference to depression and seasonal affective disorder (SAD), as can the use of full-spectrum light boxes when daylight is limited. When vitamin D is low (< 50nmol/L), as it often is during the Winter months, there is a significant risk of developing depression when compared to people whose vitamin D levels are sufficient or optimal (for more information about vitamin D, see pages 203–205).

Research shows that exercise is just as effective as taking SSRIs, though I appreciate that there are often physical and mental barriers to exercising. It's also possible that the types of exercise used in these studies had an influence on the outcomes, as the effect of exercising in a group is likely to be more substantial than exercising alone, due to the experience of connecting with others. People who experience depression are often isolated and lonely, even when living among others, so coming together as a group is a factor that should be considered and taken advantage of. Mental Health Mates, founded by journalist and author Bryony Gordon, is an international network of peer support groups run by people experiencing mental health challenges, who meet regularly to walk and talk. I highly recommend finding a walk near you or using their kit to start one up.

In one study, a 16-week programme of aerobic exercise – 30 minutes of walking or jogging – resulted in sustained raised heart rates and was found to be just as effective as taking antidepressants. Resistance training (aka weightlifting) also has a positive impact on mood. Harvard researchers reviewed 33 randomised clinical trials and concluded that resistance training two or more days a week resulted in significant reductions in participants' depressive symptoms.

Love Your Gut

If your brain is going to some interesting places, then look at what's happening in your gut, because there is a massive correlation between the health of your gut and your mental health. Your gut bacteria produce neurotransmitters such as dopamine, GABA, serotonin, acetylcholine and noradrenalin, all of which are involved in mood, ability to concentrate, anxiety, motivation and reward. Improving the health of your microbiome is a simple and effective way of supporting your mental and hormonal health.

Nutrition

Eating wholefoods, prepared and cooked at home, is big medicine. If I have a few days where I'm on the go and end up eating simple carbs and not enough protein and veg, my mood tanks pretty quickly and I find myself craving greens like broccoli and rocket.

Your brain needs fat so incorporate more healthy fats into your diet and supplement with omega-3 fatty acids. An analysis of 13 research trials found that the use of omega-3 fatty acids such as fish oil can improve anxiety and depression.

You can also up your intake of vitamin B12. We need B12 to make red blood cells and to have a healthy, regulated nervous system. Heartburn medications (aka proton-pump inhibitors) prevent you from absorbing B12 and as we age our ability to absorb it also decreases. If you're vegan, you won't be getting any B12 from your diet, which means that you *have* to supplement with it. A lot of vegans come to me for help with their hormonal and mental health, and some of them, after careful consideration, are willing to incorporate a small amount of animal products into their diet. One way of doing this that's particularly good for those who don't like the experience of eating meat is to take Mother's Best liver pills (see Resources), which are made from the livers of grass-fed, pasture-raised cows in California.

Speaking of vegetarianism and veganism ... If you suffer from anxiety, please look at whether supplementing with taurine is appropriate for you. Taurine is absent in plant foods and vitamin B12, also absent in plant foods, plays a role in the production of taurine. That means there's a double-whammy effect; you don't get it in your diet and, in the absence of B12, you're gonna have a hard time making it. Taurine can also improve your response to supplementing with iron when you're deficient as, again, vegetarians and vegans often are (and, yes, meat eaters can be too). My vegan clients who have decided to start eating eggs, and those who have – pardon the pun – gone the whole hog and started eating meat too, have noticed a significant reduction in their anxiety levels.

We also need carbohydrates. If you've taken up a keto diet, which is frequently touted as being the solution to the weight gain associated with menopause, and your stress levels have climbed up and your ability to sleep has diminished, it could be because you need more carbs. Eating starchy carbs such as rice and potatoes as part of a well-balanced meal increases production of GABA, which calms your nervous system. They also make tryptophan more available to your brain, which is a good thing when it comes to mood and sleep because a diet that's deficient in tryptophan results in poor sleep quality.

CASE STUDY

Lindsay was irritable, highly irritable. Everything and everyone was annoying her, and it didn't help that her periods were heavy AF. And it was even more annoying that they were coming more frequently and lasting even longer. Her breasts were swollen and painful, but, she told me, at least she didn't want anyone near her anyway. I reassured Lindsay that she wasn't the only 44-year-old I knew experiencing this and that it's a common scenario for my clients to find themselves in; that it's what happens when oestrogen is high and progesterone is low.

We came up with a strategy to try and improve the balance between the two hormones and reduce the heavy blood loss that was flooring her every 24 days. As she started bleeding, and every four to six hours for the first couple of days, she took ibuprofen. Her iron levels were low so she focussed on iron-rich foods and took an iron supplement too, and because vitamin C both aids iron absorption and supports progesterone production she started taking vitamin C and Vitex agnus-castus, a herb that also supports progesterone production and can help with heavy bleeding, premenstrual irritability and breast tenderness. I mentioned that micronised body-identical progesterone was an option, but that I'd be interested to see what the supplements and some acupuncture did first, so she began having acupuncture once a week for most of her cycle, twice in the week before her period was due to start, and on day one or two of her period. I also suggested that Lindsay actually voiced her frustrations somehow, instead of trying to bottle them all in, only for them to explode out of her when the pressure got too much.

Over the next few months, Lindsay's periods did lighten. Her breast tenderness and irritability also improved, and she noticed that her sleep deepened too, which she felt was having an overall positive effect. Lindsay told me that she was relieved to know that she had other options available to her, should she have need of them. She was up for taking body-identical progesterone if and when things shifted for her, and that in itself took away the weight of the situation. This is the power of knowing that you do have options.

Supporting Supplements

Supplements absolutely have their place when it comes to supporting mental health and wellbeing, but don't go out, buy all of them and hope for the best. Not only will you end up rattling, but you'll spend a small fortune too. Instead, I recommend you save that money and invest in working with a naturopath or nutritional therapist who can give you specific recommendations.

Magnesium

Magnesium is a great all-rounder for perimenopause, because it helps to calm the adrenal glands, and reduce stress and anxiety. It also supports sleep, balances blood sugar, improves insulin sensitivity, and you need it to safely process and excrete oestrogen. What's more, it's essential for energy production, muscle relaxation and bone health – 63 per cent of magnesium is in your bones and when it's low, your body can compensate by pulling it out of them, which can predispose you to osteoporosis and fractures.

Most of us don't get enough magnesium through our diets, and as a result, magnesium deficiency is common. Modern agricultural practices have depleted the soil crops are grown in, and foods that should be high in magnesium and other minerals aren't what they used to be, so there's less of it in our food supply. Like many nutrients, it's also damaged or eliminated as a result of food processing. But the issue isn't just that we're not getting enough through our diet. Alcohol, excess sugar consumption and medications such as the contraceptive pill, blood pressure medications and acid blockers all interfere with absorption. And we need more when we're stressed.

Food sources of magnesium include black beans, dark green leafy veg such as spinach and Swiss chard, pumpkin seeds, flax seeds, hemp seeds, Brazil nuts, almonds, avocado, banana, salmon and dark chocolate. When it comes to picking a supplement, magnesium oxide is cheap to make and absorption is not great. Magnesium citrate helps to improve bowel motility, which is helpful if you're prone to constipation (build up your dosage gradually to avoid loose stools). Magnesium glycinate is well tolerated and you can go to a higher, more therapeutic dosage (300 to 600mg).

Vitamin B6

Our need for the B vitamins goes up as we age – our ability to absorb them declines as a result of poor digestion, medications interacting with vitamin B and it being used up to process alcohol. Low vitamin B levels are associated with cognitive decline, low bone mineral density (a risk factor for osteoporosis and fractures), poor DNA repair and formation, and cardiovascular disease and stroke, so it's clear that B vitamins are important during perimenopause. Whilst all the B vitamins are important, the B vitamin I want to draw your attention to is B6, because it can support progesterone production, reduce inflammation, support oestrogen detoxification, and improve histamine intolerance, PMS, PMDD and other mood-related issues.

Turmeric (*Curcumin*)

Turmeric root has a strong anti-inflammatory action. One of its active ingredients is called curcumin, which can be bought in supplement form, and of course you can add it to soups and curries too. Absorption is increased when it's taken with a fat and black pepper, so some formulations include these in their capsules. Curcumin has antidepressant properties and studies have shown that it's as effective as taking fluoxetine (Prozac), and when taken alongside escitalopram and venlafaxine, it provides more rapid relief from symptoms than when they're taken on their own. It also has antioxidant, antimicrobial and anticancer properties, and can be used to lighten periods and reduce pain, making it a great option if you struggle with heavy and/or painful periods.

Taurine

Taurine is a non-essential amino acid. Non-essential means our bodies can make it from two other essential amino acids. We also get it through the consumption of animal products in our diets. Oestradiol depresses the formation of taurine, so regardless of whether you still have a cycle or you're taking oestrogen, you need more of it than men. And as I mentioned above, if you're vegan then taurine may improve any anxiety you're experiencing.

It's found in high concentrations in the brain and plays a major role in the release of neurotransmitters, including the activation of GABA receptors in the brain, and also has neuroprotective effects. Taurine is involved in memory, learning and mood, and can help to reduce anxiety and stress. It also stimulates bone formation and inhibits bone resorption, is a powerful antioxidant and can improve insulin sensitivity.

L-theanine

L-theanine is an amino acid that supports relaxation and reduces anxiety by boosting levels of calming neurotransmitters such as GABA, serotonin and dopamine, whilst lowering levels of stimulating neurotransmitters. It isn't a sedative, but it can help with sleep, because it reduces the stress that keeps you awake. L-theanine can also reduce high blood pressure and, as a result, it can interact with medications that are prescribed for high blood pressure, as well as other supplements that can lower blood pressure.

GABA (*Gamma-aminobutyric acid*)

GABA is another amino acid and it works as an inhibitory neurotransmitter in your brain, meaning that it puts the brakes on nervous system activity and calms you down in the process. It can reduce anxiety, balance mood and support sleep. Many of the other supplements that I've listed here influence GABA and act on the GABA receptors in the brain, and it can also be taken as a supplement, though there's debate around how effective it is – yet another area that needs more research! GABA interacts with high blood pressure medications and antidepressants, and it can interact with other supplements too, so this is one to speak to your practitioner about.

CBD (*Cannabidiol*)

CBD is the second most prevalent active ingredient found in the cannabis plant. The first is tetrahydrocannabinol (THC), which is the psychoactive chemical that gets people high when they smoke or ingest cannabis. Whilst CBD is a component of cannabis, it won't get you high and it can help with anxiety, depression and insomnia, though using products with a small amount of THC may work even better, especially if your insomnia has been resistant to other forms of treatment. It can also help with lots of other health issues, such as recovery from burnout, PMS, period pain, headaches, migraines and neurological disorders. If this approach interests you, try a full-spectrum CBD oil that's derived from hemp as it will contain less than 0.2 per cent THC and is legal in the UK. Dr Dani Gordon's book, *The CBD Bible*, has lots of great information on the various types of CBD products and how to use them for specific conditions.

Adaptogens

Adaptogens are herbal pharmaceuticals that help us to recover from, and cope with, physical and emotional stress. Most of them come from plants, and medicinal mushrooms are adaptogens too.

Ashwagandha (*Withania somnifera*)

Ashwagandha is best known as an adaptogenic herb; it helps you to deal with stress. It's anti-inflammatory and helps to protect against the oxidative stress that damages your cells and DNA. It can improve immunity and some research suggests it may be useful for those with neurodegenerative diseases. It can also lower anxiety levels and can be used safely alongside antidepressants.

Maca (*Lepidium meyenii*)

Maca is an adrenal adaptogen, meaning it helps you to cope with stress. It's often recommended for those with low oestrogen, which you will be after the menopause, but maca doesn't stimulate oestrogen production. It can regulate the hormonal glands in your head – the hypothalamus and pituitary – which in turn can balance your hormones levels, including oestrogen, but also your adrenals, pineal gland and thyroid. Maca can improve sleep quality and duration, hot flushes, heart palpitations, depression and nervousness, and sexual desire. Because of its regulating effect on your adrenal glands, it can also improve energy and mood. Opt for Peruvian maca and take it as a supplement or add the powder to smoothies.

Rhodiola (*Rhodiola rosea*)

Another adaptogenic herb, Rhodiola is made from the root of the plant. It can improve many of the neuropsychological symptoms of menopause, including fatigue, depression, anxiety, memory decline and stress intolerance. It's said to increase energy, improve attention and memory, and to help you deal with and recover from stress.

Holy basil (*Ocimum sanctum* aka tulsi)

Holy basil is an Ayurvedic herb that's classified as an adaptogen. It can help with stress of all kinds – physical, chemical and psychological. In fact, so much so that, because you can drink it as a tea, it's often described as liquid yoga (you can also take capsules). It has positive effects on memory, cognitive function and depression too.

Lemon balm (*Melissa officinalis*)

Lemon balm is an edible herb of the mint family. You can make a tea out of it or buy it as a supplement or essential oil. It can reduce cortisol levels and anxiety, improve memory, concentration and mood, support sleep and improve digestion.

Skullcap (*Scutellaria lateriflora*)

Skullcap is a calming herb that helps to restore the nervous system and it's often used in combination with valerian, passionflower or hops to help with sleep issues and anxiety – these often form the base for sleepy teas.

St John's Wort (*Hypericum perforatum*)

Often described as herbal Prozac, St John's Wort can help with depression, anxiety, nervousness and sleep issues, but shouldn't be taken if you're using antidepressants, the birth control pill, sedatives, pain medications, immune-suppressant medications or warfarin.

Medicinal mushrooms

Medicinal mushrooms are mushrooms that are known for their ability to support health and healing, and, no, they don't include the magic variety. There are hundreds of types, but you might have spotted two of the more common varieties in the veggie aisle of your local shop: oyster and shiitake. Most clinical trials featuring medicinal mushrooms are animal ones, but what they've discovered is promising. The different mushrooms all have their own unique properties, including an ability to calm the nervous system, boost mood, increase energy and focus, reduce inflammation, support the immune system and regulate blood sugar levels, and some may even protect the protective sheath that surrounds nerve cells.

Some can be cooked with, but they're also available as tinctures, powders, teas and capsules. I love adding a teaspoon of dried mushroom powder to my black coffee in the morning or to herbal tea in the afternoon. You can make tea either by simmering dried mushrooms in water for 30 minutes to two hours or by adding a powdered form to hot water. Some mushrooms contain compounds which can only be extracted by alcohol, so taking them in the form of a tincture is a great way to get the most out of them.

Cordyceps are known for their ability to improve energy levels and stamina. They provide high levels of antioxidants, and are said to support the adrenal glands and reduce stress too.

Lion's mane mushrooms contain two compounds that have been shown to stimulate the growth of brain cells. In animal studies, they reduce symptoms of memory loss, prevent the nerve damage associated with Alzheimer's disease, reduce depression and significantly lower blood sugar levels. Studies with humans demonstrated they can improve mental functioning in older adults with mild cognitive impairment and one small study of menopausal women found that eating them reduced feelings of irritation and anxiety.

Reishi mushrooms have been touted as an anti-ageing elixir for thousands of years and modern research has demonstrated that they have antioxidant effects, as well as influencing the immune system and nerve cell degeneration. Taken as a powder, capsule, tincture or tea, they can help to lower stress, soothe the nervous system and aid sleep.

Now, What Did I Come Up Here For?

Perimenopausal symptoms like hot flushes and night sweats are bothersome, but what impacts my clients the most is when their brains are affected by the hormonal shift of menopause. In one study of women aged 40 to 55, forgetfulness was the third most commonly reported symptom and this is certainly what my clients tell me. They lament that they frequently go upstairs to do something and by the time their knees have creaked up the stairs, they've forgotten why they went up there in the first place. Brain fog prevents the ability to concentrate and think clearly. It's like your brain's internal weather system has switched to humid – you can feel that a thought or word is there, but can't quite get to it (ironically, my period is close to starting and I'm experiencing exactly this as I type), and your brain feels fuzzy so you can't pull things into focus. Thank goodness for my editor. Highly successful women who've spent years climbing the career ladder to get to the top tell me that their cognitive function is faltering, they can't keep track of their thoughts or schedule, they're constantly worried about making critical mistakes and their sense of self is being destroyed in the process. Mums tell me that they're always forgetting things and that their family members are running out of patience with them. This is an aspect of perimenopause that is rarely appreciated or considered, and when those experiencing it go to their GP, some will unfortunately be told that they're depressed or stressed and be sent away with antidepressants or sleeping pills, when what they should be offered is hormone therapy.

CASE STUDY

Kathryn, a 52-year-old client of mine, had gone through perimenopause without much bother. The hot flushes she experienced weren't significant enough to fluster her – her years of working as an executive meant that she'd found ways to regulate her nervous system when under stress, so she was able to transfer these skills to ease her hot flushes. She'd gone up a dress size, and she felt healthy and strong at her new weight, and relished the opportunity to buy some new clothes. Kathryn told me that she felt she'd 'escaped unscathed' – until her ability to focus and remember things started to change, which was when she reached out to me. Kathryn had spent years climbing the corporate ladder and was finally in the position of leadership she'd always envisioned for herself, but she was worried that that was now under threat. Along with poor memory and being unable to concentrate, Kathryn felt a nervousness and hesitancy that was alien to her, which is why she came to me for coaching. She didn't feel like herself at all.

I asked Kathryn when her last period was and, after checking her app, she told me it had been eight months ago. Because she hadn't had a full year of no periods, Kathryn technically hadn't gone through menopause yet, but it certainly seemed that she was experiencing symptoms because of low oestrogen. Not only was her brain changing, but her knees were bothering her, pain that she'd put down to overdoing it on hikes, and she had neck strain that she thought was from too much computer work. I told her that I'd love to coach her, but that she should speak to her GP about using hormone therapy first. Kathryn had worked with coaches for years and was ready to tackle her brain, so she was shocked when I told her that whilst we could do that, I thought it was worth seeing if some oestrogen would do the trick. Slightly bemused, she agreed to make an appointment to see her GP. A week later, she was taking combined hormone therapy (oestrogen and progesterone) and it didn't take long for her nervousness to ease. Then her joints began to improve and she realised that she wasn't reaching for words like she had been. She decided she didn't need coaching after all.

Using hormones such as oestrogen and testosterone can improve mental focus and clarity, memory and sleep. Oestrogen increases levels of a protein called brain-derived neurotrophic factor (BDNF) in the hippocampus – a part of the brain involved in memory consolidation. This is why when oestrogen is low in the menstrual cycle or life cycle (post-birth, and in late perimenopause and postmenopause) you might find yourself struggling to finish a sentence or explain yourself in the way that you're accustomed to. BDNF is also involved in depression and is thought to play a role in emotional regulation, and oestrogen hormone therapy increases BDNF and improves mood and depression. So does exercise.

The stress hormone cortisol has a negative effect on memory and cognition. When researchers gave study participants oral doses of cortisol for four days that equated to the levels produced in response to physical or psychological stress, it inhibited their ability to recall information. If your life is full and you're dashing around tending to everyone and everything, then you're going to need to make some changes, because stress hormones cause and aggravate so many perimenopausal symptoms. Whatever treatment strategies you use, you can't afford to ignore what your stress hormones are up to. And that means addressing sources of stress.

The Long Goodbye

Alzheimer's disease is an irreversible, progressive brain disorder that gradually destroys memory and cognitive function, eventually leaving those who have it unable to perform simple tasks that they mastered early in life. The brain of someone with Alzheimer's looks very different to a healthy brain, because of the presence of amyloid plaques (hard accumulations of abnormal protein), tangled bundles of nerve fibres and the loss of connection between nerve cells. These brain changes result in symptoms such as memory problems, impaired reasoning or judgement, vision/spatial issues and trouble finding words.

In most people with Alzheimer's, symptoms appear in their sixties and, as such, it's a disease that we associate with old age. But the first signs of Alzheimer's actually appear in midlife. I know that you don't need anything else to keep you up at night, but this is a topic that has to be mentioned, because the decisions you make now will impact on what happens over the course of your postmenopausal years. In the final third of our lives, we don't produce the type of oestrogen that has kept our brains and bodies ticking over since we started menstruating.

Our knowledge of oestrogen's involvement in cognition comes from randomised controlled trials in which premenopausal women whose ovaries had been removed were either given a placebo or oestrogen therapy. Those taking the placebo experienced a decrease in verbal and working memory following surgery, but those taking oestrogen did not. Researchers view perimenopause as a therapeutic window in which hormone therapy may prevent cognitive decline if it's started early enough. Now, you may have read a newspaper headline that said that MHT increases the risk of developing dementia, so let's tease that one apart. The main research being referred to is the Women's Health Initiative Memory Study (WHIMS), an arm of the flawed WHI trial which has been heavily criticised for its use of older women who, at the time, were already 10 years or so past menopause. The 1,326 participants aged 50 to 55 years, who commenced hormone therapy soon after menopause, did not display any cognitive decline whilst taking hormones or in the years that followed. However, the women aged 65 to 79 at the start of their treatment did show a persistent decline in cognitive function and memory. Further studies have also concluded that when oestrogen therapy is initiated shortly after periods stop or immediately following surgical menopause, it has positive effects on memory and cognition.

Laboratory studies have demonstrated that oestrogen regulates the growth of nerve cells and that it offers protection against the damage resulting from blocked arteries in the brain that causes ischemic stroke. This is why the use of oestrogen therapy is suggested as a potential way of preventing the kind of dementia associated with Alzheimer's disease.

The Dopest Neurotransmitter

Dopamine is a neurotransmitter that plays a role in pleasure, motivation, learning, movement and even lactation. It's part of a reward system in your brain; when dopamine is released, it creates feelings of pleasure which motivates you to repeat the behaviour.

Dopamine is crucial when it comes to complex cognitive processes and too little or too much of it results in poor performance. Not enough will have you lacking motivation, enthusiasm and focus. When it's high you can feel on top of the world, but too much of it can put you into overdrive and may contribute to mania. Let's tie that into your experience of the menstrual cycle. Oestrogen increases dopamine and you'll feel its effects in the preovulatory phase of your cycle. If you have low baseline levels of dopamine, then you'll experience enhanced performance in this phase, whereas if you have a higher baseline, then performance can be impaired.

When dopamine is low, you can struggle to feel enthused and motivated, and dopamine deficiency is implicated in depression, binge-eating, addiction, Alzheimer's and Parkinson's disease. Dopamine is involved in movement and the loss of dopamine-producing nerve cells in the brain causes symptoms of Parkinson's to appear. Professor D. Eugene Redmond and his team of researchers at Yale University found that oestrogen deprivation caused the death of 30 per cent of the dopamine cells in the brain, the cells that help to protect against Parkinson's disease, but that they could be regenerated if oestrogen was administered within 10 days. By 30 days, however, it was too late and the cells appeared to be permanently lost. Redmond concluded that, 'The results of the study shed light on why men, who have less oestrogen in their bodies and more androgen to antagonise it, are more likely to develop Parkinson's Disease than premenopausal women, and why postmenopausal women are more likely then to develop the disease.' Redmond does, however, caution against using this to make a decision about the use of hormone therapy.

Now that we've covered the various ways that perimenopause itself and the challenges of midlife can impact on mental health and brain function, let's get into what you can do practically to take care of yourself and reduce the many sources of stress you're likely to be facing.

6

Where's your head at?

Menopause isn't called the change for nothing – your life is going to change. So what's your attitude towards change like at the moment? Does the idea of change exhilarate you or are you shitting it? There is an association between attitude towards menopause and experience of symptoms, with a negative attitude increasing the frequency and severity of a range of symptoms. This is fantastic news, because even if you are currently feeling all doom and gloom about menopause, you can change your experience of it by changing your thoughts and feelings about it. I want to be clear that when I'm talking about mindset, I'm not suggesting that your symptoms are all in your head. I'm saying that what your mind gets up to can have a huge impact on your experience of peri- and postmenopause. Adopting a more neutral or positive belief system about this stage of life and the decades that follow will only serve you well. This is an opportunity to radically change how you think and feel about yourself and your life.

Consider also the impact of those around you and their attitudes towards menopause. Caring less about people-pleasing and taking care of others is one of the great gifts of the menopause transition, and it may well require a shift in the dynamics of your professional and personal relationships, particularly your home life. The changes you make during this stage of life - such as prioritising your needs, desires and interests, and doing less for others – could mean that more is required of them. One possible consequence of this is that your colleagues/kids/partner may not be happy that you are less available to them and no longer at their beck and call. You might have enough resilience to handle this or it could provoke thoughts that cause you to feel guilty. Remember, you're in charge of how you think and feel, and they get to decide how they're going to think and feel. Stay in your own head and take responsibility for yourself.

I know I'm meant to tell you that this is when you should find a sense of balance within your life. It's perhaps what you aspire to as well. But balance isn't possible because it doesn't exist. One aspect of your life will always require more time, energy and money than the others. So now that we've established that balance is a load of shit, what can we work towards? Do you want to feel balanced? Do you want to feel settled? Some of you will and that's okay, but this isn't a stage of life where you have to settle down. You can also rise up.

Take a look at what your life so far has looked like and decide what you want to happen next. When the weight of responsibility is heavy in life, you might find yourself thinking about what isn't possible for you. If you were one of my clients, I would coach you hard on that belief. Instead, here are some questions for you to reflect on:

- What would you like to be possible for you?
- What would you do if you could?

Is part of you feeling nervous excitement and another part bricking it? Good! Your next step is to put this book down and take some time to picture yourself in your postmenopausal years. Seriously, I want you to stop for a moment and do this, and ideally grab a pen and paper so that you can make notes. If you're unsure how to do this, use the questions above and below to create a picture that you're happy with (you can also download some worksheets to fill in at www.maisiehill.com/perimenopausepower):

- How does your future self wake up in the morning and how do they feel upon waking?
- What does your morning routine look like and how do you greet the day?
- Where do you eat your breakfast?
- When you open your wardrobe, what's inside?
- What work are you doing and how do you approach it?
- How do you communicate with others?
- Who do you socialise with?
- How do you experience connection?
- How do you experience intimacy?
- Where do you spend your time?
- What does your home look and feel like?
- What does your social life look and feel like?
- What is your evening routine like?
- How do you feel when you get into bed and is anyone there with you?

It's totally fine to muse on these questions and I recommend returning to them frequently. Once you have a strong sense of your future self, it's time to start asking them some questions:

- What wisdom do they have for you?
- What three feelings do they experience the most in their life?
- Why do they experience them – what's going on in their life that creates these emotions?
- What have they decided to stop bothering with?
- Who have they let go of?
- What and who do they make time for?
- What have they embraced?
- What brings them pleasure?
- And perhaps most importantly, what is *not* happening that makes this future life so good?

Stressed Beyond Belief

An out-of-whack stress response is the one thing that's guaranteed to cock up your experience of perimenopause (apart from patriarchy, although patriarchy is most definitely involved in this too, surprise, surprise). There's a circuit of communication and response which runs from the hypothalamus and pituitary glands in your head, and your adrenal glands which sit on top of your kidneys. Collectively, they form what's known as the HPA axis and the HPA axis is where your hormones dance with your nervous system.

When you're stressed, your HPA axis is activated and you release stress hormones like cortisol, noradrenalin and adrenalin. This is what your body is designed to do so this isn't a problem, but sustained periods of stress and ongoing activation of your HPA axis cause problems, such as changes to the production of cortisol. Cortisol should vary throughout the day, peaking an hour or so after waking, then gradually reducing to reach its lowest level around bedtime. With HPA axis dysfunction, you can produce too much or too little cortisol in general. Produce too much in the morning or too much in the evening and other hormones, such as DHEA, melatonin and your hunger hormones, can be affected too.

HPA axis dysfunction is all too common before we even get to perimenopause and certainly during it, and it's vital that we improve HPA axis function, because it's our adrenal glands that become the main source of hormones once our ovaries shut up shop. *This is why we all need to be thinking about perimenopause long before we actually get there.*

HPA axis dysfunction can be caused by:

- Unrelenting emotional and mental stress.
- Sleep deprivation and sleep disturbances.
- Shift work and night work.
- Environmental and food allergies or sensitivities.
- Over-exercising, dieting and disordered eating, including skipping meals and calorie-depleting diets, which is why intermittent fasting doesn't suit everyone in perimenopause.
- Eating junk food.
- Using steroids such as those used to treat allergies and asthma.

Initially, HPA axis dysfunction tends towards high levels of cortisol before bottoming out, which is when cortisol production will be low and other hormones such as oestrogen, progesterone and DHEA also become depleted. The DUTCH test (see pages 261–262) can show you exactly what your HPA axis is up to, but you can also access cortisol testing through your GP – cortisol levels should be tested in the morning (before 9am), though a diurnal cortisol panel, which is taken at four points in the day, is far more helpful, because it assesses your cortisol curve. Signs and symptoms of HPA axis dysfunction include:

- Fatigue and feeling burnt out.
- Not feeling rested after sleep.
- Relying on caffeine and sugar to function.
- Struggling to feel alert in the morning.
- Brain fog.
- Feeling tired but wired.
- Finding it hard to wind down for bedtime.
- Difficulty falling asleep or staying asleep, or both.
- Feeling anxious, nervous or depressed.
- Panic attacks.
- Being easily angered, prone to yelling and/or screaming.
- Feeling distracted and not present.

- Low/high blood pressure.
- Feeling dizzy when you stand up.
- Awareness of your heart beating/palpitations even when relaxed.
- High blood sugar, insulin resistance or diabetes.
- Low blood sugar between meals.
- You catch every cough and cold flying around, and it takes a while for you to recover from illness or to heal a wound.
- Feeling unable to cope and less resilient to stress.
- Nausea, vomiting or diarrhoea, or alternating between loose stools and constipation.
- Issues with ovulation and fertility.

You can improve HPA axis function by:

- Doing something about the stuff that stresses you out, obvs. Hopefully this chapter has given you some starting points and I'd love to see your face in The Flow Collective, because this is the kind of stuff we deal with in there.
- Getting outside in the daytime to expose yourself to light, particularly if you struggle to wake up in the morning (so-called 'wake up' lights can be useful in the darker months).
- Setting things up so that you can wind down in the evening and avoid blue light from electronic devices to allow cortisol to decrease and melatonin to increase.
- Stroking a furry friend. Snuggling with pets increases oxytocin and endorphins – calming healing hormones which will dial down stress hormones.
- Avoiding processed, refined foods.
- Focussing on eating a nutrient-dense diet instead of dieting.
- Working on balancing your blood sugar by eating at regular mealtimes and eating enough protein.
- Laying off caffeine and sugar – your blood sugar could do without the wild ride.
- Watching something funny. Belly laughter is good medicine.
- You can also stimulate the release of oxytocin and endorphins by having an orgasm or by lightly stroking your upper abdomen. Close your eyes, take a few relaxing belly breaths and use your fingertips to lightly stroke downwards from the bottom of your breastbone to your belly button. This

feels nice when done through a layer of clothing (particularly if it's got a stretchy quality to it), which means you can do it anywhere, even whilst you're waiting for the bus.

- Gardening and reading both lead to a decrease in cortisol, but gardening outperforms reading. If you don't have a garden or an allotment, find someone who needs help with theirs, because generosity can decrease cortisol levels too.

Boundaries

There is a common thread in all my work with clients and that's the impact of habitual people-pleasing and an inability to give and uphold boundaries. If you want to have a positive experience of perimenopause, and if you want to take steps now to ensure your health in the decades that follow, then its paramount that you have healthy boundaries in place. Personal boundaries are what define our edges, creating a space where we can think, feel and genuinely be ourselves. They allow us to know and manage where we end and others begin, and are the key to healthy personal and professional relationships.

An absence of healthy boundaries can create anxiety, depression and exhaustion – all common complaints during perimenopause! When your boundaries are foggy or non-existent, you lose your sense of who you really are and what makes you happy. Your existence becomes entrenched in what others think and need of you, and, if truth be told, in our attempts to manipulate others. No matter the hormonal imbalance or health factors, I guarantee these issues come into play. It's what I most commonly coach my clients on so that they can prioritise their hormonal and mental health.

Anxiety, confusion, resentment, frustration and anger are often signs that our boundaries have been transgressed. This can happen when the other person isn't aware of a boundary (and until it's been transgressed you may not be aware of your own either), or when you've made them aware of a boundary and they intentionally cross that line.

We start off our lives skilled at setting boundaries. As young children, we said 'no' clearly and loudly, and with no explanation. We let our parents know when we didn't want to do something. We told them to stop if we didn't like what they were doing. We knew what we did and didn't want, and we freely expressed ourselves without caring what they, or anyone else who happened to be present, thought.

From an early age though, we are taught that we are responsible for how others feel: 'Don't do that, you'll make Mummy sad' is a prime example that most of us will have heard (and even said). But sentences like this simply aren't true. The only time we experience emotional pain is when we think a thought about what someone said or did. My son is a feisty four-year-old and lately, whenever I give him a boundary, such as 'I'm not a climbing frame – I want you to stop climbing on me,' he responds by telling me that I'm stupid and that he's kicking me out of the family. This never upsets me, because I don't have any negative thoughts about what he's told me, which means I can stay connected to him and support him through his emotions, and calmly say whatever feels appropriate, which includes addressing how he speaks to others. When I do this, I'm letting him know that I am responsible for my emotional wellbeing and behaviour. If, however, I was to withdraw or get mad, I'd be sending a signal that he is responsible for my emotional state and that he has to behave a certain way in order for me to feel good and, consequently, for him to feel safe and loved. Don't go thinking that I'm a perfect parent all the time, because I'm not, but when parents are able to stay connected during times of disagreements, they raise children who are able to experience a wide range of emotions and who can inhabit the various parts of themselves. You didn't pick this book up for parenting tips and you're probably wondering what all this has to do with perimenopause. A lot. The combination of a lack of boundaries in the places you really need them and a tendency to people-please are likely to leave you in a state of perpetual exhaustion. These are both common tendencies in those socialised as female, especially when we're producing oestrogen – my postmenopausal clients tell me how liberating it is to stop giving a flying you-know-what about what others think once their cycles stop.

By the time we arrive in perimenopause, we fulfil a dazzling array of roles in our lives: daughter, sibling, parent, taxi-driver to teenagers, colleague, boss, partner, lover, PTA member, cook, cleaner, teacher and negotiator. All of these roles require different aspects of ourselves, so we find ourselves in a position of trying to keep all the plates spinning whilst trying to look composed. We're not. We're falling apart trying to keep it together. Whilst a sudden influx of money combined with some extra hours in the day might make a difference to your life and mine, time always gets filled and money always gets spent. What is always available to you as a solution is your boundaries.

Boundaries are a way for us to communicate our needs, desires and limits to others. They are not a way to control the behaviour of others, nor are they an ultimatum. When we let someone know they've crossed a boundary, we're giving them a chance to adjust how they're behaving if they want to. They might not like or understand it, but even if that were to be the case, it's still possible to respect a boundary. If they choose not to respect the boundary, then it's on you to follow through with the consequence of that. And, of course, they'll have their own boundaries too. Ultimately, boundaries are a way for us all to express what we're okay with and what we're not. Just like you, other people get to act as they see fit and you get to decide if you're on board with it.

Although boundaries may seem to cause separation, they actually create connection. Here's why: when a boundary is violated, but it's not expressed – let's say X happens, but instead of saying something you keep quiet – then there is a disconnect. In fact, it's unlikely that you'll be able to take in anything that they say in that conversation, and you probably go on to relive the situation again and again in your mind. The issues that come up most when I'm discussing boundaries with clients are:

- Not knowing what they're okay with – or not.
- Deciding what's okay, but not communicating it to the people who need to hear it.
- Expecting people to respect boundaries without communicating them clearly.
- Using boundaries as a way to try to control other people.
- Fearing the consequences of boundary violations and not protecting them, so the boundary violation continues, most likely with you blaming the other person for what they've done, instead of being responsible for your actions or non-actions as the case may be.

Tips for setting boundaries:

1) Think of a situation where your boundaries are challenged (such as a tricky family member or co-worker).
2) Decide what you're okay with and not in that situation.

3) Form a sentence that you can use to let the other person know where your boundary is.
4) Decide what the consequence will be if they are unable to respect your boundary.
5) Let someone know when they've violated your boundary and what the consequence is or will be if they continue.
6) Follow through with the consequences.
7) Know that other people don't have to agree or understand your boundary – your boundary is for you.

For example, your parents or in-laws might be in the habit of popping by when they feel like it. For some of you, this won't be a problem. But for Amy, it was. Her mother-in-law would appear, unexpectedly, at the front door once or twice a week. A tight smile would be on Amy's face as she 'welcomed' her in and exclaimed, 'I didn't know you would be coming over today!', hoping that she would get the point. Amy would seethe inside for the duration of the visit and for many hours afterwards, often resulting in a disagreement with her wife and a level of resentment that prevented sleep. When we discussed it, I asked her if she'd ever spoken to her mother-in-law about it. She hadn't. This was a clear boundary violation for her, but because she hadn't expressed it and explained what the consequence would be if things didn't change, her mother-in-law remained clueless and kept repeating the behaviour.

When it comes to stating your boundaries and enforcing consequences, do so from a place of calm composure. If that doesn't feel available to you in the moment, then I suggest simply stating that you need a moment (or longer) before responding. When we communicate boundaries whilst filled with anger, it's unlikely that much good will come from it.

Your world will not fall apart because you have decided to communicate your boundaries. Boundaries may feel like you're creating distance, and in some ways, you are, but that allows for truth and intimacy. Pretending to be someone that you're not through habitual people-pleasing creates relationships that are built upon lies.

When you have a history of having your boundaries trampled on by loved ones, colleagues or complete strangers, then when it comes to finally expressing them it's probably gonna suck to begin with. It'll feel awkward, your chest will feel tight and your breath will become shallow, your body will stiffen up in anticipation of what your imagination has conjured up in an attempt to keep you safe. But when you don't communicate your needs, desires and limits to other people, you're not safe, so this is a muscle that you need to start flexing. It will feel liberating too, I promise – as in jump, squeal and punch the air kind of liberating. And after a while it'll become a habit and your new normal. You'll be able to let people know your boundaries without over-thinking it and it won't feel a big deal.

The Beauty of 'No'

'No' used to be such a dangerous word to me, but now it's beautiful. And if there was ever a time to embrace the beauty of 'no', it's perimenopause. That one word is capable of giving you so much time, energy, and improved mental and physical health, so think about what and who you'd love to say no to. Make a list. Seriously, stop reading and spend 10 minutes writing out all your nos. The ones you'd say if you didn't fear the other person's reaction and what they'll then think of you.

When you agree to do things that you don't want to do, or you agree with what someone's saying when, internally, you don't, you're people-pleasing. You're trying to control the other person's opinion of you and their response. You can't make someone behave a certain way and you can't make them think something either, and, quite frankly, this is a complete waste of time and energy. It's exhausting to keep up a charade and yet we are raised to consider others, be nice, be good, do as we're asked, be polite and not ask for what we want (even when the request is basic). No wonder by the time we land in perimenopause we're all so bloody exhausted. There's an expectation that if we fulfil others' needs, this will create harmony in our lives. But all it creates is resentment and rage.

When my clients are ready to embrace saying 'no', but it feels so foreign to them that they can't come up with the actual words to use, I give them this list and suggest that they pick a few to try on for size as they begin to flex their muscles:

- No.
- No, I don't want to.
- No, thanks.

- I'd rather not, so no.
- I can't give you an answer right now. Can you check in with me later on/next week/when hell freezes over?
- That's not something I'm up for.
- Maybe next time.
- I'd love to, but can't.
- I can't make it.
- I can't do that time, but how about ________?
- Sounds fun, but I'm not available.
- No thank you. It sounds great, but no.
- If there were two of me, I'd be a 'hell, yes'.
- At the moment I'm saying no to everything unless it's ________.
- I really appreciate you asking me to do this, but it's a no for me.
- I'm not sure I'm the best fit for that.
- I love that you trust me with the task of ________ /baking 100 cupcakes/organising the office party, but I'm at my capacity right now, so no.
- That sounds amazing and it's something I'd love to do, but it's not something I can commit to.
- I'm honoured that you asked me, but this falls outside of my professional remit.
- I can't do that, but I can ________. Would that help?
- I wish I could make it work, but my bandwidth is at capacity right now.
- Right now, I'm focussing on ________, which means I need to say no to this, but I appreciate you thinking of me.
- I know that in the past I've often been the one to ________, but I'm not up for doing that right now.
- That's not really my jam, so no.
- I'm sorely tempted to say yes, but I know that will end up impacting ________ so I'm going to have to say no.
- This sounds right up my street and I love that you thought of me. Unfortunately, I don't think I can give this the time and energy it deserves right now, but let me know if there's any other way I can get involved.
- I know that this behaviour is acceptable to you, but it's not to me.
- I know I/we usually ________ but this is what I'd like to happen instead.

Or:

- Yes, but I can only do it for ________ amount of time/I need to leave at ________/I'll only be able to ________.
- I'd love to do ________ but that means having to compromise/put the brakes on ________, so let me know what you'd like me to prioritise.

If it's not a clear or immediate yes, consider it a no. It's easier to change a no to a yes than to back out of a yes that you regret. If you prefer to, practise saying the nos that are easier, the ones that aren't as loaded, and build up to the bigger ones (you are coming to ours for Christmas, aren't you?). Then, once you've said it, wait. Don't fill the space that comes after that all-important sentence. If you fill it with apologies and excuses, for example, then you're weakening your no and giving someone opportunities to get you to a yes. Instead, appreciate the full stop at the end of your sentence and allow the other person to hear your no. Bask in the beauty of your no.

People-pleasing

It's not surprising that people-pleasing is so prevalent. In terms of our evolutionary history, it was only a minute ago that confrontation ran the risk of us being kicked out of our community and to do so meant risking death. This – along with our experiences in childhood – is why going against what's been asked of us feels inherently risky. It's why we people-please.

One massive benefit of perimenopause and menopause is that you stop giving a shit about what other people think of you. If this hasn't been your experience yet, then let's speed the process up so that you can use your brain and energy on more important things. When you're in a situation where you become aware that you're people-pleasing, or more likely, afterwards, ask yourself what was it that you were thinking that made you feel that you couldn't be truthful. Then decide what you're going to do to either clear things up or do differently next time you find yourself in a similar situation.

You can't feel seen, heard and connected in your relationships if you're not being yourself, so this is important. Do you want to spend the rest of your life exhausting yourself by pretending to be someone else? You may come to realise that in an attempt to please everyone, and be liked and thought well of by others, some of your personal relationships are inauthentic, created on a false foundation of people-pleasing lies. But your relationships will probably survive you deciding to be you. In fact, they may thrive. And it's possible that some people won't be thrilled with the new (old) you. Not everyone is going to like you, but a jar of Marmite doesn't worry about the people who can't stand it and nor should you.

Let Your Freak Flag Fly

You may discover that after years, decades, of people-pleasing, you've lost your sense of self. All the yeses that were really nos have chipped away at you, so that you no longer recognise what remains. Perimenopause and menopause are a time of rediscovery. The hormonal rollercoaster of perimenopause forces us to confront the truth of our lives. You might feel content and proud of what you see. But there may be grief, resentment and sadness too. The speeding-up of the cycle brings with it a fast and furious energy that you can use to work through these feelings, and finally accept and let go. You get to decide how you're going to think and feel about perimenopause and the years that follow it. You can decide what you want the next decade to be like. So, what *do* you want?

7

Going to waist

It's normal for body composition to change once we land in perimenopause and during postmenopause too. Let me say that again: it is normal for your body to change. Nothing has gone wrong.

It's common to experience weight gain, even if no other factors, such as diet, eating patterns and physical activity, have changed. Weight gain can be due to the ageing process, but an increase in weight, overall body fat and particularly abdominal fat has been independently linked to the hormonal changes during menopause, due to changes in how you burn energy. During the luteal phase of the cycle, the presence of progesterone raises body temperature, which means the rate at which you use energy goes up. But between insufficient progesterone production in cycles where you do ovulate and an increase in cycles where you don't ovulate at all, progesterone becomes increasingly absent and reduces the rate of energy consumption during the luteal phase. This appears to be one factor that leads to an increase in fat deposits during perimenopause.

Once oestrogen declines, there is an abrupt shift in the rate at which you use energy. Prior to menopause, fat would be stored in your bum and thighs thanks to the presence of oestrogen, but without oestrogen on the scene, what you get is an increase in central adiposity – the scientific way of describing a spare tyre. Less oestrogen can also cause joint pain, which makes exercise more difficult, and less oestrogen also means it's harder to maintain muscle mass. Muscle is important because it uses energy even when you're resting, so less muscle means more energy surplus, which causes weight gain.

Add to this the impact of stress hormones, inflammation, thyroid dysfunction, a decrease in physical activity, and pelvic floor dysfunction that causes hesitancy around exercising, and you can see why it's common to gain weight and for the distribution of fat to shift.

Noticing bodily changes such as these can be challenging because, from a very early age, our worth in the world has been largely determined by how we look, and society favours thinness. But being thin doesn't equate to being healthy, and most of my clients notice their health improves when they start eating more, not less. And although being overweight is associated with the conditions in this chapter, such as insulin resistance, diabetes and metabolic syndrome, they can occur in those with a lower body mass index (BMI) too. In fact, using BMI as a tool to measure size and health is flawed as body shape and build aren't taken into account – bodybuilding clients of mine have been refused IVF treatment because they were 'obese' and they barely had any body fat on them.

My suggestion when it comes to changes to your body composition is to start off with accepting and loving your body as it is. Despising the body you're in is never going to feel good, and any so-called 'improvements' that come from a place of loathing, punishment and restriction are unlikely to last, and will contribute to poor mental health along the way.

When it comes to weight loss, counting calories and fad diets rarely work. They often leave you under-nourished, tired and depleted, which not only feels like crap but also makes you more prone to 'binge-eating' because you're understandably ravenous. Which, if you're anything like me, just leaves you with a pile of shame and unworthiness to then deal with.

Instead, I suggest concentrating on feeling energised and nourished, building physical strength, and decreasing your risk of insulin resistance by reducing stress and inflammation, supporting sleep, and moving your body in ways that feel good. And that's what this chapter is all about.

Not By the Hair on My Chinny-chin-chin

If you're spending an increasing amount of time in front of the mirror, monitoring the amount of hair sprouting around your mouth and on your chin, the weight that's collected around your middle, the acne that rivals what you went through as a teenager, all whilst wondering if your hair is falling out, then insulin resistance could be to blame. Too much insulin has a negative effect on your sex hormones, causing acne, facial hair growth, scalp hair loss, irregular cycles and lack of ovulation. It's involved in many hormonal and reproductive health issues, such as PCOS, heavy periods and fibroids, and can put you at an increased risk of developing breast cancer and endometrial cancer. Signs of insulin resistance include:

- Hypertension (high blood pressure)
- Abnormal cholesterol levels
- Adult acne
- Weight gain

- Excess facial hair
- Loss of head hair (aka male pattern baldness)
- Anovulation
- Lethargy and daytime sleepiness
- Hunger
- Sugar cravings
- Difficulty concentrating (brain fog)
- Wrinkles
- Skin tags (small, soft, skin-coloured growths on your skin).

What Exactly is Insulin Resistance?

Insulin is a hormone that's made by a gland called the pancreas and it helps to regulate blood sugar levels. When you eat some food, your blood sugar level goes up and your pancreas responds by briefly secreting insulin, so that your body's cells absorb the sugar from your blood. Insulin carries any excess sugar to your liver and muscles, where it's stored as fuel for when you need it. Let's say it's been a while since you ate, because you had a manic morning trying to get out of the house on time, so your blood sugar is running low. In this situation your liver needs to release its energy stores. It's a smart system, but like all smart systems in the body, things can go wrong. And this is a system that is particularly affected by menopause.

Insulin should be released when it's needed, which means, ideally, levels should be low, but when your cells lose their ability to respond to insulin – as is often the case when your diet features refined carbs and liquid calories such as sodas, juices and energy drinks – more insulin needs to be produced to keep your blood sugar levels balanced. So your pancreas ups its game by releasing more insulin. With time, constant exposure to insulin results in your insulin receptors becoming less sensitive, hence the term insulin resistant.

Higher levels of insulin create inflammation and because your cells can't absorb glucose properly, it gets stored as fat. The influence of insulin can be felt on all your other hormones, such as oestrogen, progesterone and testosterone, which means that when insulin is out of whack, you're gonna feel it, and it will absolutely make it harder to reduce menopausal symptoms like hot flushes and night sweats, not to mention making you feel tired and low in energy.

Don't be fooled by its name and think that insulin resistance is an issue that's solely related to blood sugar levels and diabetes though. Insulin resistance leads to inflammation, oxidative stress and premature ageing, and is associated with diabetes, heart disease, stroke and dementia. Plus insulin can cause cells to grow at an uncontrollable rate. The impact of this is most notable among cancerous cells, which is one reason why the cancer rate is higher among those who are diabetic and/or obese.

High levels of insulin are also a big problem because they set off a chain reaction with your other hormones. Cortisol (the stress hormone) goes up, which is a problem, because cortisol and progesterone compete for the same hormone receptors, but cortisol pips progesterone to the post, which can lead to progesterone deficiency and oestrogen dominance and, as you already know by now, this is a common hormonal imbalance during the early phase of perimenopause. There are also insulin receptors on your ovaries and excess oestrogen makes them produce more testosterone than oestrogen, which can cause an increase in body hair and acne. Risk factors for developing insulin resistance include:

- A family history of diabetes.
- Receiving a diagnosis of gestational diabetes during pregnancy.
- A body mass index (BMI) greater than 29 (but as I mentioned, BMI needs to be taken with a large pinch of salt).
- Carrying excess weight, particularly around your middle (apple shape).
- Polycystic ovarian syndrome (PCOS).
- A diet that's high in refined carbs and sugar.
- A sedentary lifestyle.
- Use of prescribed medications such as antidepressants (especially those classified as SSRIs) and steroid medications.
- Hormonal birth control.
- Smoking.
- Inflammation.

Apple-shaped obesity is associated with an increased risk of insulin resistance and a slew of other long-term health issues. As a rough guide, if your waist circumference is more than 89cm (35 inches) then you fall into the 'apple' body shape. People who are apple-shaped are at higher risk of developing insulin resistance and metabolic syndrome – the medical term for a combination of diabetes, high blood pressure and obesity.

Testing for Insulin Resistance

Blood glucose levels aren't much use when it comes to testing for insulin resistance, because your blood sugar level can be normal and you can be insulin resistant. Instead of testing blood sugar/glucose, your doctor can order tests that specifically look for insulin resistance:

- **Fasting insulin** (aka Kraft test) simply tests for insulin and it's good at detecting severe insulin resistance. Fasting insulin should be under 8 mIU/L (55 pmil/L).
- **The insulin-glucose challenge test** is a more sensitive type of test that can pick up insulin resistance earlier on, even when blood glucose and fasting insulin levels are normal.
- **HOMA-IR index** is a calculation that finds the ratio between fasting insulin and glucose. It can show the presence and extent of insulin resistance. When HOMA-IR is low (0.5-1.4), you're sensitive to insulin and insulin is doing a good job of managing your blood sugar levels. If HOMA-IR is high (above 1.5), then this shows insulin resistance and the higher the number, the more resistant to insulin you'll be.

Insulin resistance is an issue that we all need to be aware of and requires preventative action. This is a condition that we should all be taking active steps to prevent. Not only does it have serious health and life consequences, but it costs us an absolute fortune in public health spending. The good news is that insulin resistance can be reversed, so let's get onto how.

Cut Out Sugar

You can't reverse insulin resistance without dealing with sugar in all its forms. Cakes, puddings, sweeteners, honey, syrup, agave, molasses, fruit juice and dried fruit. Yep, that means no energy balls. It also means being prepared to deal with the emotional disharmony that often causes us to crave or seek comfort in sugary foods. It's understandable if the idea of this feels overwhelming or scares you, but you don't have to do it alone. Inside The Flow Collective we have a whole programme on dealing with cravings and improving diet and in it, I really focus on dealing with what's going on inside your head (as well as your body and fridge).

Find Balance with Carbs

Simple carbs, such as bread, pastries and pasta, need to be limited in order to reduce the glucose burden that they create, and the inflammation that can drive weight gain and food cravings. Potatoes aren't the enemy, but they shouldn't be the priority on your plate either. If you eat your protein first, slowly and mindfully by chewing it sufficiently, then you'll feel full sooner than if you start with starchy veg. Starch is important, because it helps to soothe your nervous system, which can make it easier to fall asleep at night, and it can also stabilise your blood sugar overnight, which reduces night wakings. The ketogenic diet is a very low-carb diet that's often used to stimulate weight loss, the specifics of which I'll get onto in a bit. Some of my clients who've gone keto have found that their reduced intake of starch meant that their sleep got worse.

Eat Enough Protein

Many of my clients rely on sugary snacks and caffeine to prop them up throughout the day, because they're not eating enough protein. Protein helps you to feel full, stabilises your blood sugar and can also reduce sugar cravings. It also allows you to build muscle, keeps your liver happy and therefore your ability to detoxify oestrogen, and it plays a role in triggering your circadian rhythm.

You want to be eating a serving of protein (30g) at every meal, which equates to a chicken breast, three eggs, a fillet of fish or half a block of tofu. Why 30 grams specifically? Because that's the amount needed to reach the leucine threshold in order to trigger muscle protein synthesis. Leucine is an essential amino acid, a building block of protein that your body can't manufacture, which means that it has to come through diet. You need between 2.5 to 3 grams of leucine per meal in order to trigger the process of muscle protein synthesis. That means you need to consume 30 grams of protein to protect your muscles, *at every meal.*

When I look over my clients' food diaries I see that many of them are eating salads and soups, and counting them as a meal. Whilst I love salads and soups and encourage you to eat them, unless they contain adequate protein they do not constitute a meal. In fact, most of my clients don't consume a substantial amount of protein until their evening meal – no wonder they're all knackered and moody! You can't expect to build or sustain your muscles if you're only eating protein as part of your evening meal. Protein that's rich in leucine also helps to increase insulin secretion and stabilise blood sugar – another reason to eat the protein on your plate first.

If you don't eat animal sources of protein, then you're gonna need to up your game, because leucine is harder to come by in plant-based foods. You can add in a branch chain amino acid (BRAA) complex to your meals, but if you're not opposed to eating animal products then bring them back into your diet – please. Eggs are a great source of protein, but you need to eat more than one or two. Three large eggs gets you 18 grams of protein, but it's still not enough to tip the leucine scale – you'll need to eat five for that to happen.

Intermittent Fasting

Intermittent fasting (IF) can help to reset your metabolism, reverse insulin resistance, reduce inflammation, lose weight and even reduce cancer risk. To do this, you simply restrict the time period in which you eat to an eight- to 10-hour eating window, such as 10am to 6pm, 8am to 6pm or 9am to 7pm. You get to pick the eating window that suits you, but I recommend eating by 7pm as having dinner later than that means production of your sleep hormone, melatonin, can be delayed, which can prevent you from falling asleep at a decent time. Eat meals that contain all three macronutrients – protein, fat and starch – so that you feel full, satisfied and have enough energy. Regardless of life stage, it's incredible what prioritising macronutrients will do for your health, because so many of us eat big meals that lack nutrition. Outside of your eating window, you stick to drinking water, teas and coffee that don't have anything added to them, such as milk, sugar or sweeteners.

Another way to practise intermittent fasting is to fast twice a week or on alternate days. A 12-month study of insulin-resistant individuals compared alternate day fasting (where 25 per cent of energy needs were met on 'fast days' and 125 per cent on the alternating 'feast days') with calorie restriction (where 75 per cent of energy needs were consumed every day) and a control group. Whilst weight change and BMI were similar among the alternate fasting and calorie restriction groups, insulin levels and insulin resistance were greatly reduced in the alternate fasting day group when compared with the calorie restriction group. That being said, I think this type of intermittent fasting suits male bodies more than female bodies.

Intermittent fasting is not suitable for everyone though. Many of you who are in the perimenopause zone, and even those of you who are premenopausal, will be experiencing significant stress, and intermittent fasting can add to that burden, causing you to retain or gain weight and resulting in further disruption. When you're stressed, sleeping poorly, undernourished and struggling to make it through the day, intermittent fasting could do more harm than good which is one reason why I prefer to focus on eating balanced, satisfying meals at regular mealtimes (and healthy snacks if needed), and cutting out sugar whilst addressing other aspects of health.

Metformin

Metformin is a drug that's used to treat diabetes and it's sometimes prescribed to those who have polycystic ovarian syndrome (PCOS) too. It can help to improve insulin resistance, support weight loss and reduce the risk of cardiovascular disease. But, around 25 per cent of people taking it experience bloating, abdominal pain, constipation, diarrhoea and gas. Taking metformin comes with an increased risk of vitamin B12 deficiency, so you'll want to make sure that you're getting B12 through your diet and adequate supplementation. There are also other strategies that are comparable to using metformin.

Supplements to Improve Insulin Sensitivity

- Magnesium deficiency has been suggested as one potential underlying cause of insulin resistance and development of type 2 diabetes and levels of magnesium appear to be directly related to insulin sensitivity; the lower magnesium is, the more insulin resistance there is. As you might expect, magnesium improves insulin sensitivity and it can support many other aspects of perimenopause, such as energy levels, mood and sleep (see pages 147–148 for more information and a recommended dosage).
- Low vitamin D is associated with insulin resistance, so get yours checked through your GP. Make sure you enjoy short amounts of midday sun and supplement as needed (see pages 203–205).

- Zinc supports a ridiculous number of processes in the body, from the production of hormones to how your liver and immune system function. When zinc levels are low, insulin can't do its job properly and glucose remains in the bloodstream, instead of being stored. It also has an impact on the levels of leptin (the hormone that regulates appetite and hunger) and cortisol (a stress hormone), as well as levels of sexual desire. Not only that, but zinc blocks the enzyme 5a-reductase that's responsible for the conversion of androgen hormones such as testosterone to DHT, the super-potent hormone that's responsible for the acne around your chin and jaw, and all the hair loss that you're freaking out about. Zinc is an essential nutrient that's often missing from our diets and, like most minerals, there's less of it in our foods thanks to over-farming and modern agricultural methods. In supplemental form, zinc citrate or ascorbate is easier to absorb than zinc oxide or sulphate.
- Myo-inositol is a little-known vitamin-like substance that your body makes from glucose and it's often considered to be part of the B complex group of vitamins. Myo-inositol is involved in insulin-signalling inside cells and taking it as a supplement can improve insulin sensitivity, as well as supporting ovulation, which is why it's an effective treatment strategy for those with PCOS. Myo-inositol can also support mood changes in the premenstrual phase of the cycle and PMDD, and has shown positive effects when used in the treatment of metabolic syndrome in postmenopausal women. The supplemental range for taking myo-inositol is 2,000 to 4,000mg per day. Myo-inositol is also a precursor to another type of inositol, D-chiro-inositol, which plays a role in the action of insulin. A ratio of 40:1 for myo-inositol to D-chiro-inositol is recommended.
- Alpha-lipoic acid is a powerful antioxidant that your mitochondria love, because it's involved in energy production. It also improves insulin sensitivity and can support weight loss. Dietary sources include liver, kidney, spinach, broccoli and tomato. The standard supplemental range is 300 to 600mg per day.
- Consuming 3 grams (one and a half teaspoons) of cinnamon a day for 16 weeks results in significant improvements to all the components of metabolic syndrome. Taking one half to three teaspoons of cinnamon a day can improve cholesterol levels and reduce sugar cravings too.

- Fenugreek can stimulate insulin secretion, enhance insulin sensitivity and improve glucose tolerance. It also has oestrogenic activity which is why it can support breast milk production as well as reduce menopausal symptoms such as hot flushes, night sweats, insomnia, mood changes, and headaches as well as improve cholesterol levels. Crushed fenugreek seeds can be added to curries, baked in bread or brewed as a tea. The supplemental dose is 1 to 1.5 grams per day.
- Berberine is a phytonutrient that's found in several plants, such as goldenseal and barberry, and it's been used in Chinese medicine for thousands of years – whilst in China for my clinical placement, I was given barberry wafers before a large meal to improve digestion. Only later would I learn that berberine has an effect on gut bacteria and can improve insulin sensitivity. Berberine has proved to be equal to or superior to metformin at improving insulin resistance, though if you're interested in taking it, I recommend working with a naturopath/nutritionist as it interacts with some common medications and long-term use may have a negative impact on your microbiome and digestion.
- Chromium is a mineral that can improve insulin resistance. Diets that are low in chromium have a negative effect on glucose and insulin. Chromium picolinate is better absorbed than other forms and the supplemental dose is 200 to 500mcg per day.
- Ashwagandha root extract helps to reduce stress levels, which is thought to reduce food cravings and improve eating behaviours, thereby supporting weight loss.

Curb Cortisol

You've probably heard that stress can make you pile on the pounds and it does this in several ways. Cortisol increases the activity of the body's major fat-storing enzyme, lipoprotein lipase (LPL), causing an increase in abdominal fat, and abdominal fat cells also seem to be very responsive to cortisol as they have four times as many cortisol receptors on them as other fat cells. Elevated cortisol levels, which are often a feature of modern life, impacts on what insulin is up to and can lead to insulin resistance; glucose can no longer enter cells and gets stored as fat instead. And it won't surprise you to hear that when cortisol is high, we tend to crave (and have) high-calorie foods. This is yet another reason why dialling down stress is so important during perimenopause, but ideally, long before it even begins.

Inflammation

Acute inflammation is a good thing – it's the body's response to infection or trauma. Heat, redness, swelling, pain and loss of function are how your body heals and protects itself. But ongoing chronic inflammation is not helpful, and causes or contributes to many health issues, including hormonal imbalances, weight gain, diabetes and cardiovascular health.

Diet, stress, lack of sleep and toxins can all lead to systemic inflammation in which your body tries to deal with the repeated internal injuries it's being faced with. It does this by flooding your body with inflammatory markers in an attempt to put out the fire. But a continued response like this has negative consequences, like weight gain, fatigue, poor sleep, headaches, joint pain, skin issues and indigestion. Sound familiar?

Inflammation can cause or aggravate many a menstrual cycle issue, including period pain, PMS and histamine intolerance, PCOS, endometriosis and adenomyosis. It can also impact the balance of your hormones, which as you already know, are already all over the place in perimenopause.

Sources of inflammation include:

- Smoking
- Stress
- Lack of sleep
- Lack of exercise
- Environmental toxins (we'll get onto these in Chapter 10)
- Dietary sources of inflammation include:
  - Sugar
  - Processed food
  - Vegetable oils
  - Alcohol
  - Cow dairy
  - Gluten
  - FODMAPs

FODMAPs

Fermentable, Oligo-, Di-, Monosaccharides, and Polyols are a group of sugars that aren't well absorbed by the small intestine. Instead, they move slowly and attract water, then when they make it to the large intestine, FODMAPs are fermented by gut bacteria, producing gas as a result. If you're prone to bloating and IBS symptoms such as stomach pain, diarrhoea and constipation, then it's worth seeing if excluding FODMAPs makes a difference. Monash University developed the low-FODMAP diet and have excellent information on their website and their app has a traffic light system to indicate whether foods are low, moderate or high in FODMAPs. The FODMAP diet can be helpful in the short term but is not a long-term strategy due to its restrictive nature, it's therefore best followed under the guidance of a qualified nutritional therapist or naturopath who can also assess if there is an underlying issue that needs to be resolved.

You might be wondering what, exactly, that leaves you with to eat. The answer is plenty. Whilst we have been conditioned to think that a cheese sandwich and crisps constitutes lunch (and I appreciate that it's a lunch that many around the world would love to even have as a possibility), it's not exactly nutrient dense. You'll find more information about what to eat to support hormone health in Chapter 10, but in essence, it means eating protein, healthy fats and a mixture of starchy veg (potatoes, squash, parsnips, carrots, etc.) and non-starchy veg (greens, broccoli, asparagus, peppers, mushrooms, cucumber, etc.). Supplements such as omega-3 fatty acids, resveratrol, curcumin, N-acetyl cysteine, and bioflavonoids such as green tea and grapeseed extract can all help to reduce inflammation, as can exercise and sleep.

Sleep

Those of you who work shifts and night work are at greater risk of developing metabolic diseases and cancer. But you don't have to work shifts or nights to have a misalignment between your sleep-wake cycle and melatonin production. Not getting enough sleep, poor-quality sleep, disturbed sleep and obstructive sleep apnea – where the walls of your airway relax and narrow, interrupting your breathing pattern and sleep – are all risk factors for developing and worsening insulin resistance.

When your circadian rhythm is disrupted due to shift work, working nights, jet lag and lifestyle choices (i.e. staying up late watching Netflix), cognitive function is impaired and your risk of developing metabolic syndrome increases. If you're thinking one night won't hurt, it will: a single night of sleep deprivation doubles cortisol production the following morning and decreases insulin sensitivity by 40 per cent.

The odds of developing metabolic syndrome go up if you get less than five to six hours' sleep or more than eight to 10 hours, and the link between sleep duration and metabolic syndrome is greater for women than men. Though a further study concluded that shorter sleep duration was associated with an increased risk of metabolic syndrome, but longer sleep duration was not. Getting enough good-quality sleep improves blood sugar balance and insulin sensitivity, and it also helps to reduce inflammation in the body, which can also drive insulin resistance. When you're sleep-deprived, leptin – the hormone that tells you when you're full – can go down and ghrelin levels can spike, causing you to overeat and gain weight.

Hunger Hormones

Leptin and ghrelin are two other hormones that we need to consider in relation to appetite and weight management. Leptin lets you know that it's time to stop eating. It's secreted by your fat cells and when this system is functioning as it's meant to, fat cells will produce leptin, sending a message to your brain that you're not starving and that there's enough energy to go around. That means that your appetite goes down and your body can use up the energy being stored as fat. The more body fat an individual has, the more leptin they'll produce. When someone is obese, they can have too much leptin in their blood and persistently high levels of leptin leads to *leptin resistance.*

Leptin resistance is when there's plenty of leptin, but your brain is no longer sensitive to it. The message isn't being picked up, so you don't recognise when you're full. Instead, you keep eating and your fat cells keep producing more leptin, which causes further resistance. Leptin resistance slows your metabolism, so you don't burn energy at the same rate. It slows the conversion of thyroid hormones and it impacts oestrogen too, because when leptin is high it can push oestrogen down the less favourable pathways and it also slows down the enzyme that 'neutralises' oestrogen (see the diagram on page 255). When your body fat percentage goes down, leptin goes down, which is why weight loss can trigger an increase in appetite and food cravings.

Ghrelin, on the other hand, tells you when you're hungry and need to eat, and it appears to have an influence on insulin secretion too. It's produced in the gut and peaks every four hours or so, which roughly correlates to breakfast, lunch and dinner, telling your brain that it's time to eat. Ghrelin production increases as a result of dieting, which is why some people eat more and go through the rebound effect of gaining the weight they initially lost. This is why 'dieting' (and I use that term loosely, because it's not one that I like) should focus on eating nourishing foods at sensible times. Eating sufficient protein is once again key, because protein suppresses ghrelin and consuming enough fibre is also important. The ketogenic diet can work well for some people, because ketosis suppresses the increase in ghrelin that can occur with weight loss.

These hormones also apply to those of you with a lean frame and low appetite, because it could be that your leptin is low, which means you're at an increased risk for anxiety, depression and bone loss.

Going Keto

Head to any menopause Facebook group and you'll find a lot of discussion about what kind of diet improves menopausal symptoms such as weight gain, belly fat (their words, not mine) and brain fog. The two dietary patterns that come up the most are the ketogenic diet and intermittent fasting (IF).

The ketogenic diet was first used by Russell Wilder in 1921 as a way to treat epilepsy and it remains a way of managing drug-resistant epilepsy. It consists of a high amount of healthy fats (55 to 60 per cent), a moderate amount of protein (30 to 35 per cent) and a very low amount of carbohydrates (5 to 10 per cent). That means if you're consuming a 2000 kcal-per-day diet, the amount of carbs would equate to 20 to 50 grams per day. One medium sweet potato – 13cm (5 inches) long and 5cm (2 inches) wide in case you want me to be specific – contains around 20 grams of carbohydrate and if that's what's in a sweet potato then it's hardly surprising that a ketogenic diet means that bread, pasta, rice and cereals are essentially off the table. But carbs are present in lots of different foods, including fruits, so going keto means avoiding or limiting a lot of what you'd normally eat.

Carbohydrates are the main source of energy for the body and when it's deprived of carbs, insulin secretion is reduced and your metabolism shifts into a state called ketosis. In ketosis, you use fat for energy, which is why a keto diet can result in rapid weight loss.

As your body adapts to burning ketones for energy instead of carbs, you might develop what's known as 'keto flu' and experience side effects such as fatigue, headaches, irritability, brain fog, nausea, sugar cravings, dizziness and trouble sleeping. Keto flu can last for a few days or up to two weeks, sometimes longer. Staying hydrated, adding electrolyte powder to water (similar to using rehydration sachets if you have diarrhoea and vomiting), and getting adequate rest and sleep can help.

Becoming keto-adapted can take weeks or months and takes place once you've changed how you use metabolic fuel. You go from being a sugar burner to a fat burner. This kind of fat adaptation occurs as a result of the restriction of carbohydrates in your diet, but going keto isn't simply a low-carb diet. In order to achieve ketosis, most people need to consume between 20 and 50 grams of carbs per day. To put that in perspective, the Standard American Diet includes around 250 grams of carbs per day. Reducing the amount of carbs many of us consume and changing the type of carbs we eat is, on the whole, a helpful idea. The keto diet can result in weight loss, help to balance blood sugar levels and improve insulin resistance. It emphasises healthy fats and eliminates processed foods, which is no bad thing either. But it is a restrictive and rigid diet structure which involves ignoring your instincts about food in order to follow the rules. It can also increase cortisol levels (say hello to stress and anxiety), cause sleep issues, fatigue, digestive disturbances and negatively affect thyroid function – all of which can feature during perimenopause.

The keto diet can result in rapid weight loss, but whether it should be used long term is debatable and, if you're feeling angry, tired, depressed and struggling to sleep whilst on it, then maybe it's time to eat more carbs, such as rice and potatoes. Going keto can lead to an increase in eating foods such as meat and cheese, which create acidity in the body, whereas foods such as fruits, vegetables, nuts and seeds are alkaline, so going keto and getting plenty of greens can help to counteract this effect.

Metabolic Syndrome

Metabolic syndrome is a massive problem. The World Health Organization defines it as a condition that's characterised by a group of cardiovascular risk factors, including:

- Insulin resistance
- Hypertension (high blood pressure)
- Hyperlipidemia (too many lipids, or fats, in your blood)
- Type 2 diabetes
- Abdominal obesity
- Cardiovascular disease
- Stroke.

Metabolic syndrome started out in the West, but as a Western lifestyle has spread across the globe, so metabolic syndrome has spread too. It's a massive issue that costs lives and an absolute fucking fortune in healthcare spending.

Metabolic syndrome is more common in midlife women than men and it also affects us more. The precise causes of metabolic syndrome aren't clearly defined, but are linked to diet and lifestyle: being overweight/obese, having a sedentary lifestyle and insulin resistance. We hear a lot about BMI (body mass index), but when it comes to metabolic syndrome, it's abdominal fat and waist circumference that are the main predictors of poor health outcomes.

That doesn't mean those with a lean frame are exempt from developing it either though.

After menopause, levels of oestradiol (E2) drop to a very low level, sometimes to zero. This has a huge impact on metabolism, fat distribution and the action of insulin. Large studies have demonstrated that E2 has a protective effect on the prevention of diabetes and metabolic syndrome.

Slow and Low

If you feel like you're wading through treacle physically and mentally, if you've gained weight, have no energy and feel depressed, then you might be perimenopausal – or your thyroid could be the problem. Your thyroid is a butterfly-shaped gland found at the base of your neck, just below the Adam's apple (larynx). It produces hormones that control your metabolism and when they misbehave, as they often do in women and particularly as we age, you get a wide range of symptoms.

In *hypo*thyroidism (low thyroid function) you don't produce enough thyroid hormones and can experience weight gain, fatigue, more frequent periods, periods that are heavier and longer, an intolerance to cold and forgetfulness. In *hyper*thyroidism (overactive thyroid function) you produce too much in the way of thyroid hormones and can experience weight loss, restlessness, sleep problems, infrequent periods and heat sensitivity. These are really the tip of the iceberg though. Your thyroid impacts on numerous body processes, so when things go awry you feel it in all sorts of ways.

Signs of hypothyroidism (underactive thyroid) include:

- Fatigue
- Loss of ambition and motivation
- Weight gain
- Mood swings
- Depression
- Poor memory
- Reduced ability to concentrate
- Brain fog
- Feeling cold or sensitivity to cold

- Reduced sweating
- Constipation (that may be relieved by diarrhoea)
- Abdominal bloating
- Easy bruising
- Blood clotting issues
- Amenorrhoea (no periods)
- Irregular periods
- Periods that are heavy and/or long
- Anaemia
- Muscle cramps and weakness
- Pins and needles
- Joint pain and stiffness
- Carpal tunnel syndrome
- Lack of co-ordination
- Balance problems
- Dizziness
- Vertigo
- Tinnitus
- Dry skin and hair
- Loss of the outer third of your eyebrow
- Head hair loss
- Brittle nails
- Hoarse voice
- High cholesterol
- Low sexual desire
- Infertility
- Miscarriage
- Exaggerated menopausal symptoms.

Signs of hyperthyroidism (overactive thyroid) include:

- Weight loss
- Normal or increased appetite
- Heat intolerance
- Sweating
- Palpitations
- Anxiety

- Racing thoughts
- Restlessness
- Nervousness
- Excitability
- Tiredness
- Irritability
- Irregular periods
- Infertility
- Frequent bowel movements
- Hyperactivity
- Muscle weakness and loss of strength
- Tremors and shakiness
- Hair loss
- Soft nails
- Bulging eyes
- Sleep issues
- Goitre (an enlarged thyroid gland).

You can have a blood test to check your thyroid function, though your GP is likely to just test TSH, and possibly T4 too, and these tests might pick up thyroid dysfunction, but they could also miss it.

Thyroid stimulating hormone (TSH) is released by the pituitary gland in your head. It sends signals to your thyroid gland in your neck, giving it instructions on how much thyroid hormone to produce. When thyroid function is optimal, your pituitary and thyroid casually chat back and forth to keep things running as they should, but when thyroid function is sub-optimal, your pituitary gland has to yell at it in order to get it going, and it does this by secreting larger amounts of TSH. That means that a high TSH result indicates your pituitary gland is working extra hard to compensate for a not-so-great thyroid. Whereas if TSH is low, it may be that you're over-producing thyroid hormones and that you have hyperthyroidism. TSH is a great test to run, though there is debate over what counts as a 'normal' result (see box on pages 191–192) and there are other thyroid hormones to consider too.

Your thyroid produces four different types of hormone: T1, T2, T3 and T4. The main hormone produced by your thyroid is T4 – thyroxine. If your doctor orders a test in addition to TSH, it's likely to be for Free T4

(FT4), because measuring it is a good indicator of thyroid function. Most of your thyroid hormones are bound up to carrier proteins in the blood and it's only the small amount of 'free' thyroid hormones that have an effect in the body, which is why the free thyroid hormones get tested. *Free* T4 refers to the amount of thyroxine that's actually available to do its job – very different to *Total* T4, which includes all the thyroxine that's there but not available. I like to use the analogy of comparing the amount of petrol that's in your car versus what's at the petrol station. When FT4 is high, it indicates that the thyroid is overactive, whereas a low level of FT4 indicates an underactive thyroid.

But you can have 'normal' levels of TSH and FT4 and still have an underactive thyroid, because in order for T4 to become active and do its job, it needs to be converted into Free T3. Free T3 is about 10 times as active as T4 and carries out 90 per cent of thyroid function. That means T4 can be 'normal', but if it's not getting converted into T3 then you'll get hypothyroid symptoms, because you're not converting T4 very well.

There's also another inactive form of thyroid hormone called Reverse T3 (RT3) which can block the receptors for Free T3, acting like a brake – a handy mechanism in times of stress or illness when the body wants to slow your metabolism down so that you can use your energy to heal. If Reverse T3 is high, you're probably converting too much T4 to Reverse T3 and not enough to Free T3, and this results in symptoms of hypothyroidism, even though TSH and T4 come back as normal. Reverse T3 is a test that shows how much of the free and active T3 is able to bind to your thyroid receptors. In times of stress RT3 binds to your thyroid receptors, but instead of turning them on, it turns them off.

Thyroiditis is an inflammation of the thyroid gland that can lower your production of thyroid hormones. Hashimoto's thyroiditis is an autoimmune genetic disorder where the body's cells attack the thyroid gland and, with time, decrease its capacity to produce thyroid hormone. It's responsible for the majority of hypothyroidism cases, but it's rarely tested for, because this extra information won't impact how your GP treats you. You can test positive for thyroid antibodies but not get any symptoms for five to 10 years. If you test positive for antibodies but don't have symptoms, then that's great news, because you can be proactive and prevent it from developing. Some of my clients have been unwilling to focus on Hashimoto's in the absence of symptoms, but believe me when I say that if you can get a head start, you're gonna want to take it. Hashimoto's can be reversed, but why wait till symptoms develop?

If you're unable to access a full thyroid assessment through your GP, which is most likely to be the case, then you can pay to have one privately. In the UK it costs between £80 and £120 to have TSH, Free T4, Free T3 and both types of thyroid antibodies tested. Some tests also include vitamin D, vitamin B12, ferritin (a protein in the blood that stores iron) and C-reactive protein (an inflammatory marker), and if you opt to have Reverse T3 tested then the price usually goes up to around £200. For more information on which blood tests to do, where to do them and discount codes that make them more affordable, I recommend checking out the information on www.thyroiduk.org.

Key points when it comes to thyroid function:

- Thyroid dysfunction is more common in women.
- Thyroid function declines with age.
- Perimenopausal symptoms may actually be hypothyroidism.
- Thyroid dysfunction can worsen your experience of perimenopause.
- Always ask your doctor what your actual results are. Don't accept 'normal' as an answer. You need to know your numbers.
- You may need to invest around £100 in private blood tests to get a proper picture of what's going on.
- What matters most is how you feel. Your numbers can be 'good' and you can still feel like shit.
- Conventional thyroid medication can make a massive difference or barely any. There are other medications that can be used alongside it or instead of it.
- There are lots of ways to support thyroid health and even reverse your symptoms. See Resources for my suggestions for further reading.

Normal vs. Optimal

When I ask clients if they've had their thyroid function checked, they often tell me yes and it was normal. When I ask them to request the actual lab results, their TSH result is often a number between 2.5 and 4.5, which is classified as 'normal' according to conventional lab ranges. But when scientists set these lab ranges, they base them on what the average is across the population, which for them includes elderly patients and those with undetected decreased thyroid function. The 'normal' range is therefore overly generous and it certainly isn't optimal. A range of 0.5 to 2 (2.5 in the elderly) has been suggested as a normal TSH and this tighter range is particularly important if you're trying to conceive.

Test name	Standard reference range	Optimal reference range
TSH	0.4–4.5/5.5 mIU/mL	0.5–2 mIU/mL
Free T4	9–23 pmol/L	15–23 pmol/L
Free T3	3–7 pmol/L	5–7 pmol/L
Reverse T3	11–21 ng/dl	11–18 ng/dl
TPO antibodies	< 35 IU/mL	< 2 IU/mL
TG antibodies	< 35 IU/mL	< 2 IU/mL

What matters most is the absence of symptoms. If your numbers are optimal but you still feel like the walking dead, then trust how you feel.

Ways you can support your thyroid include:

- Food sensitivities can be a root cause of Hashimoto's and symptoms often improve when you remove gluten, dairy, grains, eggs, soya, seeds and nightshade vegetables from your diet, either short term or long term. I always recommend that my clients who have hypothyroidism work with a naturopath or nutritional therapist who knows what they're doing, because diet has to be addressed.
- Eat a nutrient-dense diet and chew your food. Nutrient deficiencies can be caused by eating nutrient-poor foods and/or an inability to digest and absorb nutrients. Not chewing food, low stomach acid, a deficiency in digestive enzymes and certain medications such as the birth control pill can all result in nutrient deficiencies that cause or exacerbate hypothyroidism. The nutrients we're particularly concerned with are selenium, vitamin

B12, vitamin D, ferritin (the protein that stores iron), magnesium, zinc and thiamine (B1). Private thyroid function tests often include vitamin D, B12 and ferritin, which is great, because you want to know if you're depleted in them before supplementing with them.

- Iodine is crucial for thyroid health – too little is an issue, but as is the case with a lot of nutrients, too much is also problematic. Iodine deficiency is one of the main reasons for hypothyroidism in some parts of the world, but in Western countries that's not usually the case. In Western countries, thyroid autoimmunity (Hashimoto's) is the problem, and high doses of iodine can trigger an autoimmune attack on the thyroid, particularly in those who are deficient in another nutrient called selenium. Iodine is processed by the thyroid gland and during this process, a free radical called hydrogen peroxide is released, which can cause further damage to the thyroid. But if you have adequate levels of selenium then it will neutralise the hydrogen peroxide. This is why supplementing with iodine is controversial. It's also another great reason to work with a nutritional therapist or naturopath who is experienced in thyroid issues.
- Balance your hormones. Too much oestrogen can suppress thyroid hormone and increases our need for TSH. This is why those who have hypothyroidism and are taking some types of oestrogen therapy may find their need for thyroid medication and support goes up. Progesterone, on the other hand, stimulates thyroid hormone. When you have a hormonal imbalance of excess oestrogen and low progesterone, as many of us do, either during perimenopause or earlier in life, then that sets the scene for hypothyroidism.
- Improve your digestive function. A leaky gut – a condition in which the lining of your intestines becomes more permeable, allowing molecules to escape from the gut and into the bloodstream – can cause thyroid problems, so cut out problematic foods and have some bone broth to help it heal.
- Get off your mobile phone – just two hours of use per day can raise TSH and lower T4.
- Practise good sleep hygiene (see pages 246–253), because getting less than six hours' sleep is associated with a reduction in TSH and T4.
- Address HPA axis dysfunction (see page 160), because both too much and too little cortisol can affect thyroid function.
- Avoid caffeine.

- Avoid endocrine disruptors in the environment (see pages 276–280).
- Get your vitamin D level tested and supplement if it's low. Vitamin D deficiency is associated with an increase in thyroid antibodies in Hashimoto's patients.
- Exercise can help to restore thyroid function, but overtraining can raise cortisol which, in turn, will negatively impact thyroid hormones.
- On that note, look at how you can reduce sources of stress and take action.
- Test and address for any infections.

8

Bad to the bone

Right now, you're probably focussed on your hormonal symptoms such as mood changes, disturbed sleep, issues with temperature regulation, and what your vagina and vulva are up to. And why wouldn't you be? These issues are demanding your attention now. But I want you to think 30 years into your future and create a picture in your mind of what you'd like your life to be like. Imagine where you'll live and what your home will look and feel like. Picture yourself looking at the fantastic clothes in your wardrobe and enjoying having time to get ready in the morning. Maybe you have a garden that you enjoy tending to and socialising in (all old people love gardening, right?). More than anything, you love the freedom that's come with reaching retirement (if that even exists by the time you and I get there). Now imagine what a fractured hip would do to your life. Recovering from one takes several months to a year, and rehabilitation is hard work. Some people recover well from hip surgery, but for others life is never quite the same. You might not only struggle to get up and down the stairs, but you could have a hard time getting up and out of the chair you sit in. I'm painting a dire picture here, because I really want you to consider the health of your bones. Just like your pelvic floor, we take bones for granted and don't give them much thought until something's up with them.

Dem Bones

We tend to think of bones as solid, static body parts that don't do much other than hold us upright and protect our vital organs. But bone is a dynamic living tissue that stores nutrients, minerals and fat, and our bone marrow produces red blood cells, white blood cells and platelets. Our bones even play a role in the fight-or-flight stress response.

Bone undergoes a continuous process of self-renewal, known as bone turnover or remodelling. As adults, remodelling is taking place in approximately 15 per cent of our bone surfaces at any one time – that's the equivalent of one room in a house always being done up and the process is similar too.

In the same way builders would come into your home, look for areas of damage, and knock them down and remove them along with anything that you want to be updated, the bone remodelling process involves the activation of osteoclasts, whose job it is to break down and absorb bone tissue that's been damaged as a result of repeat loading. Once their job is done, osteoblasts arrive on the scene to do the slower job of forming new bone – or installing new kitchen cabinets. After that, minerals fill the newly created bone. This remodelling cycle takes three to six months and, amazingly, no loss of bone mass takes place whilst it's happening. Up until now, the odds are that your skeleton has been fairly stable – as in the amount of bone mass you have has been stable – but once your periods stop, the health of your bones changes significantly.

When you were a child and throughout adolescence, your skeleton grew rapidly in terms of size and density. The amount of bone tissue in your skeleton is known as bone mass and, as you grew up, your bone mass grew too. By the time you were 18, you'd acquired up to 90 per cent of your bone mass, and by your late twenties your bones reached their maximum strength and density, which is known as peak bone mass. Peak bone mass is affected by a number of factors: genetics, sex, race, nutrition, smoking, physical activity and hormones. Regular periods are a good indication that there is sufficient oestrogen being produced to build and maintain bone mass during our cycling years. Low body weight, excessive exercise and disordered eating can cause a condition called hypothalamic amenorrhoea, in which your body reaches a point where it decides that times are tough and that energy shouldn't be wasted on reproducing, so you stop ovulating and menstruating. In this low-hormone state, bone mass suffers.

Bone mass stays relatively stable in your thirties, but once you hit your forties you start to slowly lose bone mass. Loss of bone mineral density picks up pace a year before your final period and this phase of rapid bone loss continues in the two years that follow your last period, at which point the rate of loss becomes less steep but continues throughout your remaining years. This is because oestrogens have a major role to play in the bone turnover process in women (and in men too), so when oestrogen declines, bone resorption increases and exceeds the rate at which new bone is being formed, leading to bone loss. It's like the builders are always knocking stuff down, but you still have no cupboards, which is why in the five to seven years that follow your last period, you can lose as much as 10 to 20 per cent of your bone mass. In addition to this, during the first five to 10 years after menopause, the space between the vertebral discs of the spine – which has protective, shock-absorbing properties – progressively decreases, which can increase the risk of fractures to these bones.

The abrupt loss of hormones that takes place as a result of surgical menopause is associated with an increased risk of fragility fractures, but receiving oestrogen therapy prevents this bone loss.

Osteoporosis

Osteoporosis is a disease of the skeleton that's characterised by a reduction in bone mass and changes to the architecture of the bone, leading to bone frailty and an increase in fractures. It's a disease that disproportionately affects females and the risks associated with it increase as we age. One in three women over the age of 50 will experience a fracture due to osteoporosis. Risk factors for developing osteoporosis include:

- Being postmenopausal
- Early menopause
- Amenorrhoea (an absence of periods not related to menopause)
- Low body weight and eating disorders
- Lack of physical activity, specifically weight-bearing exercise
- Smoking
- Excessive alcohol intake
- Coeliac disease
- Prolonged use of some medications, such as those used to treat asthma, thyroid dysfunction and seizures, and long-term use of contraceptive injections.

A reduction in bone mass puts you at risk of developing osteoporosis, a disease which weakens your bones and increases your risk of fracture.

> Although it's a condition which primarily affects 'old' people, it's something we should be taking measures against in our teens and certainly in our forties, if we haven't done so already. That's if you want to be independent, mobile and enjoy your later years, which you do, right?

The Thigh Bone's Connected to the Hip Bone

At the top of your thigh bone (the femur) is the 'ball' that sits in your hip socket. Just below the ball is the neck of the thigh bone, known as the femoral neck, and this is the most common site of hip fractures associated with osteoporosis. As you can imagine, scientists are very interested in what happens to the femoral neck during the menopause transition and they've discovered that it gets bigger at a rate of 0.4 per cent per year. You might be thinking that this is a good thing, an in-built way for the skeleton to compensate for the loss of bone density. And it's a good attempt. But bigger doesn't mean better. In fact, it comes with a cost; it increases the likelihood that your thigh bone will buckle. Indeed, the buckling ratio increases at a rate of 2 per cent per year in the three years surrounding your last period.

An increase in body weight is common during perimenopause, particularly when oestrogen declines, and your periods become infrequent and eventually stop. That means there's more load on your bones at the same time that they experience a loss in density and therefore strength. Even though women with a high BMI have a higher bone density than those who aren't overweight or obese, this doesn't mean much, because the increase in load outweighs bone strength.

Can I Find Out if My Bones are Okay?

Given the massive impact osteoporosis and fractures have on health and quality of life, I think it's worth considering that you will get it and doing all you can to prevent it. So, let's talk about what you can do.

A bone-density scan can be used to measure how much bone you have and you might be referred for one if you've broken a bone, have symptoms or risk factors for osteoporosis, or if your bone health is being reviewed to assess how well medication to improve bone density is working. This kind of test uses a type of X-ray that emits a low-radiation dose called dual energy x-ray absorptiometry (DEXA or DXA scan).

DEXA provides information about how much bone tissue you have and it can pick up any deformities of the spine at the same time, but *it's not capable of detecting changes in bone architecture or telling us how strong your bones are.* This last point is important because those who are told that their bone density is low, putting them in the much-debated osteopenia range, will often think that their bones are weak and liable to break, so they hold off on doing the very exercise that they need. A friend of mine was told in her early twenties that she had osteopenia, so she avoided exercising with weights because she was fearful about breaking a bone at a time in her life that was crucial to building bone mass and resilience. Those who are told that they have osteopenia may rapidly change how they see and think of themselves, and that in itself has huge consequences. How do you imagine thinking of yourself as frail would impact your life – would you go grab some weights or wrap yourself in cotton wool?

The results of a DEXA scan are given as a 'T score', which compares your bone density to that of a young and healthy person:

- +1 to -1 means that your bone density is in the normal range for a young and healthy person.
- -1 to -2.5 means your bone density is below the normal range and classifies you as being in the osteopenia range (i.e. you have a relatively minor loss of bone density).
- -2.5 and below is the osteoporosis range.
- -2.5 or less with a fragility fracture is the severe osteoporosis range.

Being in the osteopenia or osteoporosis range doesn't mean that you'll break a bone, it's just one way of assessing bone density and, whilst low bone density is a major risk factor for fracture, it isn't considered to be sufficient in itself to assess risk. This is why the World Health Organization supports the use of the fracture risk assessment tool (FRAX), which is a question-based assessment tool that can be completed online.

Doing Something About It

The risk of osteoporosis is immense during our postmenopausal years and it's frequently underestimated by the public and healthcare professionals.

This is going to sound dramatic, because it is: once you fracture your hip, you're 10 to 20 per cent more likely to die than someone else your age who hasn't fractured their hip.

A hip fracture can lead to a rapid decline of physical and mental health, loss of independence and social connection. Recovery from hip fracture is slow and often incomplete, and it can lead to seeing out your years in a nursing home. I realise I'm hammering home the point, but it's one that needs to be made long before you're in the position where it's become an issue. It may feel like there's nothing to be done, and you might look back on your teens and twenties and wish you'd been more (or less) physically active, but there's no point spending time arguing with the past. Focus on the present and your future instead, because it's not too late to take action. Your bones are changing constantly; old bits are continually replaced with new bits, which means that you can influence the health of your bones. Don't accept that this is yet another lot in life for those of us who are female. Just because it's prevalent, doesn't mean it has to be your fate.

The European Society for Clinical and Economic Aspects of Osteoporosis and Osteoarthritis (ESCEO) recommends the following for women over the age of 50:

- 1–1.2 grams of protein per kilogram of body weight per day
- 20–25 grams of high-quality protein at each main meal
- 800IU of vitamin D
- 1000mg of calcium (though the World Health Organization recommends 500mg which is in line with recent research findings)
- Physical activity three to five times a week
- Eating protein after exercise.

Protein

To maintain musculoskeletal function, you need to consume a *minimum* of 1 gram of protein per kilogram of body weight. So if you weigh 70 kilograms, you'd eat at least 70 grams of protein per day at least. That doesn't mean eating 70 grams *of a* protein, which would equate to a paltry half a chicken breast, it means the amount of food which equates to 70 grams of protein, which would look like a three-egg omelette for breakfast, a chicken breast for lunch and a salmon filet for dinner. You can find around 20 grams of protein in the following portion sizes:

- Three large eggs
- One salmon fillet
- One chicken breast
- Half a block of tofu (150 grams).

It's not just your bones that are supported by oestrogen, your muscles are too. When oestrogen declines, muscle mass and strength are lost, as well as the ability of muscles to repair after an injury and regain the mass that's lost as a result. Regular exercise and consuming an appropriate amount of protein is crucial in order to maintain bone and muscular strength. Make sure that post-exercise you consume a high-quality protein meal with an adequate amount of carbohydrate within one to two hours. Ideally this would be a regular nutrient-dense meal along the lines of salmon with sweet potato and some greens, or grilled chicken and roasted veg, but if you're short on time then three scrambled/boiled eggs with some avocado or veg will do. Try to stay clear of protein bars and shakes that are sugar-loaded.

Heavy Load

The Hutterites are a branch of the Anabaptist movement who originate from Austria and South Germany, and now reside in Western Canada and the US. Hutterite women have a larger bone size and bone density than other US females. What's so different about Hutterite women? Hutterites live in isolated, self-sufficient, largely agricultural communities with a high level of physical activity and from the age of 15 girls carry out strenuous physical tasks, the kind of tasks that are great for bones – weight-bearing and resistance exercises.

Weight-bearing exercise includes walking, jogging, running, tai qi, dancing, tennis, netball and similar sports. How effective these are at maintaining bone loss depends on the frequency and intensity of them, as well as how many months and years they're done for. Although there are many benefits to walking and walking can improve the bone mass density of the femoral neck (the section of thigh bone before the 'ball' that goes into your hip socket), it only provides a modest load on the skeleton, that it appears to be the only site it affects. Low-density exercise, even when performed for longer periods of time, does not result in an increase in bone mineral content and bone mass density in the way that high-impact exercise does, which is why weight-bearing exercise that includes jumping, such as volleyball, basketball, netball and martial arts, seems to have a greater impact on bone mass density.

Strength/resistance training exercises are ones in which your joints are moved against some kind of resistance, which may be supplied as free weights, gym machines, tubes or your own body weight. These kinds of exercises are excellent at increasing bone density to site-specific areas, such as the lumbar spine and neck of the femur – the areas prone to fractures. Rather than going for a low load and lots of repetitions of these exercises – which can reduce the rate of bone loss of the spine but not result in favourable changes to bone bass density – go for high load and low repetitions at least three times a week. If this is all new to you, then start with a lower load and build up to larger weights gradually.

Biking and swimming can be great for cardiovascular exercise and mental health, but they don't provide adequate loads to the bones of the hips; swimming is non-weight bearing due to the buoyancy of the water and biking compresses the pelvis but not your actual hip joint.

One study found that after 18 months of high-impact exercise, premenopausal women aged 35 to 45 years experienced a significant increase in the bone density of the femoral neck. But don't take that to mean that if you're older, then there's no point. In postmenopausal women between the ages of 50 and 70, doing high-intensity interval training (HIIT) for a year prevented the rate of bone loss that was seen in the control 'no-exercise' group. But the benefits didn't stop there. The HIIT group gained muscle mass and strength, better balance and improved rates of physical activity, all of which can reduce your likelihood of falling and fracturing a bone. Not to mention improving just about every other possible parameter of health.

A two-year study of women aged 49 to 65 demonstrated that improving back strength helps to prevent the hunched-over posture that's common with ageing and osteoporosis. This is a group of women who were oestrogen-deficient, so imagine what impact you can have on your bone and posture if you start doing strength training whilst you have oestrogen on your side.

The positive impact of weight-bearing and strength exercises on building bone density and bone resilience is well-documented during our *pre*menopausal years, but this does not continue after menopause unless you're supplementing with oestrogen. Now, that doesn't mean to say that if you can't, or decide not to, take MHT that you shouldn't do these exercises, just don't expect them to have the same effect on the health of your bones as they would if you were on MHT.

Your bones need you to use them, because although they're very sensitive to not being used, they're also sensitive to vigorous activity and heavy loads. Now is the time to start high-load resistance training that specifically targets the areas where osteoporotic fractures are common: the hips and spine. Get yourself some kettlebells and get lifting.

Calcium

There is a huge emphasis on calcium intake for the health of our bones, particularly in women of a certain age, but the Harvard Nurses' Health Study, which followed over 70,000 women for more than 12 years, found that those with higher intakes of calcium in their diet were just as likely to suffer a fracture as those with low calcium intake. The World Health Organization has reduced its recommended intake of calcium and is promoting exercise instead.

Nonetheless, calcium continues to be recommended – more than half of menopausal women are supplementing with calcium and annual worldwide sales are several billion dollars – but we should be cautious about how much we take, because higher intakes of between 1000 and 2000mg of calcium per day are associated with a higher risk of fracture. Plus excessive calcium intake of more than 1500mg per day may lead to an increased risk of kidney stones and cardiovascular disease such as heart attack. Once oestrogen declines, the risk of cardiovascular disease already goes up, so we don't want to add more risk factors.

The World Health Organization recommends 500mg a day and good food sources of calcium that are both high and readily absorbed by the body include sardines, white beans, Chinese cabbage, Brussels sprouts, kale and mustard greens.

Vitamin D

Vitamin D is known as the sunshine vitamin, because your body makes it when your skin is exposed to the sun. But it's not a vitamin, it's what's known as a *prohormone*; a substance that the body converts into a hormone. That being said, let's stick to calling it vitamin D for the sake of simplicity. Vitamin D helps your body to absorb calcium, which is why it's so crucial for bone health, and it supports your immunity and hormone health too.

Here's the problem: we only manufacture it when our skin is exposed to the sun at a certain wavelength. For vitamin D to be made, the sun must be high enough in the sky for your shadow to be shorter than your body. Depending on where you live or, more specifically, how far away from the equator you live, you could miss out on making vitamin D this way for the majority of the year. For example, in the UK the sun is low in the sky for a lot of the year (October to May), making it nigh on impossible to make vitamin D. It also means that when the sun is higher during the Summer months, but you're following guidance to avoid midday sun in order to prevent skin cancer, you may be missing out on making vitamin D, which can actually result in increased rates of skin cancer. All of which means that there's a balance to be had: excessive sun exposure increases the risk of skin cancer, but sun exposure is required in order to maintain adequate vitamin D levels. Reducing rates of skin cancer though is incredibly important, but a sensible amount of sun exposure is needed too. That does not mean lying out in the sun. Walking to the shops or eating your lunch outside will provide enough opportunity – the NHS recommends 13 minutes, though this advice, as with much in medicine, is based on someone who is fair-skinned. If you are Black or Brown then up to a couple of hours' exposure may be needed. The Summer months allow your body to stock up on vitamin D as our bodies can use stores of it for 30 to 60 days when levels are adequate. Our vitamin D levels peak in September, thanks to all the sun exposure that's taken place over the Summer, then they reach a low in February (this is for those of you in the Northern Hemisphere, at a similar latitude to the UK). That means supplementing from October to April, or thereabouts, is gonna be a good idea for a significant number of people (it's estimated that 50 to 70 per cent of adults in developed countries don't have enough) and your GP can run a simple blood test to see if you're deficient. I recommend taking vitamin D3 drops, which also contain vitamin K2 as it helps to get vitamin D where you need it – in your bones.

We can also get vitamin D through our diet. Oily fish, eggs, meat and fortified foods such as dairy and non-dairy milks, but these are only likely to contribute up to 5 to 10 per cent of what we need and you need to eat foods that are rich in vitamin D along with fat, because this allows it to be better absorbed into your bloodstream. People who are most at risk for developing vitamin D deficiency include those who:

- Wear concealing clothing where very small areas of skin are exposed to sunlight.
- Have darker skin tones.
- Spend a lot of time inside. If you think this only applies to people who are housebound, consider how much time you spend outside every day.
- Are obese.
- Are older.

In fact, 50–70 per cent of adults living in developed countries don't have enough vitamin D, and it's an important one for both peri- and postmenopause for the health of your bones, but also because it can improve insulin sensitivity and regulate your stress hormones. Vitamin D deficiency is also linked to cancer and cardiovascular disease.

Medications

MHT

The decision to take MHT (or not) is usually based on menopausal symptoms such as hot flushes, mood and cognitive changes, joint pain and vulvovaginal changes. I encourage you to think beyond your current experience of menopause to the decades in front of you. Strong, resilient bones mean freedom to move your body and independence in all areas of life. And MHT, in combination with strength training, not smoking or drinking excessively, and adequate nutrition will enable that.

Long-term use of oestrogen can decrease the process whereby bone is absorbed and broken down, and increase bone formation, and even short-term use of oestrogen can decrease the fracture risk associated with osteoporosis. But once it's discontinued, the effects are lost (good job there isn't a 'limit' on how long you can take it for). The International Menopause Society (IMS) recommends 'MHT [menopausal hormone treatment] as one of the first-line therapies for the prevention and treatment of osteoporosis-related fractures.'

The use of progesterone also slows the rate of bone resorption, so the combination of oestrogen and progesterone together decreases the rate of bone loss and promotes bone formation, suggesting that each has a complimentary role in the preservation of bone mass. In the discussion around MHT, progesterone is usually seen as only important for the health of your uterus, so if you've had your uterus removed via hysterectomy then some medical professionals will see no point in taking it, but here we have a clear example of why its use should be considered in those without a uterus as long as there's no clear reason not to take it. Given how woeful the other treatment strategies are, it's likely that MHT will eventually be presented as an option anyway. So why wait?

Bisphosphonates

Bisphosphonates are a class of drug used to prevent the loss of bone density associated with osteoporosis. They work by slowing down the rate at which the cells which break down bone (osteoclasts) work, allowing the cells which build bone (osteoblasts) to do their thing. The combination of these two actions can help to strengthen your bones and reduce the risk of fracture. Bisphosphonates are usually prescribed as tablets, though they can be given by injection. However, because the process of building bone doesn't happen overnight, an improvement in bone density isn't usually seen until you've been taking them for six to 12 months. How long you should take them for is up for debate. Current recommendations are three to five years, with concern that taking them for longer than five years may do more harm than good and increase the risk of fracture.

Bisphosphonates can cause fatigue, headache, abdominal discomfort, joint or muscle pain and flu-like symptoms including fever. Two rare but serious effects of taking them are kidney damage and the development of osteonecrosis of the jaw – a condition where the jaw bone becomes exposed, and pain and infections develop. They also remain in your skeleton once you stop receiving treatment; as long as 12 to 15 years has been suggested. 'Drug holidays' may sound like a trip to Ibiza that you may or may not have been on, but it's recommended that you take a break from bisphosphonate treatment, usually after five years of use.

Bisphosphonates are usually only prescribed to those with osteoporosis who have already sustained a fracture or those who have a clear risk of fracture, and calcium and vitamin D levels need to be adequate to support the use of bisphosphonates, though these supplements shouldn't be taken on the same day of the week that you take your bisphosphonates. The point is, bisphosphonates can be useful in those with osteoporosis, but there's a lot you can do to reduce or delay your need for them.

Tibolone

Tibolone is a synthetic steroid that's used as an alternative to oestrogen to relieve common menopausal symptoms and it appears to be effective in preventing bone loss of the spine and femur bone, though there's insufficient data on how successful it is in reducing fracture risk. Tibolone can have a negative effect on lipid metabolism and insulin resistance, and it may increase the risk of stroke.

Selective estrogen receptor modulators (SERMS)

SERMS such as raloxifene and bazedoxifene act against oestrogen in some tissues of the body by blocking it, but they can act like oestrogen in others. Because oestrogen can fuel the growth of hormone-receptor-positive breast cancer, SERMs can be useful in lowering breast cancer risk in postmenopausal patients – you might have heard of one called tamoxifen. They're also used in the treatment of osteoporosis due to their ability to increase bone density.

Raloxifene reduces the risk of fractures to the spine, but it does not reduce the risk of non-spinal fractures, such as to the hip. Bazedoxifene can reduce the risk of fractures to the spine and other bones. It's common for those using SERMS to report the occurrence of menopausal symptoms such as hot flushes and vaginal dryness, and using them also increases the risk of venous thromboembolism (blood clots) and fatal stroke.

9

Whip it out

Your ovaries and uterus might start getting up to no good during menopause or they might have already been giving you grief for years and suddenly decide to up their game. You might be considering if it's worth hanging on to them or whether it's time to call it a day. Your doctor has possibly already discussed treatment strategies, including their removal, with you. And your family and friends probably have an opinion about what should be done, especially if they're used to witnessing you flood through your clothing or doubling up in pain.

This chapter is a guide to the most common menstrual cycle issues and reproductive conditions that we're faced with during the menopause transition. I'll explain what they are and some of the treatment strategies that can be used to manage or resolve them. You'll see that some conditions are aggravated by the hormonal shifts of perimenopause, but ultimately improve postmenopause, so in knowing that this is to come your focus might be on getting through the rough patch as best you can. You might also decide that you can't wait and you'd rather be done with it. There's no judgement from me. You know your symptoms, and how they impact your health and quality of life. My hope is that the information here helps you to make an empowered decision, whatever that may be, and lets you know that there are alternatives to whipping it out.

Hysterectomy refers to the surgical removal of the uterus, though I'm hoping that 'hysterectomy' will be retired in favour of the medically accurate uterectomy. Hysteria (read: being emotional) was once believed to be a mental disorder that could be attributed to being a woman, the source of which was having a uterus. The cure for hysteria was to remove the source of these uncontrollable emotions – the uterus – and the surgery was named a hysterectomy. Fascinatingly (and I use that word with much sarcasm), uterectomy is used to describe the removal of the uterus in animals, but not in women.

What is removed depends on the condition that led to the uterectomy being necessary; other parts of your reproductive system, such as your ovaries, cervix or uterine tubes may need to be removed in addition to the uterus. Uterectomy may be advised because of:

- Periods that are painful, heavy or frequent and which do not improve with other medical treatments.
- Endometriosis, a condition in which tissue that is similar to the lining of your uterus grows in locations outside the uterus, often causing severe pain (see pages 236–237 for why a uterectomy may not be appropriate).
- Adenomyosis, where the endometrial tissue that lines the uterus encroaches into the muscular wall of the uterus, usually causing severe cramps and heavy bleeding.
- Uterine fibroids – non-cancerous growths.
- Uterine prolapse.
- Severe, recurrent or untreatable pelvic infection.
- Cancer of the vagina, cervix, uterus, uterine tubes or ovaries.
- Though the occurrence is rare (0.05 to 0.1 per cent), uterectomies are also performed as a life-saving measure when severe bleeding from the uterus cannot be controlled following childbirth (which includes caesarean births).

Types of Uterectomy

- Total uterectomy is an operation in which your uterus and cervix are removed. The ovaries aren't usually removed, but if they are, along with the uterine tubes, then this is referred to as a total uterectomy and bilateral salpingo-oophorectomy. The NICE guidelines recommend that the ovaries should only be removed if there's a significant risk of them causing problems – for example, if there's a history of ovarian cancer.
- Subtotal uterectomy involves the removal of most of your uterus, but not your cervix. This type of hysterectomy isn't common as leaving the cervix in place means there's a risk of developing cervical cancer, though some patients prefer to keep as much of their reproductive system as possible.
- Radical uterectomy is where the uterus, surrounding tissue, uterine tubes, ovaries, part of the vagina and lymph glands are removed. This type of uterectomy is usually performed when cancer is present.

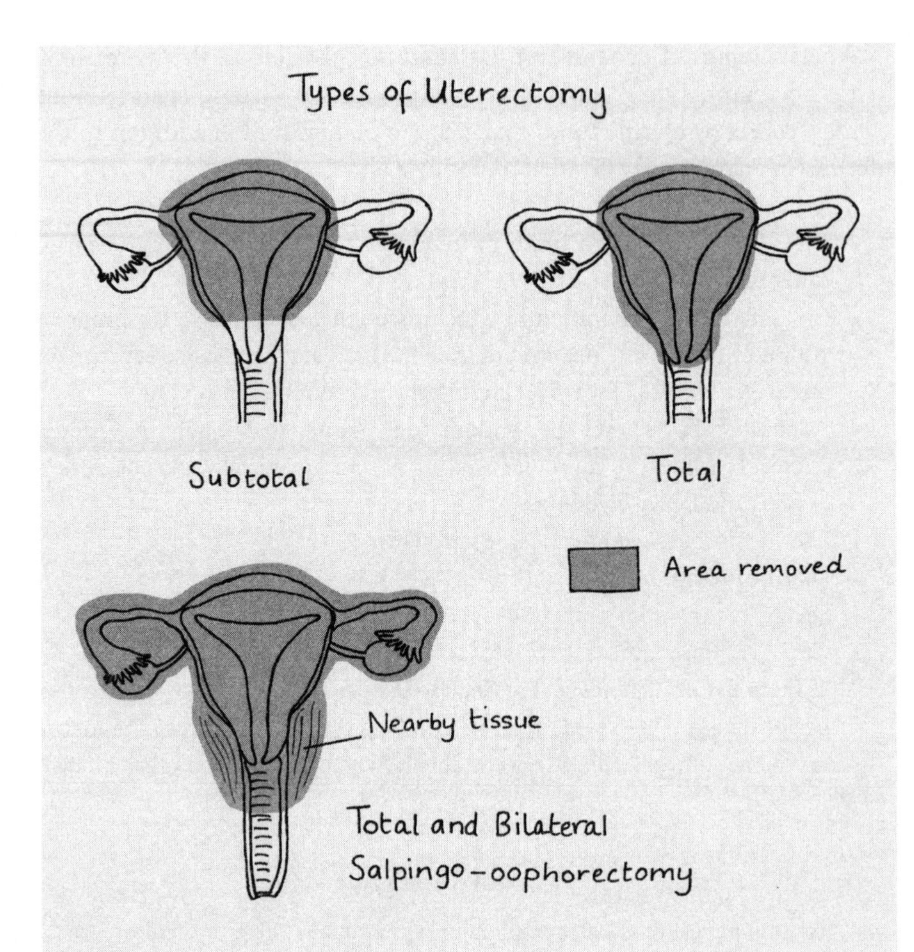

There are three ways a uterectomy can be performed:

1) **Laparoscopic uterectomy** is also referred to as keyhole surgery. Laparoscopic uterectomies are carried out under general anaesthetic and during the procedure small cuts are made in the abdomen. This allows a tiny video camera to be inserted, so that your surgeon can see what they're doing, and for surgical instruments to be inserted to remove the uterus and any other reproductive organs via the vagina.
2) **Vaginal uterectomy** is when the uterus and cervix are removed through an incision that's made at the top of the vagina. This allows

the surgeon to detach the ligaments that hold the uterus in place. Vaginal uterectomy may be carried out using a general anaesthetic, local anaesthetic or spinal anaesthetic.

3) **Abdominal uterectomy** is when an incision is made in your abdomen, usually along the bikini line (similar to the kind of incision performed in a caesarean birth), but sometimes vertically from your belly button to bikini line. Though both laparoscopic and vaginal uterectomies are less invasive and have shorter recovery times when compared to abdominal uterectomy, an abdominal uterectomy may be recommended if your uterus is enlarged due to the presence of fibroids or tumours, which, due to its size, prevents it from being removed vaginally.

You won't have periods or be able to conceive after a uterectomy, which may come as a relief, but you may also feel sad – allow yourself to feel all the feels. If you still have your ovaries then you'll still experience cyclical changes until you reach menopause, which may take place sooner than if you hadn't had a uterectomy because the removal of the uterus can impact on the ovaries left behind. For some, having a uterectomy will cause ovarian hormones to decline and menopause to be initiated, either immediately following surgery or years later. One study found that 14.8 per cent of those who'd had their uterus removed went through menopause within four years of having a uterectomy (compared to 8 per cent of the control group who didn't have any surgery). And another study concluded that those who've had a uterectomy are likely to go through menopause four years earlier than they would have if they hadn't had the surgery. The point is, if you've been advised to have a uterectomy or you've already had one, then it's even more important that you make decisions now about how you can support your health, as well as considering using hormone therapy if it's recommended and any other treatment strategies.

After a uterectomy you no longer need to consider contraception, but you do still need to consider protecting yourself from sexually transmitted infections (STIs).

Removing the ovaries at the same time reduces your risk of ovarian cancer, simply by the fact that they aren't there any more. But when the ovaries are removed before reaching natural menopause, you stop producing sex hormones such as oestrogen and testosterone immediately. That means that you enter menopause and begin experiencing hot flushes, sleep disturbances, mood changes and genito-urinary symptoms following the surgery. When this happens it's called surgical menopause and it's recommended that you start menopausal hormone therapy straight away, because otherwise cognitive changes take place that cannot be reversed, even if you begin MHT later on (see page 156).

Preparing for a Uterectomy

Experience of recovery from a uterectomy varies and will depend on the type of surgery performed, the reason for the surgery, how fit and well you are, whether you smoke or not and how smoothly the operation goes. The great news is that there's a lot that can be done before you walk into hospital for your operation. So much consideration and effort is put into preparing to get married – particularly how we'll look at our wedding – but imagine if, as a population, we put even just 10 per cent of the same time and effort into preparing for surgeries.

Speak to your doctor before the operation about using menopause hormone therapy. You can speak to your GP, but I recommend speaking to the doctor who will be carrying out your operation and/or a menopause specialist, so that you can get this organised before your surgery. When speaking to your GP, be sure to take a copy of the NICE guidelines as, unfortunately, in my experience they may not be aware of the importance of hormone therapy following ovarian surgery. There are some circumstances where MHT isn't appropriate and if your ovaries were removed but not your uterus then you'll need a progestogen as well, in order to prevent the lining of your uterus from building up.

You can prepare for surgery by:

- Stopping smoking – smoking increases the risk factor for any surgery (hypnosis and acupuncture can really help with cravings).
- Cardiovascular exercise such as walking, running, cycling.

- Strengthening exercises so that your upper and lower body are ready to compensate for what your core isn't able to do whilst your abdomen recovers.
- Pelvic floor exercises are important before and after surgery. Actually, they're always important (see pages 68–70).
- Batch-cooking meals to eat whilst recovering – prioritise proteins such as red meat, chicken, fish, and beans and pulses.
- Focussing on improving gut health. Not only is strong gut function the foundation of a healthy immune system, but you'll also receive IV antibiotics during surgery, which are completely necessary, but they will have an impact on the healthy microbes in your gut.
- Asking a friend or family member to be there when you wake up. Many of my clients have had abdominal surgery and uterectomies, but not remembered anything that they were told afterwards because they were under the influence of anaesthesia. They've expressed frustration and sadness that they couldn't remember what they were told, because they were still out of it. Knowing and understanding how the surgery went and any relevant findings is important following any kind of surgery, but particularly if the uterectomy was performed because of endometriosis or cancer. So make sure there's a family member or friend present when the medical team comes to discuss how your surgery went, and to film what they say as well as taking photos of any images they have, such as photos of endometriosis lesions.
- Some of my clients have felt unperturbed about their uterectomies, others have felt conflicted and sad about them. Either way, something I offer them before the operation is a parting ceremony. This provides an opportunity to express the thoughts and feelings that come up for them prior to the surgery and is a way to say goodbye that isn't about the surgery. I encourage them to write a letter to their womb and ovaries, talking about the troubles they've had together and recounting the good times too. They may choose to share their letter with me by reading it out loud. Then I give them a nourishing ATMAT treatment based on the ancient Mayan technique of abdominal massage (see page 259), and leave them to have an Epsom salts bath before getting into bed. Creating some kind of ceremony is a lovely way to honour your body and all it's been through, as well as acknowledging and respecting the decision to have a uterectomy.

Recovering from a Uterectomy

Most people are admitted on the day of their operation and will leave one to five days later, depending on the type of surgery, how it went and their overall health. Initially, you'll have a catheter in place. This is a small tube that drains urine from your bladder into a collection bag. You may also have a drainage tube if you had an abdominal uterectomy. Once these have been removed, you can get going with pelvic floor exercises, which will aid your recovery. It can feel challenging to locate and activate your pelvic floor when you're under the effects of anaesthesia, so imagine that a fart is about to escape and you're trying to stop it from coming out.

You'll receive painkillers whilst in hospital and once you're at home too. Forgetting to take them at the recommended frequency means that it can take a while for the painkilling effects to work adequately again. Setting an alarm on your phone will help to remind you to take them at the frequency you've been advised.

It's very common to have light vaginal bleeding after a uterectomy and this can last up to six weeks. If you experience heavy vaginal bleeding, start passing blood clots or notice a foul-smelling discharge then speak to your GP immediately.

Following a uterectomy, you may also experience:

- Temporary pain from the operation.
- Reduced strength and cardiovascular fitness.
- Swelling around the wound.
- Temporary bruising around the wound.
- Temporary loss of sensation around the wound.
- Bladder and bowel changes such as constipation and UTIs (staying hydrated and eating plenty of fruits and fibre will help counteract this – and I don't mean the cereal Fruit 'n Fibre).
- Vaginal dryness, particularly if your ovaries are removed and you don't start hormone therapy.
- Emotions: relief, sadness, shock, grief, depression, joy.

Ask your healthcare team if they have an enhanced recovery protocol and whether it would be appropriate for you to follow it. Enhanced recovery is an evidence-based approach to helping people to recover quickly following major surgery. Many hospitals now have enhanced recovery programmes in place following surgical procedures and it's sometimes referred to as rapid or accelerated recovery. The focus of it is to get you back to full health as soon as possible. Research shows that the sooner you're up and moving following surgery, and eating and drinking again, the shorter your recovery time will be. General principles of enhanced recovery include:

- Staying active – you might walk to the operating theatre instead of being wheeled there, but why not dance and shimmy your way down the corridors instead?
- Drinking clear fluids or carbohydrate drinks up to two hours before your operation. In contrast to the traditional nil by mouth approach, this is a feature of enhanced recovery programmes, because patients who are hydrated up until their surgery and who start drinking fluids after their operation report lower pain scores than those who have longer periods of fluid abstinence before and after.
- Carbohydrate-loading with fluids containing glucose can reduce anxiety and hunger before your operation, and reduce loss of muscle mass afterwards.
- Mobilising as soon as you're able to after your surgery. That's the scientific way of saying standing and walking.
- Eating a healthy diet. Food is medicine, after all.

Staying hydrated after your operation is also really important as it helps to reduce the risk of forming a blood clot in the major veins of your legs, known as deep vein thrombosis (DVT). It also supports wound healing, prevents infection, helps to flush out anaesthesia, energises you and helps to prevent constipation – this is not a time to be straining to poo! If you're feeling nauseous then it might feel counterintuitive to drink, but it will actually help. In this case, regular small sips will get you going.

Protein is especially important following any kind of surgery. General protein recommendations are to consume 1 gram of protein per kilogram of body weight, so if you weigh 60 kilograms then you'd eat 60 grams of protein per day. But following surgery this should increase to 1.5 grams per kilogram of body weight, so if you weigh 60 kilograms then you'll eat 90 grams of protein per day. Now, if you've ever had the pleasure of eating hospital food then you'll know that achieving this kind of protein intake is going to be challenging, so ask loved ones to bring protein smoothies and protein-rich meals to you every day. You could also cook some chicken and bone broth soup in advance as it's perfect recovery food, thanks to the protein and gut-healing properties of bone broth.

You can feel relieved and positive about the surgery *and* feel sad that you needed it, but whatever your emotions about it are, let them surface. It doesn't have to be a case of either/or. The effects of the anaesthesia will emphasise how you're feeling anyway, so speak to whoever is supporting you about how they can support you emotionally. You might want to ask them to encourage you to express your feelings, but remind you that you're likely still experiencing the effects of the anaesthesia. If your ovaries are removed, then the suddenness of entering surgical menopause can't be underestimated physically and emotionally, which is why, even if you don't plan on taking MHT long term, it's worth considering using it in the interim whilst you adjust and recover.

Why Have a Uterectomy?

Let's look at some of the reasons why a uterectomy might be recommended and what other treatment strategies you could use.

Abnormal Uterine Bleeding

Abnormal uterine bleeding is common during perimenopause and is an umbrella term that encompasses heavy periods and bleeding between periods. Basically, it's any bleeding that changes in regards to frequency, regularity, duration or volume. You should speak to your GP about these changes, because although abnormal uterine bleeding is often a consequence of the hormonal shifts of menopause, other more sinister causes need to be ruled out. In the vast majority of cases, abnormal bleeding patterns are not because of cancer, but you must get any changes checked out by a healthcare professional. I can't tell you how many people send me DMs about changes to their usual pattern of bleeding who haven't contacted their GP. Even if you think it's unlikely that you'll want to follow their recommended treatment strategy, this is something that your GP needs to know about.

Once you're in your forties, your usual pattern of menstrual bleeding can become more irregular and heavier. The hormonal rollercoaster of perimenopause means that you'll go from cycles in which oestrogen is low and you won't ovulate, to cycles in which oestrogen is higher than it's ever been before. In these high-oestrogen cycles, ovulation either lacks oomph or doesn't take place at all, resulting in little or no production of progesterone, which means that oestrogen production is unopposed and you don't get the stabilising impact of progesterone on the lining of your uterus or the ability of progesterone to lighten periods.

It's important to keep track of blood loss: when you're bleeding, what the volume is like and how long you bleed for, as well as any other symptoms. That way you can spot any changes and give your GP and any other healthcare professionals the data they need.

When you go to your GP, they will ask you questions about your symptoms as well as your menstrual history and probably perform a pelvic exam. They will likely refer you for a transvaginal ultrasound (TVU), during which your reproductive organs will be assessed using an ultrasound probe with a condom placed over it, which is then placed inside your vagina so that any abnormalities can be noted. It's important to stress that it's quite normal for something to be found during an ultrasound, regardless of how old you are. Growths like ovarian cysts and uterine fibroids are common across the reproductive years and unless they're giving you grief, most of the time we have no idea that they're even there until someone looks for them.

They may then suggest: a sonohysterogram (SHG), which is a special kind of ultrasound in which saline fluid is inserted into your uterus via your cervix to enable a clearer image; a hysteroscopy, where a small camera is inserted into your uterus via your cervix under local or general anaesthesia; a biopsy, where a small tissue sample is taken from your endometrium or polyp (if a growth like this is present) to be analysed. Other investigations include a cervical screening test and screening for sexually transmitted diseases. An endometrial biopsy may be performed, though if the lining of your womb is less than 4 or 5mm then it may be considered unnecessary, because the risk of endometrial hyperplasia (see pages 226–227) or cancer is low.

Heavy Periods

Long and/or heavy periods are one of the most common complaints that I hear from my perimenopausal clients and friends. They're a big issue in perimenopause, not just because of what's required in terms of managing blood loss, but because the unpredictable timing of periods can leave you feeling on guard and unable to trust your body, which has huge consequences for how you see yourself and for how you live your life. Then there's the exhaustion factor, because blood loss leaves you vulnerable to anaemia and, rather ironically, anaemia can also cause heavy periods. This can turn into a vicious cycle that gets harder to claw your way out of, but I want you to know that there are things that can make a huge difference – and we'll get onto those in a moment.

When it comes to defining heavy periods, we don't need to get into exact measurements of how many millimetres you need to bleed in order to be classified as having a heavy period. You already know if you have heavy periods or not, because you:

- Soak through pads and super tampons quickly.
- Have to get up and change them in the night.
- Might have to double up and use tampons and pads or period-wear at the same time.
- May flood.
- Have large clots in your flow.
- Find it hard to leave the house, because it's easier to manage your flow if you're at home and near the bathroom.
- Are really tired from the excessive blood loss that's associated with anaemia.

You're probably wondering why the hell we get them in the first place. You might also be wondering why your teenager is having them too and if this is some kind of cruel joke. The answer is all to do with anovulatory cycles, and the balance between oestrogen and progesterone.

During adolescence and perimenopause, you're more likely to have excess oestrogen in relation to progesterone, because you ovulate less frequently and therefore don't produce sufficient progesterone. In adolescence this is because the brain and ovaries are getting used to communicating with each other. In perimenopause it's because they're tired of communicating with each other and progesterone production is winding down. Low progesterone means that you don't get the period-lightening effect of progesterone, but, thankfully, you can take body-identical progesterone instead. The excess oestrogen that's often behind heavy periods is also linked with conditions such as endometriosis, adenomyosis and fibroids, so they're all important factors to address as well.

Heavy periods can also be a sign of hypothyroidism, which, as we covered in Chapter 7, is common during perimenopause. They're also more common if you have a copper IUD or use the Depo-Provera shot for contraception. Prolonged periods can indicate an anovulatory cycle and having a heavy period when you don't usually get them could also be because you were pregnant and are miscarrying.

People with excessive menstrual bleeding also tend to have an increased rate of prostaglandin production in the lining of their uterus as a period starts. Prostaglandins are a good thing. They help the uterus to contract and expel its lining, but in excess they cause inflammation and pain, which is why people with heavy periods are prone to bad cramps too. It also explains why non-steroidal anti-inflammatory drugs (NSAIDs) and following an anti-inflammatory diet (such as the one outlined on page 182) can help to reduce excessive flow and relieve period pain. Using NSAIDs such as ibuprofen and mefenamic acid can reduce blood loss by 20 to 40 per cent. Mefenamic acid is stronger than ibuprofen, so must be prescribed and comes as a capsule or tablet.

If you've always had heavy periods, and especially if you have a history of prolonged bleeding after dental work or heavy blood loss after giving birth or having surgery, ask your GP to test for a blood clotting disorder called von Willebrand disease, thrombocytopenia, and platelet function defects, as coagulation defects (the inability of your blood to clot) such as these are not as rare as is generally thought – von Willebrand disease accounts for around 20 per cent of cases of heavy periods.

When you get your period, your body has to strike a balance between keeping your blood liquid enough so that it can flow out, and clotting enough so that you don't bleed excessively. It achieves this by releasing anticoagulants that stop blood from clotting, or, if blood loss is heavy, clots will form to limit blood loss. These can be numerous and shockingly large in size. They can also occur when blood pools in the vagina (if you've been lying down sleeping, for example) or in your uterus (if a condition like adenomyosis interferes with the ability of the uterus to contract, or a growth such as fibroids or polyps, which can intrude on the uterine cavity, obstructs flow), but if you feel you're clotting excessively, speak to your GP.

Hormonal birth control such as the pill and the Mirena® IUD are often suggested as ways of treating heavy periods, and although they can reduce blood loss (by up to 90 per cent with the Mirena®), they don't treat the cause of them and won't be helpful if you can't or don't want to use hormonal contraception. Some people who use hormonal birth control find that their periods are heavier and that they experience breakthrough bleeding, which is when you bleed outside the time when you have your withdrawal bleed, so although these methods are frequently used to manage heavy bleeding, they can sometimes *cause* heavy bleeding.

Tranexamic acid, a medication which is taken in pill form during your period, helps your blood to clot and prevent heavy blood loss, but it's controversial as it also increases your risk of developing a blood clot (the sort that can block a blood vessel and end up travelling to your lungs or brain), which is why they're not used in people taking hormonal birth control, which has its own risk factor for blood clots.

In cases of severe anaemia and especially if fibroids are present, hormonal medication described as a gonadotropin-releasing hormone agonists (GnRH agonists – see pages 224–225) may be prescribed. This works by halting the production of sex hormones and suppressing ovulation, resulting in what is essentially a temporary menopausal state.

Endometrial ablation, where the lining of the womb is scraped away or destroyed, results in reduced bleeding 80 to 90 per cent of the time, but comes with a 25 to 50 per cent chance of developing amenorrhoea (the loss of periods), which is less of a problem when you're coming towards the end of your reproductive years. Endometrial ablation isn't recommended for those who are at an increased risk for endometrial cancer.

Uterectomy is a very final treatment choice and should only be considered as a last resort. I've had several clients come to me for treatment, because they've received a date to have a hysterectomy, but between the treatments they've had and the dietary and lifestyle changes they've made, we've managed to get their bleeding under control. I've also had clients for whom these strategies haven't worked well enough and that's meant that they've had a uterectomy, knowing that it was absolutely the right choice for them, and they've received crucial support as they worked towards acceptance of their hysterectomy. My client Bella had been experiencing heavy periods for some time, but what prompted her to get in touch, really out of desperation, was that she'd had an episode of flooding that was so severe that the ear drum in her left ear had been deprived of its blood supply and her hearing had been affected. Using acupuncture and nutritional support we were able to reduce her heavy flow so that her iron levels could recover.

Plan for Dealing with Heavy Periods

- Taking ibuprofen during your period can reduce heavy flow by half, making it a very simple and useful intervention, especially when you're waiting for other interventions to have a preventative effect. Take one 200mg tablet as soon as you start bleeding and every four to six hours that you're experiencing heavy bleeding thereafter. Ibuprofen shouldn't be taken on an empty stomach, so take it alongside breakfast, lunch and dinner.
- Body-identical micronised progesterone (see page 100) can have an incredible effect on heavy periods. Dr Jerilynn C. Prior, Scientific Director at the Centre for Menstrual Cycle and Ovulation Research, recommends 300mg before bedtime (or 10mg of medroxyprogesterone acetate, which is a synthetic progestogen) for 16 days per cycle (days 12 to 27) or, in those who are already anaemic and/or experiencing other menopausal symptoms, such as sleep issues and night sweats, these doses should be taken daily for three months.
- Supplementing with iron can help you to recover from heavy blood loss and prevent further excessive loss. Anaemia can come about as a result of heavy blood loss, but can also cause heavy blood loss, making dietary changes and iron supplementation a great first line treatment option. Before supplementing, ask your GP to do a blood count as well as a test for ferritin, which shows how much iron you have stored.
- Try supplementing with curcumin, the active ingredient in turmeric, as it reduces heavy periods and can also relieve menstrual cramps. It comes in capsule form and consuming it with a fat such as avocado or coconut oil will aid absorption, which is why some companies include a source of fat in their formulations.
- One study found that taking a herb called shepherd's purse outperforms the NSAID mefenamic acid in reducing blood loss.

- Many clients find ATMAT (see page 259) is a massage therapy that helps to restore the body to its natural balance and many of my clients find it really beneficial.
- Moxibustion (aka moxa) is a gentle form of heat therapy used in traditional Chinese medicine which involves burning the dried leaves of a herb called mugwort on or above acupuncture points in order to stimulate them. A Chinese medicine practitioner can show you how to do moxa at home, so that you can use some points to prevent heavy blood loss during your period and other points to build you back up from deficiency to nourished.
- Stock up on menstrual underwear, aka period pants, as they are often designed to cope with heavy flow and can be used alongside other menstrual products.

Postmenopausal Bleeding

Postmenopausal bleeding refers to a period of bleeding after 12 months of none. This type of bleeding *always* requires investigation. Although the odds of it being due to uterine cancer are low, it's important for it to be investigated so that it can be ruled out. Besides, you don't need something else to worry about, so speak to your doctor and get it checked out.

Fibroids

Fibroids are benign (non-cancerous) tumours. A staggering 77 per cent of us will have a fibroid, or several, at some point in our lives. Most people with fibroids do not experience abnormal bleeding, which will be a shock to those of you who come close to bleeding out every time you have a period. Whilst they can be the cause of heavy bleeding, other possibilities for bleeding should be explored. It's thought that their location is what determines whether they result in heavy bleeding or not. Fibroids that are in the uterine wall are less likely to cause heavy blood loss, but fibroids that grow into the uterine cavity or underneath the endometrium (lining of your womb) are more likely to, because of their impact on the surrounding blood vessels. In essence, they push against them, causing them to bleed quite extensively.

Uterine fibroids are abnormal growths of muscle tissue that form in, or on, the walls of the uterus. Most grow in the uterine wall and are referred to as intramural. If they project into the uterine cavity, they're called submucosal, and if this type is attached to the lining of the uterus by a stalk, then they are referred to as pedunculated. When they grow outwards from the uterus and into other places in the pelvis they are described as subserosal. They're the single most common reason for someone to have a uterectomy, though up to 50 per cent of people with them don't have any symptoms and won't know that they have them until they have an ultrasound scan.

Problems that they can cause include: heavy and/or painful periods, dysfunctional uterine bleeding between periods, iron deficiency anaemia, pelvic pain, needing to wee frequently if the fibroid presses against the

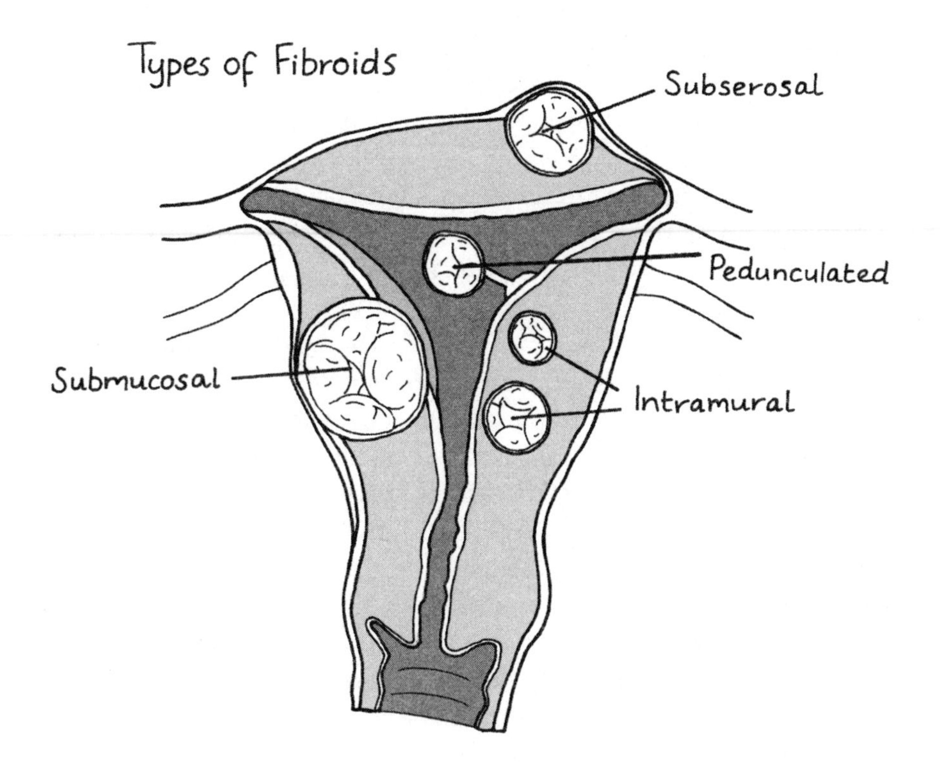

bladder and constipation if it imposes itself against the colon or rectum. Fibroids are associated with hormonal imbalances such as excess oestrogen and they can shrink after menopause when hormone production diminishes. They're more common in people whose family members have them and in those with an African ancestry. If you're Black then you're not only more likely to have fibroids, but you're also more likely to receive shit medical care to take care of them too.

A transvaginal ultrasound (TVU), where an ultrasound probe with a condom over it is placed inside your vagina to assess your reproductive organs, can identify fibroids and polyps, and provide information such as their size and location. It's common for them to be spotted during ultrasounds for other reasons, such as other menstrual irregularities, and during pregnancy.

Medical management includes non-invasive procedures that cut off the blood supply to the fibroid, such as uterine artery embolisation, in which a tiny tube called a catheter is inserted into an artery in your leg. This is guided through the arteries that supply the uterus with blood until the artery that supplies the fibroid is reached, at which point some very small particles of plastic are injected via the catheter to deprive the fibroid of blood.

Surgery can be performed to remove problematic fibroids. A myomectomy is minimally invasive and involves the removal of the fibroid through either keyhole laparoscopic surgery to the abdomen, or abdominal surgery if the fibroid(s) is quite large, but in severe cases a uterectomy may be suggested.

However, unless they're particularly large or causing problems, a watch-and-wait approach is usually adopted. You won't be surprised to hear that medications used to treat the symptoms of fibroids include hormonal birth control and hormonal suppressants, such as gonadotropin-releasing hormone (GnRH) agonists (brand names include Zoladex and Prostap). GnRH agonists may be recommended to those with severe anaemia as a result of heavy bleeding, as well as those with significant uterine fibroids. They can provide temporary relief from heavy bleeding, but are usually prescribed as a precursor to surgery as it gives you a chance to recover from anaemia, reducing the likelihood of needing a transfusion during surgery. It can also shrink the size of any fibroids that are present by up to 50 per cent, which can mean that they can be removed via your vagina rather than through abdominal surgery. However, use of GnRHa can decrease the size and firmness of fibroids, making their removal via myomectomy more difficult.

Taking GnRH agonists induces temporary menopause due to the state of low oestrogen that's achieved, meaning it can reduce your bone density and you can get symptoms such as hot flushes. And once you stop taking it, fibroids usually grow back to their former size anyway, which is why it's not a long-term treatment strategy and usually just a pre-surgery one. You might be offered another medication called ulipristal acetate (Esmya is a brand name), which is taken orally as an alternate short-term strategy to shrink fibroids and reduce bleeding prior to surgery.

Fibroids usually have receptors for oestrogen and progesterone on them and once the influence of ovarian hormones wanes after menopause, fibroids usually shrink and disappear, though some can become calcified, turning into a hardened mass. Calcified fibroids don't require treatment unless they're large enough to press upon the bladder or bowel and cause problems such as incontinence.

There's also a lot that you can do to help yourself, including:

- Supporting oestrogen detoxification (see pages 253–257). Oestrogen, as much as we love it, contributes to the growth of fibroids, especially when we don't get rid of it after we've used it. Supporting your liver and gut health so that you can safely process and excrete oestrogen before it has a chance to be reabsorbed can help with fibroids as well as other 'oestrogen dominance' symptoms.
- Eat a diet that's low in red meat and high in green vegetables.
- Get plenty of omega-3 fatty acids in your diet by eating fatty fish or by supplementing with fish oil or algae if you don't consume fish.
- Reduce alcohol intake as there's a strong association between alcohol consumption and fibroids.
- Use castor oil packs, ATMAT (ancient Mayan abdominal massage – see page 259), acupuncture and Chinese herbs to improve flow through the pelvis and reduce the size of the fibroids.

Polyps

Uterine polyps are abnormal growths that are found on the endometrium – the lining of your uterus – so they are sometimes referred to as endometrial polyps. They occur as a result of the overgrowth of cells from the endometrium and can be as small as a sesame seed or as large as a golf ball. They become more common with age, particularly in the perimenopausal and postmenopausal years. Whereas fibroids tend to improve after menopause, polyps can become problematic and, though rare, some can become cancerous.

Polyps cause symptoms such as irregular bleeding between periods, and periods that vary in length and heaviness, both of which are also common features of wonky perimenopausal cycles, which is why tracking your cycle and symptoms is incredibly important. The more data you collect, the more helpful it is. Some polyps do go away on their own, but if polyps are found your doctor may suggest non-invasive surgery called hysteroscopic excision. GnRH agonists are sometimes prescribed, though, as I mention above, how useful they are is up for debate, so they may be offered as a pre-surgery treatment strategy.

Endometrial Hyperplasia

This is a condition in which the endometrium (lining of your uterus) proliferates and thickens due to high levels of oestrogen during perimenopause, often causing abnormal bleeding. Endometrial hyperplasia can be described according to the degree to which it has progressed (mild, moderate or severe), and there are two types:

- Endometrial hyperplasia without atypia is where the cell number has increased and they're crowded together, causing the endometrium to thicken, but the cells are all normal. With this type there is a 2 to 3 per cent risk of uterine cancer developing. It's sometimes referred to as simple hyperplasia.
- Atypical endometrial hyperplasia is where the cells are not normal. With this type the risk of it progressing to cancer is higher at 8 to 30 per cent. Your doctor may describe it as complex hyperplasia.

Progesterone is the hormone which keeps oestrogen in check, which is why it's recommended that a progestogen is prescribed in addition to oestrogen during HRT – that way endometrial hyperplasia is less likely to develop.

When endometrial hyperplasia is diagnosed, progestins are often prescribed to treat it, usually for a period of six months. These can be taken in tablet form (such as Provera or norethisterone) or via a levonorgestrel-releasing intrauterine system such as the Mirena® coil. Both appear to

Endometrial Hyperplasia

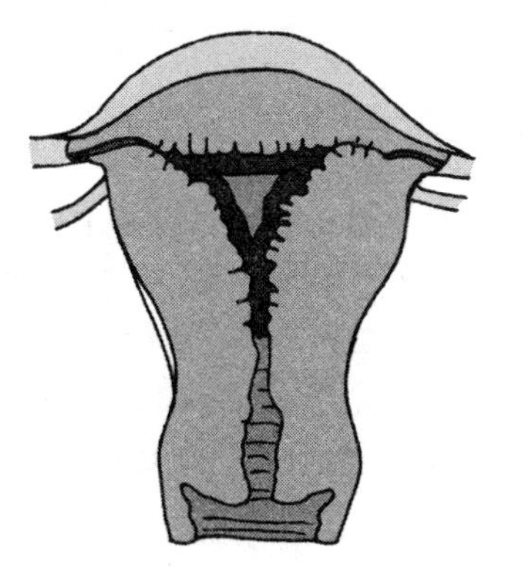

Endometrial Hyperplasia

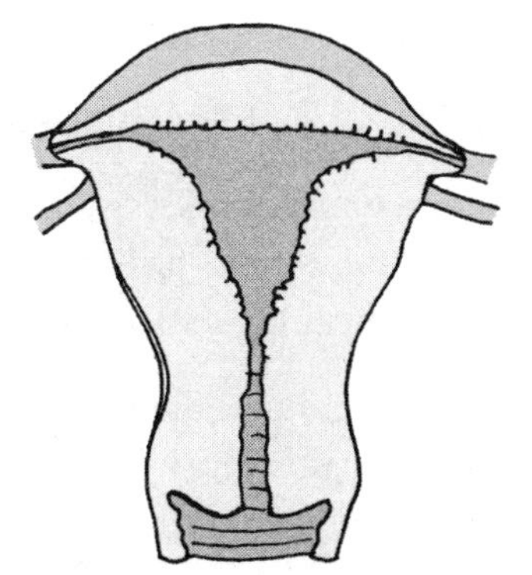

Normal Endometrium

work equally well in cases of simple endometrial hyperplasia, but there is some evidence that the Mirena® coil is superior to oral progestins when the hyperplasia is atypical.

Occasionally, a watch-and-wait method may be suggested, though this is usually only if an obvious risk factor can be discontinued, such as stopping taking oestrogen-only hormone therapy.

The Big C

There are five gynaecological cancers: uterine (womb), cervical, ovarian, vulval and vaginal. I recommend being aware of the signs and symptoms of these cancers, because in my experience most of the general population have no idea that these common symptoms can relate to gynaecological cancers. That's not to say that if you do have these symptoms that you have cancer, but your GP needs to be aware of them so that they can be investigated.

Uterine cancer is the most common of the gynaecological cancers and the fourth most common cancer among those of us with wombs. It becomes more common with age and is most common in those who are postmenopausal, but a quarter of those diagnosed with it are *pre*menopausal.

Around 10 per cent of people experiencing abnormal bleeding will go on to be diagnosed with uterine cancer.

Signs and Symptoms of the Five Gynaecological Cancers

Ovarian cancer: Persistent bloating, persistent pelvic/abdominal pain, difficulty eating, feeling full easily or nauseous, a change in bowel habits, needing to urinate more.

Uterine cancer: Bleeding between periods, postmenopausal bleeding, bleeding after sex, heavier periods, vaginal discharge that's pink, watery or brown in colour.

Cervical cancer: Bleeding between periods or after sex, pain during sex, an unpleasant-smelling vaginal discharge.

Vaginal cancer: Bleeding between periods, postmenopausal bleeding, bleeding after sex, pain during sex, bad-smelling or blood-stained discharge, a lump in your vagina, persistent vaginal itch.

Vulval cancer: A lasting itch, pain or soreness, changes to the skin of your vulva, such as thickened, raised, red or white patches, or the presence of a lump on your vulva.

The Eve Appeal is the leading UK charity for funding research and raising awareness into the five gynaecological cancers. They have an Ask Eve information service where you can speak to a specialist nurse about unusual symptoms you're experiencing or a diagnosis you've received, as well as a supportive community.

Do Genes Matter?

Hollywood actress Angelina Jolie has a strong family history of breast and ovarian cancers, and when she discovered she carries the BRCA1 genetic mutation which puts her at risk of developing these cancers she made the decision to have risk-reducing surgery: a double mastectomy in 2013 in which both of her breasts were removed, which was followed by a salpingo-oophorectomy in 2015, where her ovaries and uterine tubes were also removed.

Most breast and ovarian cancers are not associated with a genetic cause though, and only around 5 per cent of breast cancers and 15 per cent of ovarian cancers are due to an inherited gene mutation. We all carry the BRCA1 and BRCA2 genes. Their job is to repair DNA that's been damaged and suppress tumours, but if you have a genetic mutation in your BRCA gene, as 0.25 per cent of people do, then you're less able to repair damaged DNA, so your risk of developing certain cancers goes up. A 2017 study which looked at the risks of breast and ovarian cancer in BRCA1 and BRCA2 mutation carriers found that the lifetime risk of developing ovarian cancer goes from 1.3 per cent to an estimated 44 per cent in those with the BRCA1 mutation, and around 17 per cent of those with the BRCA2 mutation will develop ovarian cancer by the age of 80. Around 12 per cent of the general population will develop breast cancer at some point during their lives. In those with the BRCA1 mutation this goes up to 72 per cent and in those with the BRCA2 mutation it's estimated that around 69 per cent will develop breast cancer before the age of 80.

Because the presence of BRCA genetic mutations is rare (one in 300 to 400 people) most experts recommend that testing for them should only be carried out in those whose own medical history, or family medical history, suggests the possible presence of them, such as:

- Breast cancer diagnosed before the age of 50.
- Cancer in both breasts in the same woman.
- Both breast and ovarian cancers in either the same woman or the same family.
- Multiple breast cancers in the family.
- Two or more primary types of BRCA1- or BRCA2-related cancers in a single family member.
- Cases of male breast cancer.
- Ashkenazi Jewish ethnicity.

Ovarian Cysts

The term functional ovarian cyst describes cysts which are perfectly normal. You might be wondering how on earth a cyst can ever be normal, but they just form when either a developing follicle fills with fluid or when the corpus luteum, which forms after ovulation, fills with fluid or blood (a blood-filled cyst is called a haemorrhagic cyst). Both these types can grow to 6cm across, but many don't actually cause symptoms and *most resolve themselves without treatment within a few menstrual cycles*. When I was told that I had one, I was really worried, cried a lot and lost a lot of sleep over it. I wish someone had told me that these kinds of cysts are normal and that it would most likely just disappear of its own accord, which is why I'm telling you that now.

The prevalence rate of ovarian cysts in postmenopause is around 14 per cent. When cysts do cause symptoms, these include: pelvic pain or discomfort; sudden severe pain if a cyst bursts or if it develops a stalk which twists and stops the cyst's blood supply; pain if the cyst is large enough to impinge on nearby organs and structures like your bladder or rectum; difficulty emptying your bowels; pain during penetrative sex; a frequent need to urinate; changes to your cycle or period; and feeling full and bloated.

They're diagnosed by ultrasound or MRI, often when other conditions are being investigated, and a watch-and-wait approach is most common as most cysts disappear of their own accord. If they don't and they're sizable and/or causing symptoms, then non-invasive keyhole laparoscopic surgery may be suggested. Sometimes traditional surgery is required.

Dermoid cysts (sometimes called ovarian teratomas) tend to be quite large – up to, and occasionally beyond, 15cm across. They develop from the type of cells which go on to form eggs and, because eggs have the potential to form a multitude of tissue types and structures, dermoid cysts can contain hair, fat and parts of teeth or bone. Weird, right? This kind of cyst accounts for up to 20 per cent of non-cancerous ovarian growths. They don't usually produce any symptoms, are often discovered incidentally and are usually removed by surgery.

Cystadenomas develop from cells that cover the outer part of the ovary and there are two main types: serous cystadenomas, which are usually small, and mucinous cystadenomas, which can grow very large (up to 30cm across) and exert pressure on other organs, such as the bladder and bowel, resulting in digestive issues like constipation and pain, and a frequent need to urinate.

Cysts are diagnosed by ultrasound and checks are usually repeated a few months later to determine if the cyst has resolved itself. Your GP may suggest testing your blood for a protein called CA125, especially if you're postmenopausal, as an elevated level of it is a marker for ovarian cancer (around 5 per cent of ovarian cysts are cancerous). If you get recurrent functional cysts, ask your doctor to test your thyroid as thyroid dysfunction can be the root cause of them. You don't have to do anything to treat cysts as they usually take care of themselves, but ATMAT (see page 259) and castor oil packs can help, and are supportive of overall reproductive function, so in my book they're always worth doing.

Polycystic Ovarian Syndrome (PCOS)

Up to 15 per cent of us have PCOS, making it the most common hormonal disorder. Although some people with PCOS, and some of the doctors who treat them, might think that with the reproductive years drawing to a close in perimenopause, PCOS will become less of an issue, unfortunately that's really not the case, because although your cycles may become more regular, PCOS is linked to other health issues that already dominate the peri- and postmenopausal landscape, such as insulin resistance and cardiovascular disease.

Before we get onto why, let's talk about what PCOS actually is. Historically, you would receive a diagnosis of PCOS if a collection of cysts – often described as looking like a string of pearls – were spotted on your ovaries during an ultrasound. These cysts form when the group of follicles that are put forward for the job of ovulation in each cycle don't end up with a leader, or dominant follicle, and so ovulation doesn't happen. Instead, the underdeveloped follicles form tiny cysts which remain on your ovaries. The thing to remember is that polycystic ovaries are very common and are seen on the ovaries of around 20 per cent of those who do not have PCOS. Plus, you can have PCOS and not have any cysts on your ovaries, all of which makes the presence or absence of cysts as the sole diagnostic criteria entirely unreliable. Some of my clients who have cysts are told that they have PCOS when there is no other suggestion of it, and some of my clients who exhibit all the typical signs of it are told that they can't have it because they don't have any cysts.

Instead of just going by how the ovaries appear, it's recommended that physicians use something called the Rotterdam criteria, in which two of the following three criteria must be met in order to make a diagnosis: ovarian dysfunction (lack of, or infrequent, ovulation, which is classified as less than 10 periods a year); clinical and/or biochemical signs of excessive amounts of a group of hormones called androgens, which can produce acne and hirsutism (excessive growth of body hair) or high levels of androgens in the blood; and polycystic ovaries. When we consider that a significant quantity of androgens are made by the adrenal glands, it becomes clear that the high levels of androgens which are associated with PCOS are not just an ovarian issue, so adrenal function must be assessed and addressed too.

PCOS is a syndrome that people have a genetic predisposition to and it can manifest itself in many ways, thanks to its myriad symptoms, which include irregular or long menstrual cycles, excess weight gain, resistance to weight loss, subfertility, acne, excess hair growth on parts of the body where you probably don't want it, such as your chin, arms, chest and abdomen, and hair loss where you do want it – on your head. People with PCOS are also at risk of insulin resistance and high blood pressure, which, as we've already covered, become more prevalent during the peri- and postmenopausal years.

If you have PCOS then menopause itself may take place several years later than if you didn't have PCOS and your cycles may become more regular as you approach menopause, because the increase in follicle stimulating hormone (FSH) that occurs with age balances out luteinising hormone (LH), which is high in those with PCOS. That means that you're fertile for longer and need to take precautions if you don't want to conceive.

The good news is that if you have PCOS then you're less likely to get hot flushes during the menopause transition, but you're more likely to experience increased hirsutism and develop hypothyroidism. Insulin resistance, abdominal weight gain and cardiovascular disease are all common during the peri- and postmenopausal years, and even more so if you have PCOS, because PCOS on its own is linked to diminished fertility, insulin resistance, type 2 diabetes, gestational diabetes, abdominal weight gain, unhealthy cholesterol levels, high blood pressure, cardiovascular disease, depression and diminished confidence.

Before you sink into depression, please know that PCOS is highly responsive to simple diet and lifestyle interventions, and by taking charge of your health you will be able to significantly reduce your symptoms, and improve your cycle, your fertility, your skin and your overall health.

PCOS is commonly 'treated' by prescribing the pill and, whilst the intention is there – 'let's regulate your cycle' – the pill cannot regulate your cycle, because it works by preventing ovulation and with PCOS you really want to be ovulating, because it's ovulation that will lead to menstruation and it's important for your reproductive health that the lining of your womb is shed regularly. The hormonal shifts of perimenopause can help to regulate the cycle somewhat, but if you're on the pill then this won't happen. The pill can help to prevent the build-up of the endometrium by giving you withdrawal bleeds, but it can also impair insulin resistance after just three months of taking it. People with PCOS already have an issue with this and are more susceptible to it during the menopause transition. It can also contribute to weight gain which is unhelpful in the case of PCOS as it can further exacerbate hormonal imbalances and the symptoms you experience, and the oral contraceptives most commonly used to manage PCOS are the ones with the highest risks for developing blood clots (if you've got PCOS, you're already at an increased risk of getting them).

If you've developed PCOS after coming off the pill, this may just be down to the transitionary period that follows rather than what we could call regular PCOS. This is because when you come off the pill it can sometimes take months or even a couple of years to start ovulating again and during this time cysts can appear on your ovaries, as eggs try to ovulate but don't quite make it and accumulate on the surface instead. When you come off some birth control pills you may also experience a short-term surge in androgens, which can also contribute to what's described as post-pill PCOS.

Metformin is a medication that's often prescribed to treat the insulin resistance associated with PCOS, in which your body's cells don't respond properly to the hormone insulin, potentially leading to type 2 diabetes. It can help to lower blood sugar levels, but may produce side effects of nausea and vomiting, diarrhoea, bloating and abdominal discomfort, so whilst it's certainly an option (and in my opinion a better one than the pill), using other interventions such as diet and supplements to improve insulin resistance is preferable (see pages 173–178).

Don't be fooled into thinking that PCOS is just an ovarian issue. Your adrenal glands produce roughly the same amount of testosterone and androstenedione as the ovaries, as well as producing the majority of DHEA and all the DHEA-S, so adrenal function is vital too, and you have to look at ways of reducing and managing stress, particularly in perimenopause.

Around half of your testosterone is made in your body fat, which is why losing excess body weight can result in an improvement in the signs of excess androgens, such as acne and hirsutism. Even though 30 to 75 per cent of people with PCOS are obese, not everyone with PCOS is overweight. In fact, some people with it can have a thin stature and are described as having 'lean PCOS'.

Investigations used to confirm PCOS and rule out other conditions that present with similar signs and symptoms include:

- Fasting insulin or a glucose tolerance test.
- Haemoglobin A1c test, a blood test which gives your average blood sugar level over the past two to three months.
- FSH, LH and oestradiol test, preferably on day 3 of your period (admittedly this can be tricky if you only have two periods a year, in which case a random day is fine).
- Progesterone test (preferably mid-luteal phase – again, timing this can be tricky).
- 17-hydroxyprogesterone test, a hormone that can indicate a glandular disorder that can result in insufficient cortisol production and excess androgen production.
- Prolactin test, to look for a hormone that can suppress the menstrual cycle.
- Testosterone, SHGB, androstenedione and DHEA-S test.
- Full thyroid panel – TSH, T3, T4, thyroid antibodies and reverse T3 (see pages 187–192). In my experience GPs tend not to order a full thyroid panel, but it's important with PCOS because an underlying thyroid issue can interfere with all your hard work to improve your symptoms.
- Diurnal cortisol test. This measures cortisol in your saliva at four points in a day – upon waking, a couple of hours later, before dinner and at bedtime – giving a more thorough picture of what your adrenal hormones are up to over the course of a day rather than at one point.
- Fasting lipids, to test your cholesterol and other fats in your blood.
- Serum vitamin D test. Up to 85 per cent of people with PCOS are deficient in vitamin D, which is associated with obesity, and metabolic and hormonal imbalances, so testing for it and supplementing with it, if necessary, is wise.
- Transvaginal (internal) ultrasound to assess the ovaries for cysts.

Plan for Dealing with PCOS

- It's crucial that you focus on preventing or reversing insulin resistance. It's really important to strike a balance between weight loss (if it's appropriate for you to lose weight and if you decide you want to), managing insulin secretion and stabilising your blood sugar, all of which can be tricky, so a naturopath is the best person to help you do this. I can't emphasise enough the value of working one-on-one with a qualified naturopath or nutritional therapist. They can help you to figure out what the best diet and exercise plan is for you (see also pages 142–143). Different things work for different people and that's especially true when it comes to PCOS and the variety of ways in which it can manifest.
- Get a full thyroid panel, including tests for thyroid antibodies as people with PCOS are at greater risk for hypothyroidism and Hashimoto's autoimmune thyroiditis (see also pages 187–188 and pages 190–191).
- Generally speaking, an anti-inflammatory diet is highly beneficial (see page 182).
- Address stress, because it can result in high cortisol and elevated androgens, and PCOS can be an adrenal gland issue.
- Improve gut and liver function.
- Exercise: strength training can improve insulin sensitivity by 24 per cent – try HIIT, yoga or Pilates. Lots of cardio to try and lose weight can result in a stress response, which can cause further hormonal dysregulation, so slow and steady might be more appropriate (see pages 280–283).
- Abdominal castor oil packs (instructions can be found on my website).
- Micronised progesterone can be useful in the treatment of PCOS as taking it can slow the pulses of LH that are too high in people with PCOS as well as instigating withdrawal bleeds. It's generally supportive during perimenopause too.
- Supplements to consider: myo-inositol and D-chiro-inositol, berberine, N-acetyl cysteine (NAC), omega-3 fish oil, chromium, green tea (specifically, the compound epigallocatechin – EGCG – that's in it) or drink several cups a day, magnesium, B vitamins, vitamin D, zinc, white peony, liquorice, Vitex agnus-castus, dong quai, melatonin, reishi mushroom, probiotics ... the list goes on and on. There are a lot of ways to improve PCOS through diet and supplements, and although having so

many options might feel overwhelming to you, it's actually really good, because it means that there are specific ways to support the symptoms that you get. However, it does mean that hunting down a naturopath or nutritional therapist who loves to work with PCOS is your best way of finding which ones are most appropriate for you.

Endometriosis

I'm hoping that by the time you reach perimenopause those of you who have endometriosis know that you have it. But I also won't be surprised if a significant number of you have it, but still haven't been diagnosed, let alone received specialist treatment and support. After all, it takes an average of six to 12 years to be diagnosed after presenting with symptoms, which include chronic pelvic pain, painful periods, painful sex, back pain, infertility, gastro-intestinal symptoms, pain with bowel movements, pain with exercise, bladder pain and urgency/frequency, fatigue, exhaustion and depression.

Those of you who have it may have been told, unhelpfully, that endo (as it's often referred to) will magically go away once you go through menopause. Unfortunately, that's not always the case. People with endo can continue to experience symptoms during perimenopause and, in fact, they may heighten due to the balance of oestrogen and progesterone, which is often already off-kilter in those with endo. Some people's symptoms do improve postmenopause, but it's not always the case and to tell people with endo that it will go away once their periods stop is unrealistic and cruel. It also minimises their experiences – can you imagine a male patient being told to just wait the pain out? – and can result in a delay in treatment and years of suffering.

If you know or suspect that you have endo, then at this point you might be thinking, 'Oh FFS, I'll just have a hysterectomy – I'm done with this shit,' and I get where you're coming from. Unfortunately, hysterectomy rarely improves endo symptoms, and I've spoken with many an endo warrior who's told me they had no idea that they'd keep experiencing pain and other symptoms after having their uterus removed. To explain why this can be the case, let's go back to basics and talk about what endo actually is.

Endometriosis describes the presence of tissue that's similar to the lining of the uterus that's found *outside the uterus* (consider this your big clue as to why uterectomy rarely improves endo symptoms). This endometrial-like tissue can exist in places such as the ovaries and fallopian tubes, the ligaments that hold your uterus in place, or any of the spaces between the organs in your pelvis and abdomen. That means it can be on your bladder, uterus, vagina, bowels and rectum. Endo can also exist in more remote locations, such as your diaphragm, lungs and, in rare cases, the heart, eyes and brain.

Endometrial tissue responds to hormones, causing inflammation that results in an increase in blood supply and congestion, which in turn stimulates an immune response, as well as causing scar tissue to develop. The organs that are suspended in the pelvis by ligaments and tissues are supposed to move around to a degree, but when they get bound by scar tissue, any movement – during ovulation, sex or a bowel movement – can result in excruciating pain.

Endometriosis lesions produce oestrogen and they also respond to it – oestrogen makes things grow, including endo lesions. They also aren't great when it comes to responding to progesterone, which is a shame because progesterone is what counteracts oestrogen. And finally, endo lesions also produce large amounts of prostaglandins – the hormone-like substances that cause painful cramps.

An estimated 11 per cent of us have endometriosis, but whilst your healthcare provider might detect things that make them suspect endo during pelvic exams and scans, the only way to find out for sure if you have it or not is to have laparoscopic keyhole surgery, during which a fibre optic instrument is inserted through a small incision in your abdominal wall so that your internal organs and tissues can be viewed. This should ideally be performed by a skilled excision surgeon so that if any endo is removed it is done so in the most appropriate manner. If you have any kind of endo-related surgery, please ask a loved one to be with you post-surgery and get them to video the surgeon's explanation of what they found. You're likely to be out of it and it's important that you understand their findings and surgical approach.

When it comes to surgical management, there are two options: excision surgery, where the endometrial tissue is cut away, and ablation, where it is burnt away. Generally speaking, excision surgery performed by a highly skilled surgeon is the gold standard. Over the years I've had many clients who've undergone multiple ablation surgeries in which endo is burnt off, but they haven't reduced their symptoms and pain for very long, and commonly caused more scar tissue and problems, so I'm a big believer in one surgery, done well, where possible. That means finding a highly skilled surgeon, finding a way to be treated by them on the NHS (you can request to be referred to a specific surgeon's clinic via the Choose and Book scheme on the NHS) or under your insurance plan (excision surgery is often out of network) and travelling to them if they aren't local. It may require the involvement of more than one surgeon if, for example, you have endo on your bowels or diaphragm, which is not within the remit of your gynaecologist to remove. To give you an idea of how tricky this can be, it's estimated that there's only a handful of gynaecologists in the UK who are skilled enough to carry out this surgery and only around 150 out of over 400,000 gynaecologists in the USA. To find a list of skilled excision surgeons and other incredible resources I highly recommend joining the Nancy's Nook Endometriosis Education group on Facebook to educate yourself about endometriosis and your treatment options.

Your surgeon may tell you that your disease is minimal (stage 1), mild (stage 2), moderate (stage 3) or severe (stage 4), but this staging system doesn't actually mean much, because you can have 'severe' endo but experience minimal symptoms, or you can have 'minimal' endo and be in pain to varying degrees most of the time. Also, it can't predict your symptoms or how you'll respond to treatment, it just describes the number of lesions, their location and how deep they go, along with the presence of any adhesions.

Pregnancy does not 'cure' endometriosis and neither does uterectomy or menopause. Uterectomy is only appropriate in a select number of cases, because when endometriosis exists outside the uterus, as it frequently does, it's logical that it cannot be cured by removing the uterus. Countless people undergo unnecessary uterectomy every year because of this outdated understanding and approach to the disease, only to find that their symptoms remain. It's truly unfortunate when surgeons believe that removing the uterus and ovaries is the definitive way to 'treat' endometriosis and as such they don't remove the endo lesions.

It makes sense that the medications typically prescribed for endo target your hormones, because it's an inflammatory disease that responds to your hormones, but medication won't get rid of it, and whilst some of these medications can suppress some symptoms in some people with endo, it only acts as a band-aid. Now don't get me wrong, I'm completely on board with symptom relief and endo warriors are usually in dire need of some respite. However, medication such as the pill – which is often prescribed to those with endo – doesn't control the growth of endo and some people will find that their endo progresses whilst on the pill, so even if their symptoms are reduced whilst on it, they're a lot worse once they come off it. Drugs such as Lupron, which suppress the ovaries, essentially instigating a menopausal state, can cause horrible side effects, can't be used long term and, again, don't actually treat the endo. The press recently celebrated that the FDA have approved elagolix (brand name, Orlissa), the first new endo drug to come on the market for a decade. Orlissa is manufactured by Abbvie, the same pharmaceutical company which holds the patent for Lupron, which, perhaps not so coincidentally, after being on the market for a decade, is about to expire. When it does, generic forms of Lupron will become available, which will be cheaper, thus Abbvie's need to create an updated, 'better' drug that they could hold the patent to.

To be clear, hormonal methods may improve symptoms, but don't treat the actual endo. Any hormonal treatment to suppress endo may make it harder to find during surgery to remove it and you should speak to your surgeon about their use long before you actually have surgery, so that they can advise you when to stop taking them.

If you're wondering why the F we get it in the first place, you're not the only one; the cause of endometriosis is unknown. If you have endo, you may have read somewhere or been told that it develops when menstrual blood flows upwards into the pelvis and ovaries. This theory, known as retrograde menstruation, was developed by Dr John Sampson back in 1927 and, despite being a flawed theory, it's still touted as the reason for the existence of endo. It's flawed because endometrial lesions only *resemble* the lining of the womb, but their structure is different and they behave differently to endometrial tissue too. Plus, 90 per cent of people with periods experience retrograde menstruation, but the prevalence rate for endo is only 11 per cent. Doesn't quite add up, does it? And although being born female is the biggest risk factor for developing it, it has also been seen in males. The retrograde menstruation theory continues to confuse and complicate treatment strategies, and is one reason why uterectomy continues to be offered unnecessarily.

Other theories include: problems occurring during embryonic development; the migration of stem cells which regenerate the lining of the womb in each menstrual cycle to other areas of the body; and the dysfunction of particular genes. There is certainly a genetic link – if close family members have it then you're more likely to – and one study found endometriosis in 9 per cent of female foetuses, suggesting that it's a disease that individuals are born with which is then triggered by multiple factors later in life, such as onset of menstruation and environmental exposure to chemicals such as dioxins (see page 278) and xenoestrogens (see page 280).

It can feel like a dismal situation, but there are things that can help. Check out Endometriosis UK's website (www.endometriosis-uk.org), and get a top-notch team to support you (Nancy's Nook surgeon, naturopath, acupuncturist, physical therapist).

Plan for Dealing with Endometriosis

- Endometriosis can only be diagnosed by keyhole laparoscopic surgery and if endo is found during the surgery it will be removed, so you really want to have it carried out by someone who is skilled in excision surgery. You can find a list of surgeons in the file section of the Nancy's Nook Facebook group, as well as vast amounts of information on hormonal medications and hysterectomy, and how to prepare for and recover from surgery.
- The suggestions in the painful periods section (see pages 30–31) also apply to the treatment of endo, and it's crucial that you address oestrogen excess and reduce inflammation as endo both creates and is exacerbated by excess oestrogen and inflammation.
- Research suggests that the use of CBD oil (see page 150) may be a particularly helpful strategy for people with endo, because of its ability to treat pain as well as the proliferation of the disease.
- Low levels of vitamin D have been linked to endo and a blood test will show whether you should supplement with vitamin D or not.
- Removing all sources of gluten from your diet can dramatically improve symptoms. One study of 207 women with endo who had not been diagnosed with coeliac disease – a severe allergy to gluten – were put on a gluten-free diet for one year and 75 per cent of participants reported significant pain relief.

- Stay clear of meat and dairy that's full of hormones. Balancing your own hormones is tricky enough without adding in the hormones that are in produce that comes from hormone-laden animals. Opt for grass-fed organic meat and dairy.
- Supplements to consider include omega-3 fatty acids, curcumin, magnesium, N-acetyl cysteine (NAC), B vitamins, zinc, and resveratrol.

Adenomyosis

Adenomyosis is a condition of the uterus in which tissue that's normally only found in the lining of the womb (the endometrium) is found in the deeper muscular layer (the myometrium) causing symptoms such as pain and abnormal bleeding. Unfortunately, it often co-exists alongside endo and, just like endo, the hormonal imbalance of high oestrogen and low progesterone during perimenopause is likely to aggravate symptoms such as heavy or prolonged menstrual bleeding, severe period pain, chronic pelvic pain, pain during sex, an enlarged uterus, and abdominal pressure and bloating.

It's estimated to affect as many as 20 to 35 per cent of people with uteruses, but it's unclear exactly how prevalent it is as a definitive diagnosis is hard to come by. Like endometriosis, adenomyosis can be suspected from ultrasound or MRI results, but some people who have adeno will have images from these tests that appear completely normal, so they aren't a reliable way of diagnosing it. Other diagnostic methods include removing a sample of endometrial tissue during a biopsy to examine it for signs of adenomyosis, but this relies on removing a piece of tissue from an affected area – if the sample doesn't show adenomyosis that doesn't mean it doesn't exist elsewhere (and the procedure itself is a risk factor for developing adenomyosis). Surgical excision, where the area affected is removed, may be suggested in some cases when the disease is clearly defined by ultrasound or MRI, but this is a highly skilled surgery that can lead to severe blood loss and poor outcomes in terms of reduced pain.

The other, and very final option, is to have a uterectomy so that all of the uterus can be examined, and if you're experiencing these symptoms you might well be more willing to consider this option than you might have been earlier in life anyway.

The cause of adenomyosis is unclear, but risk factors for it include having uterine surgeries, a termination or a caesarean birth, as well as having excess oestrogen, though it's worth pointing out that there are plenty of teens who have never had sex let alone been pregnant who have been found to have adenomyosis, so it's not always caused by surgery or terminations.

Medications which suppress hormones, such as the combined birth control pill, Mirena® IUD, high-dose progestins and other forms of hormone suppressants can be used to relieve some symptoms, but as with endo, they frequently cause side effects and some can't be used long term.

There is hope, though, because many of the dietary, lifestyle and treatment suggestions in the period pain and endometriosis sections can help with improving symptoms. I've had clients with extreme flooding and pain get to a place where they don't need to take any painkillers and can even take leisurely strolls during the first few days of their periods.

10

Hormone rehab

Your hormones and your particular sensitivity to them, along with whatever you have happening in your life, will dictate your experience of perimenopause. You might decide you want to use hormone therapy to improve your symptoms and wellbeing, you might opt not to. Either way, it's crucial that you support your hormonal and mental health using a well-rounded approach, and that's what this chapter is all about.

Making decisions about your health is an ongoing process. What works fantastically now may not further down the line. The key to this process is to develop resilience; your capacity to adapt in the face of hormonal fluctuations, health challenges and life stressors. Perimenopause will work you like you've never been worked before, but it's possible that this hormonal and psychological transition will give you exactly what you need in order to be equipped for your remaining years. It's an opportunity for you to let go of everything that no longer serves you; to drop all the heavy stuff you've been carting around for years. Perimenopause is the perfect time for you to refine and redefine your life; an opportunity to reclaim joy and pleasure; to come into a deeper relationship with yourself; to unlearn putting others first.

The menopause transition is frequently viewed as something that's gone wrong and therefore needs to be fixed, but what would perimenopause look like if you trusted the process? Perimenopause is when we are faced with ourselves and confronted with the reality of our lives. Then we get to decide what we want to keep and what we want to do away with. Like a snake shedding the skin of our oestrogen years, we can let the people-pleasing niceness of oestrogen drop away. Once that happens, you can pick up whatever interests or serves you. The postmenopausal years can be liberating, not just because of the freedom that comes from not having to worry about pregnancy, but because, as amazing as the menstrual cycle is (you know I'm a fan!), the decisions we make are often steered by what our hormones are up to and the loss of the cycle can come as a relief.

Take a look at everything you've made decisions about and committed to over the years – where you live, who you live with, your relationships (romantic, familial, friendship and professional), your working life and any areas of interest – and consider if you want to recommit to them or leave them. By the way, it's possible to do this without self-judgement or guilt.

When it comes to having a positive experience of perimenopause, as well as setting the foundation for the decades beyond menopause, I recommend that you prepare by focussing on the things that you can control:

1) Simplify and streamline your life
2) Set boundaries
3) Improve sleep
4) Address alcohol consumption
5) Support oestrogen detoxification
6) Avoid endocrine disruptors (see pages 276–280)
7) Eat a nutrient-dense diet
8) Move and strengthen your body
9) Spend more time outside
10) Build your support crew.

It's also time to decide what your non-negotiables are and make adjustments to your schedule so that how you're living is in line with them. Only you know what's important to you, but here are some suggestions:

- Sleep and rest
- Health appointments (cervical screening, dental appointments, blood tests, acupuncture, etc.)
- Opportunities to move your body (exercise classes, walking, running, dancing)
- Time alone
- Connecting with others
- Networking
- Time outside
- Food and nourishment
- Intimacy
- Pleasure

- Learning
- Working hours
- Working conditions.

These things aren't optional, they're necessary. It's time to decide what's more important – picking your kid up and giving them a lift or lifting weights to build bone density to reduce your risk of hip fracture? Sometimes what's being asked of you will be more important, but I'm willing to bet that this happens way less frequently than you tell yourself it does. You might have some thoughts and feelings about doing less for others. Maybe you tell yourself that in prioritising your needs and desires, you'll let others down, or that they'll think certain things about you. That you're unreliable, unhelpful, incapable, untrustworthy, selfish. I mean, how dare you be selfish by caring for yourself in what's likely to be very basic ways most of the time?!

Your Future Self

Focussing on your non-negotiables is something that your future self will thank you for. Picture yourself in five years' time, then 10 and 20. Think about this future version of yourself. What are the things that they'll thank you in the future for doing now? Going for a run when you weren't in the mood. Keeping your brain active instead of mindless scrolling on screens. Creating downtime that soothes your nervous system and restores your energy. Saying 'no'. Laying off caffeine and sugar. Lifting weights. Having the conversations you've been avoiding. Making changes. What's your list like?

A Woman's Work is Never Done

When it comes to emotional labour and unpaid work, much of what we end up doing is silently agreed between us and other people. Think about household tasks and office jobs that you do on a daily and weekly basis. How many of them did you explicitly decide to take responsibility for? Have you discussed what needs to be done in your home and workplace with those you live and work with, and made agreements about who will do what?

When I took stock of everything I have taken responsibility for versus what my partner was doing, I was shocked. My list comprised of doing most of the food shopping, cooking and the dishes, cleaning the fridge, cleaning the cooker, doing the laundry, watering the houseplants, mowing the lawn, dusting, general household cleaning, doing the nursery run in the morning and afternoon, and childcare during the three months a year that my son's nursery was shut. All whilst running an online business, writing a book and treating clients. Talk about a recipe for burnout and relationship breakdown. My boyfriend's? Taking the bins out and doing the dishes (if I was prepared to leave them overnight). At no point had I verbally agreed to this arrangement and whilst I did waste a considerable amount of time stewing over this, I subsequently realised that only I was responsible for taking on these roles. My mentor Lisa Martinello also pointed out how much emotional labour I'd created for myself along the way #mindblown.

Beauty Sleep

Women experience sleep differently to men and it's the onset of menstruation that stimulates the main differences in sleep between the sexes. As oestrogen and progesterone begin their cyclic ebb and flow, they regulate the sleep-wake cycle and, as you transition through each phase of your life, you're increasingly likely to experience a sleep disorder. Once we're in the perimenopause zone, sleep becomes more elusive thanks to changing hormone levels and life stressors. In our perimenopausal and postmenopausal years, 53 per cent of us will be having poor-quality sleep, trouble falling asleep, trouble staying asleep, and trouble getting enough sleep. Night sweats, needing to wee and restless leg syndrome all impact on our ability to get a solid night of sleep, as does the radiating heat of someone sleeping next to you and sharing a bed with someone who snores. Then there's the situation that you're stewing about and replaying over and over again in your mind in which you're having imaginary conversations that are stimulating a stress response that's telling your body to fight or run away, and that's keeping you awake.

Lack of good-quality sleep causes problems with DNA repair, which accelerates ageing – they don't call it beauty sleep for nothing. Getting less than seven hours' sleep is associated with less clearance of the amyloid plaques found in Alzheimer's disease. Getting less than four hours sleep a night? Come on, I know that's the case for some of you. Well, we've got to sort that out, because less than four hours reduces your natural killer cells – the ones that kill cancerous cells – by 70 per cent. Poor sleep and not enough of it doesn't just leave you feeling like shit, it increases inflammation and stress hormone production, interferes with blood sugar regulation and lowers your immunity. It also raises your risk of metabolic disease, neurological disease and cancer, and makes you less resilient to stress, moody as hell and tired AF.

This is why sleep is critical during peri- and postmenopause. When I treat someone who has sleep issues, no matter what other health issues they've got going on, improving their sleep is at the top of my list of treatment aims, because without sufficient good-quality sleep all our other results will be limited. My aims are for clients to:

- Fall asleep easily within half an hour of winding down and getting into bed.
- Be horizontal by 10pm at the latest.
- Sleep soundly for seven to nine hours (less than that is associated with a whole host of negative health outcomes).
- Be free of night sweats and dreams which are disturbing or exhausting.
- Wake up feeling refreshed and restored in the morning.

Right now, that may feel like a tall order to you, but I promise you that it's possible with the right support and the substantial list of strategies I've got coming up shortly, but first I want to talk about the hormones that are involved in our sleep-wake cycles: cortisol and melatonin.

Cortisol is what helps us to feel alert in the morning. It should be at its highest in the morning and then gradually decline throughout the day before reaching its lowest level in the evening. Melatonin is the Dracula of hormones, because it only comes out at night. Melatonin is secreted by the pineal gland in your head. During the day it's inactive, but when the sun goes down and it becomes dark, the pineal gland gets going and begins to produce melatonin. This is then secreted into your blood and it tells your body that it's time to hit the hay. Melatonin levels should stay high throughout the night, peaking between 2 and 4am, and then when morning rolls around melatonin levels drop to almost nothing, which is why it's generally easier to feel alert in the mornings during the Summer months, because we are exposed to sunlight earlier than in the Winter. If you're someone who struggles to get going in the morning, open your curtains and let light in as soon as you wake – let your pineal gland know that it's time to get going.

Production of melatonin is what precedes feeling sleepy, but when one study compared premenopausal women to postmenopausal women, researchers found that there was a delay between melatonin secretion and feeling sleepy in those who were postmenopausal. Melatonin production also generally decreases with age and by the time we're in our sixties, its production can be negligible. Melatonin is also affected by high oestrogen, cortisol and inflammation – all of which can feature in perimenopause. Then there's the problem of blue light from the screens that most of us are glued to of an evening, which also delays production of melatonin and stimulates cortisol production, both of which keep you awake.

Elevated cortisol in the evenings can make falling asleep just about impossible, so it's worth looking at what is stressing you out. You might have to rethink that 7pm spin class that you love. Sure, it's great exercise and all that sweating helps you to excrete oestrogen, but what is it telling your adrenal glands? That you've got something scary to cycle away from – your body thinks that your instructor barking at you through a microphone, and you pedalling and sweating away, means that what's actually going on is that a sabretooth tiger is after you, so it ramps up cortisol secretion and, despite being absolutely beat by the time you wobble home and into bed, sleep eludes you.

Your body likes to keep to a schedule. Eating, exercising, waking and sleeping at set times all let your body know what's coming up next, which means that your pineal gland will know when to start secreting melatonin, so it will release it at the same time every day, which is important because melatonin initiates the sleep cycle hours before you actually fall asleep. Being asleep by 10pm results in optimal production of melatonin and using screens in the evening can dramatically delay production of this sleep-inducing hormone. Some medications, such as beta-blockers and NSAIDs, may suppress melatonin production if they're taken in the evening, so speak to your GP about adjusting the time at which you take them if you feel they could be impacting on sleep.

Melatonin also has an influence on the menstrual cycle and reproductive function. Some research also suggests that there's a link between melatonin and ovulation, cycle regularity and progesterone production in the second half of the cycle. It's thought that melatonin may play a role in menopausal transition, with the age-related disruption of circadian rhythm leading to an irregular cycle and amenorrhoea, and also because a drop in core body temperature accompanies the onset of sleep and is strongly linked to melatonin secretion, but in postmenopausal women this drop is lessened.

Sleep is crucial for the health of your brain. Brain derived neurotrophic factor (BDNF) is a protein that's abundant in your prefrontal cortex – that's the part of your brain responsible for executive function such as memory, self-control and cognitive flexibility. Taking a warm bath or shower before bed has been shown to elevate BDNF. The rapid cooling process once you get out also helps you to nod off as a drop in your core temperature acts as a signal to your circadian rhythm. The key, especially if you're having temperature regulation issues, is not to use really hot water and to make sure the ambient air is cool. So if you have a bath, leave a window or the door open so that air can circulate. If you're getting hot flushes or struggle to cool down after a warm bath or shower, try a lukewarm shower or a footbath instead. Adding some Epsom salts, which are rich in relaxing magnesium, or essential oils to the water will up the ante.

Improving quality of sleep is crucial when it comes to improving short- and long-term health and improving quality of life, so let's move on to how you can do that. Try these approaches to improve your sleep:

- Speak to your GP about using micronised progesterone as it can improve sleep and reduce symptoms such as night sweats.
- Don't consume caffeine after 2pm.
- Expose yourself to bright light during the daytime and get outside as much as possible.
- Ensure your room is dark at night. Blackout blinds can really help to block out streetlights.
- Replace stimulating LED lightbulbs with incandescent bulbs which emit a softer light.
- Keep your room cool and well ventilated.
- Use a cooling pillow and mattress pads. These gel-filled pads are cooling at room temperature and are even cooler once they've been refrigerated. The cooling effect lasts for hours and, because they're filled with gel, they're comfortable to lie on.
- If you share a bed with someone, consider separate bedding so that duvet fights or differences in temperature don't become a problem. Sleeping separately doesn't have to negatively affect intimacy and your relationship unless you (or your partner) choose to make it mean something that it isn't. In fact, sleeping separately can create intimacy.

- Avoid alcohol and sugar before bed as it disrupts the ability to sleep well. Alcohol blocks REM sleep – the phase of sleep where we dream and where memory consolidation takes place – and although you might think that it helps you to fall asleep, it actually results in disrupted sleep where you toss and turn and wake up, and this can even be without you realising it.
- Eat enough protein and fat during the day so that your blood sugar is balanced, and if you're prone to wake-ups because of low blood sugar have a snack before bed that has protein and fat in it.
- If, on the other hand, you don't have any problems with waking up in the night because your blood sugar has dipped, then avoid eating two to three hours before bedtime as eating later not only has the potential to disrupt your circadian rhythm, but it can also result in weight gain.
- Eat eggs. Eggs are rich in choline and choline is a nutrient that's essential for the production of a neurotransmitter called acetylcholine, which plays a crucial role in REM sleep.
- Got a dodgy digestive system? There's evidence to suggest that the gut microbiome interacts with the genes which regulate your circadian rhythm and sleep patterns. The fact is 90 per cent of serotonin is produced in the gut and serotonin is a precursor to melatonin, the sleep hormone which helps you to fall asleep and stay asleep. That means that when your gut is healthy, deep restful sleep is supported.
- Deal with any bladder dysfunction that's interrupting your sleep.
- Avoid napping during the daytime. If you find yourself feeling tired in the afternoon, make sure you're eating enough nourishing food and experiment with some gentle movement or seated yoga nidra (see page 282). If those don't revive you, then stick with a short 20-minute nap.
- Exercise does improve sleep, but sleep is more important than working out, so sleep should be your priority and if stimulating evening workouts are preventing you from winding down, replace them with calming ones such as restorative yoga.
- Consider using supplements such as magnesium, vitamins B6 and B12, melatonin, L-theanine, GABA and glycine.
- Consider using herbs such as valerian, skullcap, passionflower, hops, lavender and chamomile.
- Consider using essential oils such as lavender and clary sage.
- Incorporate Epsom salts baths or foot baths into your pre-bed routine. Epsom salts are rich in magnesium, which is absorbed by your skin and

soothes your nervous system and aids sleep. It can also help if you're prone to restless legs at night.

- Using cannabidiol (CBD) helps to boost anandamide in your body – it's the chemical compound that gives you runner's high and it also helps to induce slow wave sleep and REM sleep. (Side-note: caffeine blocks anandamide.)
- Listen to a guided meditation either before getting into bed or once you're tucked in.
- Stop ruminating by getting your thoughts out of your head and onto paper. Keep a notebook by your bed and do a brain dump before settling down to sleep.
- Don't use stimulating electronic screens before bed.

Blue Light

You know when you're in a dark room with someone and they're on their smartphone and their face is lit up with a creepy blue light? That blue light screws with your hormones in a very big way. Your sleep-wake cycle is regulated by exposure to light, which means that any time you're on your phone, e-reader, laptop, tablet or even watching television – anything with a digital screen – your body is receiving instructions that despite it being 11pm, it's time to be awake. Blue light in the evening and at night increases alertness. It also delays and lowers production of your sleepy hormone, melatonin; reduces the amount and timing of REM sleep (that's the phase of deep, restorative sleep that's important for making and retaining memories); and makes it harder for you to feel alert in the morning.

Another reason to limit mobile phone use is that it's associated with a decline in production of thyroid hormones, which of course we don't want given that you're more likely to experience thyroid dysfunction because of your sex and age. Here's what you can do to help:

- Turn your phone off for portions of the day. Put it in a drawer and focus on what's in front of you or at least have it on silent and set not to vibrate. You could even leave it at home when you go out.
- Keep your devices away from your body – in a bag or corner – and certainly out of your bedroom.

- Stop using digital devices two hours before you go to bed. So many members of The Flow Collective have been shocked at how just doing this has impacted their health positively.
- Failing that, invest in some glasses which block blue light (such as Swannies or TrueDark) and wear them in the evening when you're using electronic devices to prevent disruption to your circadian rhythms.
- Install *f.lux* on your computers and devices. It's software which adjusts your screen's colour temperature to match the time of day.
- Read an actual book, instead of one on your e-reader.
- Use incandescent bulbs in lamps for evening use as they produce less blue light.

Alcohol

Limit alcohol or stop drinking it altogether. Alcohol increases body temperature (hello hot flushes and night sweats) and raises your resting heart rate (hello hot flushes and palpitations). It also disrupts your production of melatonin and screws up your circadian rhythm.

Moderate alcohol intake also lowers progesterone, which is probably already in short supply. It also increases the amount of oestrogen that's in circulation, because it increases an enzyme called aromatase that converts testosterone and androstenedione into oestrogen. It makes you less likely to convert the potent oestradiol (E2) into the less potent oestrone (E1), so you've got more of the strong stuff going around town. And it can increase DHEA, which, when we follow its conversion pathway, creates more E1 or E2. So now that alcohol has resulted in extra oestrogen it needs to be detoxified and excreted. But oestrogen detoxification relies upon your liver and that's a bit busy dealing with alcohol. Detoxing booze also requires the same nutrients that you need to detoxify oestrogen.

Alcohol also acts as a toxin to those precious mitochondria and depletes you of glutathione, an antioxidant which means that your ability to create energy and sex hormones is impaired, so the ageing process is accelerated.

Most of my perimenopausal clients reluctantly tell me that they can't tolerate alcohol any more, but there are some who are unwilling to look at their alcohol consumption. I encourage all my clients to get honest with themselves about why they're drinking. Sometimes a glass of wine is just that. Other times it's an automatic but ineffective coping mechanism and an attempt to avoid how you're feeling, which is why dealing with the underlying urge and the uncomfortable feelings that are driving it are so important. If we don't, then those feeling just pop up in other areas. Instead of another glass of cabernet sauvignon, you'll be overeating, seeking out sugar or losing time that you'll never get back scrolling on social media.

Detox Like a Pro

Oestrogen does amazing things for us, but we don't want it recirculating around the body, because it causes issues: breast/chest pain, irritability, heavy periods, fibroids, ovarian cysts, even some reproductive cancers. You want to use it and lose it, and the process by which we do this is called oestrogen detoxification. Oestrogen detoxification is important throughout life, particularly during early menopause when oestrogen is usually high and even once oestrogen declines during late perimenopause. My clients with low oestrogen often ask if there's a case for slowing down oestrogen detoxification in the hope that if it lingers for longer in the body it will have a positive effect, but this isn't the case. Once we've used it, that's it, and the best thing we can do is to excrete it safely.

It's your liver that's in charge of this process, but don't take that to mean that you should go on what I would term as an extreme spring clean – the green juice 'cleanses' that can end up doing more harm than good. To do its job well, your liver needs year-round support, because oestrogen detoxification takes place continually in your body. Hormones such as oestrogen are fat-loving, so they don't dissolve in water, which is a problem when one of the ways you get rid of oestrogen is through your urine. The body's solution is to handle this in two phases. During phase one it breaks the oestrogen down into smaller units called metabolites and in phase two it changes the metabolites from fat-loving molecules into water-soluble metabolites, which means you can then pee/poo them out. Smart, right? The trouble is, there are different pathways that the oestrogen metabolites can go down. Some are healthy, but some are associated with heavy periods, tender breasts, PMS and hormone-dependent cancers, so it's important to encourage the favourable pathways. That's the short and extremely simplified version of oestrogen detoxification. Here's the more detailed picture of each phase.

Phase 1: Preparation

In this phase your liver does the prep work by breaking oestrogen down into smaller units. It takes oestradiol and oestrone (the two main forms of oestrogen in your body), and converts them into one of three oestrogen metabolites: 2OH, 4OH and 16OH. But let's just call them routes 2, 4, and 16. Of these pathways, route 2 is the healthy route that we want to encourage. Route 4 *can* be okay, but it has a fork in it and it's only an okay route if it goes down the correct branch. If it goes down the quinone enzyme pathway then your risk for oestrogen-based cancers goes up. Route 16 is the pathway to avoid, because it's associated with heavy periods, clots, tender breasts and an increased risk of oestrogen-based cancers such as breast cancer. It's the pathway that makes things grow – the lining of your womb, your boobs and cancerous cells.

Nutritional deficiencies, low protein intake, drinking alcohol, heavy metal build-up and using medications like paracetamol can all get in the way of this prep stage. Eating cruciferous vegetables like broccoli, kale and cauliflower which contain diindolylmethane (DIM) can support phase one. DIM promotes healthy oestrogen detoxification by reducing the formation of the 16OH metabolites (the 'bad' guys) and increasing the 2OH metabolites (the good guys), and it can also be taken as a supplement. Other supplements which can support this phase include liposomal glutathione, N-acetyl cysteine, resveratrol and quercetin.

At the end of phase 1 you're left with smaller units of oestrogen, which you now need to get rid of before they recirculate and cause problems. To do that, a reaction needs to take place and that's what phase 2 is all about.

Phase 2: Addition (Methylation)

In phase 2 the fat-soluble oestrogen metabolites from phase 1 are added to – and Dr Carrie Jones has a useful analogy for this: think about filling a bathtub up with water, pouring oil into it and then pulling the plug. What happens? The water goes out, but the oil remains on the side of the tub and doesn't go down the drain. In this phase, the oestrogen metabolites gain a water-loving molecule, which means they can swirl down the plughole or leave the body via your urine. During methylation they go from being 2OH and 4OH into 2Methoxy and 4Methoxy, the change in name simply reflecting that they are now water-soluble. Don't worry though, I'm not going to be testing you on the science at the end of this section so all you need to know here is that the smaller bits of oestrogen can now mix with water.

In order to reduce symptoms of oestrogen dominance and reduce your risk of developing oestrogen-dominant cancers, both pathways need to be working optimally – the right water should be filling your tub up *and* your drain should be able to get rid of it. When phase 2 isn't working as well as it could, oestrogen metabolites can't leave the body and the 4OH metabolite goes down the less desirable pathway. Genetic factors can impair this process so genetic testing of these markers can help you to understand how you methylate your hormones. Limiting exposure to environmental chemicals in your food, personal care products, and home and workplace is important, because they impact on your liver's ability to do its job well. Reducing dust, mould and other indoor air pollutants

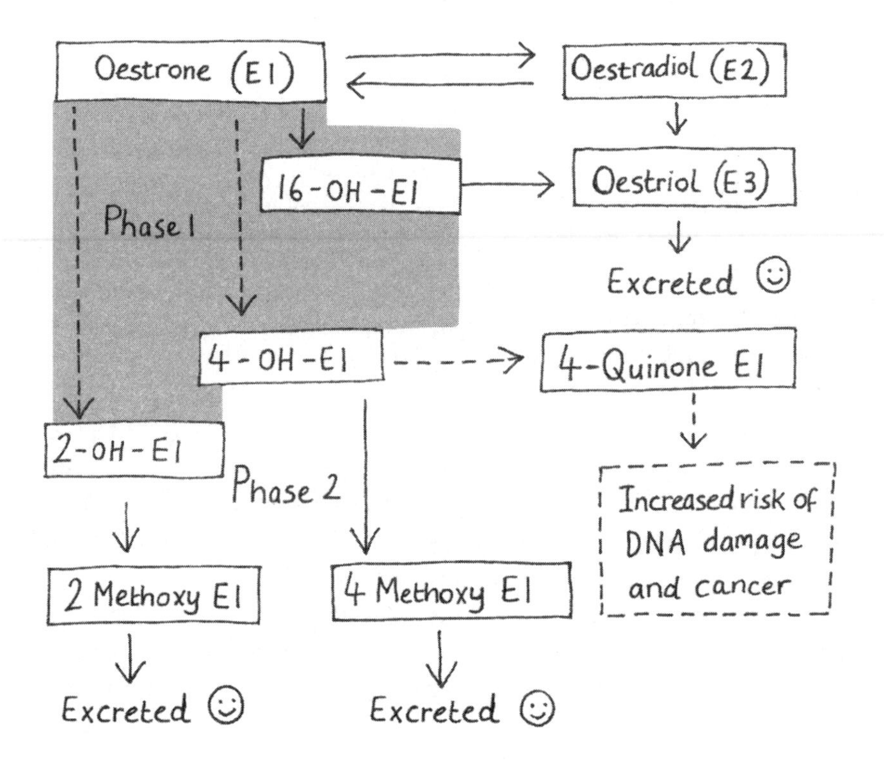

improves detoxification (I recommend that you think of air fresheners as air pollutants), as does regular exercise, sweating (one benefit of hot flushes, at least) and eating organic food where possible to avoid pesticides, herbicides, hormones and antibiotics.

Sulphur-rich foods such as eggs, garlic, onions, leeks, mushrooms and cruciferous vegetables, as well as supplements like S-adenosylmethionine (SAMe), magnesium and methylated B vitamins can support the methylation process. And the simple act of staying hydrated will clearly help you to excrete the metabolites, because you'll have more opportunities to pee them out.

As you'll have discovered in the previous chapters, oestrogen plays a role in a vast number of processes in the body (over 400!) so oestrogen isn't the enemy, we just don't want it sticking around causing trouble, because problems with oestrogen detoxification are going to worsen your experience of perimenopause and negatively impact your long-term health too.

Oestrogen Outlet

Oestrogen, along with other hormones and toxins, is also excreted through your bile – a fluid secreted by your liver – and into your intestines, where it's packaged up by an enzyme called beta-glucuronidase, which enables it to escape your body in the form of poo, which is why constipation can cause symptoms of oestrogen dominance. This wonderful process gets mucked up when the bacteria in your gut are imbalanced – from inflammation, use of antibiotics and a poor diet. This enables oestrogen to escape the enzyme package that's holding it in order to get it out of you, which means that it ends up recirculating in your body.

Think about how smoothly food exits your body. Do you poo regularly or are you backed up? Healthy elimination means having at least one satisfying and complete bowel movement per day, that's a four on the Bristol stool chart (like a sausage or snake, smooth and soft). Constipation is improved by increasing your intake of water and fibre (that means veggies), and by movement, either by moving all of your body or using manual therapies such as abdominal massage. It's no wonder that so many of us are constipated – we're sat down all day, dehydrated, and our diets lack sufficient fibre. And that's before we add in being scared to poo in the workplace.

Getting enough fibre (see page 274) supports oestrogen detoxification, because fibre binds to oestrogen in the intestine so that you excrete it out before it can be reabsorbed. Fibre is crucial to keeping your gut happy and diets that lack fibre are linked to colon cancer, unhealthy cholesterol levels and diverticulitis, a condition in which small, bulging pouches (diverticula) form along the wall of your intestines, leading to infection and inflammation. You cannot expect to have balanced hormones when your gut and liver are struggling.

The Wild Child

In an ideal world, and hopefully for most of your cycling years, oestrogen and progesterone have had a balanced relationship with each other – oestrogen has done her thing, but her BFF progesterone was by her side to keep her in check. During our forties, but often in our thirties too, progesterone production just isn't what it used to be, which means that wild child oestrogen is no longer being reined in. When this happens you can experience signs and symptoms of both excess oestrogen (see page 97) and low progesterone (see below). You can also have low oestrogen, but if it's still high in relation to progesterone, you can get signs of excess oestrogen – it's all about the relationship between the two hormones.

Low progesterone (see page 26 for symptoms), which can usually be confirmed by a blood test, can be caused by:

- Ageing.
- Perimenopause and menopause.
- Taking the birth control pill and/or lack of ovulation. If you recall, it's the follicle left behind after ovulation – your corpus luteum – that produces and releases the vast majority of the progesterone you produce (your adrenals also produce a tiny amount), so if you are not ovulating, you're not producing progesterone.
- A diet lacking in nutrition or nutritional deficiencies in magnesium, vitamin A, vitamin B6, vitamin C and zinc (these are all common deficiencies to have after using the pill).
- Low thyroid function (hypothyroidism), which becomes increasingly common as we age.
- An insufficient LH surge just before ovulation.

- High prolactin.
- High cortisol levels brought about by sustained periods of stress.

You can improve low progesterone by:

- Dealing with the sources of stress in your life.
- Supplement with vitamin B6 as it supports the development of the corpus luteum after ovulation, which is essential for progesterone production. Your liver also needs it to safely process oestrogen once you've used it, so it can help with excess oestrogen, and it can make a real difference to period pain, PMS and PMDD (premenstrual dysphoric disorder) too.
- Try taking Vitex agnus-castus (aka chasteberry) – this herb contains compounds that are dopaminergic, so they act on the dopamine receptors on the pituitary gland and inhibit prolactin. This action causes the corpus luteum to develop and grow at an increased rate, which increases progesterone production and secretion, which is why it's so popular on both fertility and perimenopausal forums and Facebook groups. It's used for irregular menstrual cycles, PMS, PMDD, breast/chest tenderness that's cyclic in nature and infertility (especially in those with high prolactin levels). Take your recommended dosage in the morning so that it's in sync with the diurnal rhythm of your pituitary gland. It can take a few months to see the impact of using it. Is it for everyone? No, it's not. Herbal medicine may be natural, but it can also be strong, which is why working with a qualified and licensed practitioner such as a medical herbalist or naturopath is a good idea.
- Using supplements such as vitamin B6, vitamin D, vitamin C, vitamin E, Vitex agnus-castus, maca and melatonin.
- Taking micronised body-identical progesterone from ovulation to the start of your period (see page 100).
- Acupuncture and pelvic massage such as ATMAT can improve blood flow to your ovaries and support progesterone production.
- Hanging out with your mates. Research has shown that enjoying the company of women can raise progesterone.

ATMAT

ATMAT – or to give it its full name, the Arvigo Techniques of Maya Abdominal Therapy – is founded on the ancient Mayan technique of abdominal massage. As a practitioner, I am biased, but in all honesty, ATMAT is a treatment that I love giving and receiving, and I'd love every single one of you reading this to experience one session.

Practitioners primarily use massage to improve the flow of blood, lymph, nerve and energy through the pelvis, which can help to improve reproductive and digestive function, making it a great treatment option for menstrual cycle issues such as pain, heavy bleeding, irregular bleeding, ovarian cysts, endometriosis, fibroids and fertility issues. It's an amazing treatment to receive during perimenopause, because it's a way to give your ovaries and uterus some love before your periods stop and they shrink, and it's a treatment that I love giving clients before they have a hysterectomy, though if we start treating soon enough the need for surgery often goes away. ATMAT can also gently encourage organs that have shifted position – such as a tilted or prolapsed uterus – back into an optimal position, and it's a lovely way to care for yourself after fertility challenges, miscarriage, termination or a traumatic birth, even if they occurred years ago.

When you see a practitioner, they'll also teach you how to massage yourself, so that you can spend five minutes a day giving your belly some TLC and getting to know your changing body. This is a practice that, once a practitioner has got your started, you can do on your own for the rest of your life, which makes it not just highly effective but inexpensive too. For more details and to find a practitioner, head to www.arvigotherapy.com.

Oestrogen imbalance (for the signs and symptoms of excess oestrogen see page 97) can be caused by:

- Anovulatory cycles (common during teen years and perimenopause, which is why you and your teen are experiencing similar issues).
- Polycystic ovarian syndrome (PCOS).

- Impaired oestrogen detoxification.
- Poor diet.
- Histamine intolerance.
- Gut issues like constipation.
- High levels of cortisol competing for and blocking progesterone receptors.
- Environmental toxins such as BPA and phthalates that are commonly found in plastics which mimic oestrogen and interfere with its action in the body.
- Alcohol consumption.
- Weight gain and obesity (because fat cells produce oestrogen).
- Diabetes.
- Some autoimmune conditions.

You can address oestrogen imbalance by:

- Supporting liver detoxification and improving gut function.
- Increasing your intake of dietary fibre to support oestrogen detoxification via your colon (and poo).
- Increasing your water intake to support oestrogen detoxification via your wee.
- Getting some decent shut-eye. There's a relationship between a disruption to the circadian rhythm and the incidence of breast and colo-rectal cancer, which is thought to be because of reduced melatonin secretion and an increase in light exposure at night.
- Reducing alcohol intake – keep your liver freed up to deal with oestrogen.
- Exercising, particularly types which are high intensity and make you sweat.
- Improving body composition.
- Eating broccoli sprouts. You can sprout them at home in three days, which makes them a very affordable way of supporting your health, just make sure they don't have mould on them before you eat them. They contain the highest concentrations of glucoraphanin and sulforaphane, which encourage oestrogen metabolites that are going down the unhealthy quinone 4OH pathway to head back to the start of the pathway, so that they have a chance of going down a better route. Sulforaphane also has antioxidant, antimicrobial, anticancer, anti-inflammatory and anti-diabetic properties, and can help to protect against cardiovascular and neurodegenerative diseases.

- Using supplements such as calcium D-glucarate, vitamin B6, magnesium, iodine (which makes oestrogen receptors less sensitive), vitamin D, N-acetyl cysteine (NAC) and resveratrol.

If you want to know what's going on with oestrogen in your body (which we all do), DUTCH testing offers the most accurate and comprehensive insights into your oestrogen levels and which pathways your metabolites are going down.

Go DUTCH

DUTCH is an acronym that stands for dried urine test for comprehensive hormones. It's a simple but incredibly comprehensive method of testing your hormones, as well as showing how you process and metabolise them. The collection is easy; all you have to do is wee on a series of pieces of filter paper over the course of your day and/or your menstrual cycle, depending on which specific test you do, send them to Precision Analytical (the lab which created the test) for testing, and your results are sent to your healthcare practitioner so that they can explain them to you and come up with a suitable treatment plan. This isn't a test that you can interpret on your own and, as it's a private test that you pay for, your GP is unlikely to know what to do with the results. If you're considering doing the DUTCH test, you need to work with a naturopath, nutritional therapist or functional medicine practitioner who is familiar with it.

The level of detailed information that you get from DUTCH testing is unparalleled and you get a heck of a lot more information than you would from a sample of blood or saliva. It doesn't just look at what your hormone levels are, it looks at your hormone metabolites and the pathways that they're going down, which is particularly relevant when you want to understand how you are processing and excreting oestrogen, and also when assessing other hormones.

It gives an accurate representation of what's going on with cortisol and cortisone (the deactivated form of cortisol). By testing cortisol and cortisone at four points throughout the day, your cortisol curve – which should be higher in the morning and lower as the day goes on – can be assessed to see if you follow a healthy curve or vary from it, which is really important when it comes to understanding fatigue, anxiety, stress, depression, libido and problems with sleep. It also assesses melatonin levels, which is important not just in assessing sleep issues, but because melatonin is an antioxidant and optimal levels of it are associated with a reduced risk of breast cancer.

The DUTCH test can help you get to the bottom of why you're struggling with:

- Symptoms of perimenopause
- Mood swings, depression, anxiety
- PMS
- Low sexual desire
- Irregular menstrual cycles
- Fertility issues
- Fatigue
- Insomnia.

Though some insurance companies will reimburse you, the DUTCH test costs around £400, so it's a financial investment, but it truly speeds up the diagnosis process and enables the most appropriate treatment plan to be developed, saving you time and money that's potentially wasted exploring different avenues before arriving at an answer and a solution. You can find a healthcare provider who uses the DUTCH test through the website www.dutchtest.com.

Could Histamine Intolerance Be Behind Your Weird Symptoms?

If you struggle with issues such as PMS, PMDD, period pain or a whole host of other weird allergy-type symptoms, then histamine intolerance could be causing or aggravating what's going on. Histamine is the chemical produced when you have allergies and it causes an immediate inflammatory response. Taking an antihistamine drug like Piriton or Benedryl provides relief, because it dials down the inflammatory response created by histamine by reducing histamine's action. But if your body doesn't break down histamine properly, you can develop a condition called histamine intolerance in which eating foods which are rich in histamine or which cause a release of histamine results in an annoying bunch of symptoms, including:

- Headaches and migraines
- Nasal congestion and sneezing
- Hives
- Eczema
- Flushing and sweating
- Difficulty breathing
- Dizziness or vertigo
- Tinnitus
- Anxiety
- Insomnia
- Tiredness
- Brain fog
- Hypertension
- Abdominal cramps
- Diarrhoea
- Gas
- Nausea and vomiting
- Swelling
- Breast tenderness
- Period pain
- PMS
- PMDD.

It's a hard condition to spot because its symptoms are varied and not many people know about it. I had symptoms of it for 10 years before I learned about histamine intolerance and the penny finally dropped – and I work in the field and have been treated by plenty of practitioners in that time. It's also a frustrating condition, because, as you'll see shortly, loads of food and drinks that are meant to be really healthy for you actually cause symptoms, which is incredibly frustrating when you're putting a lot of money and effort into improving your diet.

Symptoms of histamine intolerance often show up when oestrogen is high in the cycle, because oestrogen stimulates the release of histamine and it also suppresses the action of diamine oxidase (DAO) – the enzyme that breaks down histamine – and it triggers inflammation. Histamine then stimulates the cells in your ovaries to secrete more oestrogen. The more oestrogen that's produced, the more histamine is released. More histamine means more oestrogen, trapping you in a thoroughly unpleasant vicious cycle. People who get headaches in relation to the cycle and from painful periods are often histamine-intolerant.

Some people experience symptoms as soon as oestrogen appears in the cycle. Mine emerge on day 3, so although I feel a surge of energy and positivity, if I eat something that triggers a histamine response, like a banana, then I'll feel tired and headachy, and I can even have palpitations. A friend of mine experiences vertigo from day 3 of her cycle until she ovulates, so although her mood is better in the first half of her cycle, the constant sensation that the world is moving makes life with two small children incredibly challenging. The vertigo then disappears as soon as she ovulates. For Kirsten, a member of The Flow Collective, her main symptom is the annoying appearance of hives on her skin in the days before her period is due.

If you experience PMS or have PMDD, then I encourage you to consider if histamine intolerance could be part of what's going on. As someone who has histamine intolerance and PMDD, I can tell you that I've found there's a massive correlation between how on top of my histamine intolerance and my PMDD symptoms I am. Although it's not the cause of PMDD, when histamine is at bay, the second half of my cycle transforms and the irritability, rage and violent thoughts greatly diminish.

I imagine that if you suspect histamine could be a problem for you then you're wondering how to figure out if it is and what can be done about it. You can test for histamine intolerance by following an elimination diet that excludes the food and drink listed below and then reintroducing them to see how you respond to them. Take a deep breath because the following list may well be a list of your favourite foods and drinks. Are you ready to say goodbye to avocado and bacon on a slice of sourdough (and champagne)? Gulp, here goes. Histamine-rich foods include:

- Fermented food and drink such as wine, champagne, beer, kombucha (a fermented tea which has a slight fizziness to it), kefir (a fermented drink traditionally made with milk which has the consistency of a drinkable yoghurt), sauerkraut, sourdough, sour cream, buttermilk, yoghurt, soy sauce.
- Bone broth.
- Vinegar (apple cider vinegar, wine vinegar, pickles, mayonnaise).

- Cured meats (bacon, pepperoni, salami, prosciutto).
- Dried fruit (apricots, figs, prunes, raisins).
- Most citrus fruits.
- Some vegetables (aubergine, avocado, spinach, tomatoes).
- Some nuts (cashews, walnuts).
- Smoked fish and some species of fish (mackerel, tuna, sardines, anchovies).
- Aged cheese.

Histamine-releasing foods include:

- Alcohol
- Bananas
- Chocolate
- Cow's milk
- Papaya
- Pineapple
- Shellfish
- Strawberries
- Tomatoes.

Alcohol, energy drinks, and black and green teas can all block the action of DAO so that it's harder for your body to break histamine down, so add them to your list as well. And I'm afraid to say that dark chocolate should be avoided too. Whilst dark chocolate is low in histamine, it contains compounds that are histamine triggers.

Your doctor can also test your blood for histamine levels and for DAO, though blood testing should be done when you've been eating histamine-rich and histamine-producing foods, not after you've eliminated them, and the results aren't necessarily conclusive – mine were normal despite the fact that I react to everything on the list. As well as avoiding foods that trigger it, supplements such as magnesium, vitamin B6, SAMe, quercetin and DAO can be used to treat it, and supporting regular ovulation is important because progesterone stimulates production of DAO, which is why symptoms often improve as progesterone levels increase after ovulation. If oestrogen is high, which it's likely to be in perimenopause, then supporting oestrogen detoxification will also help (see pages 253–257). Due to the high amount of progesterone that's produced in pregnancy, which stimulates

DAO production, symptoms often get better or disappear entirely during pregnancy and then reappear afterwards.

High histamine levels can be caused by allergies, SIBO (small intestinal bacterial overgrowth), leaky gut and being deficient in DAO – the enzyme which helps to break histamine down. Low DAO can be caused by gluten intolerance, leaky gut, SIBO, Crohn's disease, ulcerative colitis, inflammatory bowel disease and some types of medication such as NSAIDs, antidepressants, and antihistamines.

Diet

What we should and shouldn't eat is a loaded topic, and whilst I do have some general recommendations for you, let's start by looking at where you eat, who you eat with and how you eat. Here are my recommendations:

- Eat away from your desk and any screens, and don't eat on the go. You might try to deny that you do this, but I'm onto you! Where you eat influences how you eat and digest food, so pick somewhere to eat where you'd be willing to invite someone else along, such as a table, bench or the grass.
- Slow down before you actually eat – meals aren't something to race through, despite how the males in my household eat theirs. Hit pause before you start eating and give your nervous system a chance to move from fight or flight to rest and digest. All that means is taking a few deep belly breaths or simply sitting down and letting your shoulders drop before you start eating.
- Be present and eat mindfully so that you can recognise when you start to feel full. If you're eating whilst scrolling, you're not going to pick up on your body's signals and if you eat in front of a screen you're likely to eat 25 per cent more calories than you would if you weren't glued to one.
- Eat till you're 80 per cent full. Your brain needs up to 20 minutes to catch up with your stomach and receive the signal that you're full. Eating slowly is not only beneficial to digestion, but gives your brain and stomach a chance to communicate before you overeat.
- Eat when you're hungry, but don't wait till you're on the verge of passing out or biting someone's head off.

- Don't nibble your way through the day as this messes with your hunger hormones and leads to weight gain. If you're prone to blood sugar instability and need to eat something (and by something, I mean protein) every three to four hours, then by all means do that. If that's not you, then stick to regular mealtimes.
- Use your teeth. They're there for a reason. Chewing your food properly means you'll extract more nutrients from it. It helps to maintain a healthy weight, prevents digestive upsets, and it's good for the health of your teeth and jaw too.
- Put your utensils down between bites to help you slow down, chew and really enjoy your food.
- Eat protein first, then veg and see if you have room for all those carbs you thought you needed to feel satisfied.

Before I get into the juicy topic of what foods to prioritise and what food to limit or avoid, let's start with some overall aims for you to always come back to. Your diet should be:

- Enjoyable to eat.
- Nutritionally rich and diverse.
- Providing you with enough fuel to feel energised throughout your day.
- Addressing any digestive complaints or food sensitivities you may have.
- Supporting the health of your microbiome.
- Stabilising your blood sugar and keeping insulin at a healthy level.
- Targeting any specific health issues that you have.

What to Eat

Breakfast

Whether breakfast is an essential meal or not is fiercely debated and, whilst I'm sure there are some people – probably males – whose constitutions and lifestyles are suited to skipping breakfast, I'm of the belief that females need a decent breakfast. My clients who skip it do so because they're stressed and 'too busy' in the mornings, or because they want to lose weight and have read that doing this is the 'easy' way to do so, but eating breakfast *supports* weight loss, and skipping it causes more physical and emotional stress. Something else I've noticed is that clients have a tendency to take care of everyone else's breakfasts in the morning, but neglect their own. Cereal, by the way, does not count as breakfast and neither does toast with jam. Breakfast needs to include a protein – eggs, salmon, nut and seed butters.

My favourite fast food for breakfast is eggs, because they're so quick to cook and you can use up whatever you have in the fridge to add to scrambled eggs or an omelette, and having some watercress or salad leaves on the side is a great way of getting a portion of greens in before you've even left the house. If you're really pressed for time, then make a vegetable frittata the night before so that it's ready to go the following morning (and the one after).

Oats are a good source of carbs and fibre, so making porridge is a good option. Just be sure to add a cup of fresh or frozen fruit (raspberries, blackberries and pear are all rich in fibre), and some healthy fats and protein in the form of nuts or nut butters or you might find yourself needing to eat a second breakfast an hour or two later.

If you're really not a breakfast person, have protein smoothies and make sure that you're not eating your dinner too late (eating earlier in the evening often stimulates your need to eat in the morning). Lean towards complex carbs which provide a sustained release of energy and are a source of fibre.

Regular meals

On the whole, three satisfying square meals a day and no snacks works well for most people, but if you're prone to low blood sugar, anaemic, stressed and sleep-deprived, then you may need to eat more frequently than that, perhaps eating every three hours until you're more nourished. Whatever camp you're in, just don't skip a meal, because your blood sugar levels will suffer. And bear in mind that you are not a cow – you don't have eight stomachs to deal with grazing all day long, so don't nibble continuously. A helpful visual to have in mind when planning your meals is for protein to take up a quarter of your plate (a palm-sized portion), another quarter should be taken up by starchy carbs, and fill up the remaining half of your plate with veggies (and I don't mean half a plate of mashed potato).

Eat the rainbow

Eat eight to 10 servings of vegetables and – to a lesser extent – fruit per day, making sure that you consume a variety of colours. Fruit and veg are actually good sources of carbs and are more nutrient-dense than a loaf of white bread. They're packed with vitamins, minerals, and phytonutrients that are essential to health, and eating a variety of colours means that you're getting more nutrients.

Vegetables are packed full of a massively diverse range of nutrients that help to prevent and treat most of the diseases that we get. They're also a rich source of fibre and help to keep your bowel movements regular and easy. Many of my clients share how they always eat a salad for lunch, which is great, but they often forget to add a protein to those lovely leaves and veg. The wonderful thing about salads is that most protein, be it fish, lentils, halloumi, beans or chicken, all taste good in a salad. And roasted veg is a great addition too. There are two types of veg: non-starchy and starchy.

Non-starchy vegetables are rich in vitamins and minerals, fibre and water, and they have a low glycemic index, which means you can go wild and eat loads of them. Non-starchy veg includes leafy greens, cruciferous vegetables such as broccoli and kale, cucumbers, celery, carrots, green beans, mushrooms, garlic, onions, artichokes, aubergines and peppers (though these can cause an inflammatory response in some people).

Starchy vegetables are a great source of carbohydrates, so they tend to be more filling than their non-starchy companions, but they can also have a higher glycemic index, which means you should have smaller amounts of them than most of us are used to. That being said, they're a far better source of carbs than those that come from grains such as bread and pasta, and starch helps to calm the nervous system and support sleep. Starchy veg includes sweet potato, white potato, squash (including butternut, acorn, spaghetti and pumpkin), parsnips, plantain, corn (though as a highly genetically modified crop, it's not one to go wild with and best if you can stick to non-GMO) and beetroot.

Crucial Cruciferous

Vegetables from the cruciferous family include broccoli, cauliflower, Brussels sprouts, bok choy, cabbage, collard greens, kale, rocket, watercress and radishes. These are important to include in your daily diet because they help to reduce inflammation, and because they're high in fibre they can regulate blood sugar and help reduce oestrogen excess. If you find they give you gas, experiment with different cooking techniques and make sure you chew them properly. And if you have a thyroid condition, be sure to eat them cooked as eating them raw can cause your intestines to release goitrogens, which increases your need for iodine and can damage the thyroid gland.

Berry, berry good

Berries are nutrient-dense superfoods that are loaded with antioxidants, which have anti-ageing properties. They're high in fibre, can help to fight inflammation, lower cholesterol levels, protect against cancer and even slow cognitive decline, so be sure to include them in your diet.

Fruits are full of nutrients and fibre, and are a healthy source of carbohydrates. They also contain substantial amounts of natural sugars, so it's better to eat more veg than fruit. Natural sugars aren't a problem when you eat whole fruit, because you're also getting fibre from the pulp and skin, but when you juice fruit you miss out on the fibre, which has implications for blood sugar levels.

Buy organic

I'm a big believer in buying the best food that your budget allows and I find it eternally frustrating that foods with low nutritional value are so cheap. When you're considering what organic foods to splurge your hard-earned money on, prioritise the Dirty Dozen, a list of the most pesticide-laden foods that's produced every year by the Environmental Working Group (EWG). It changes slightly every year, but commonly features strawberries, spinach, peaches, nectarines, cherries and apples. The EWG also produces a Clean Fifteen list of the fruit and veg that tend to have the lowest amount of pesticides on them, or in other words, produce that needn't be organic unless your budget allows for it. Current entries include avocados, asparagus, broccoli, mushrooms, pineapple and kiwi.

Fat Doesn't Make You Fat

Fat isn't the evil ingredient that we've been led to believe it is. It's been blamed for obesity and clogged-up arteries for decades, yet evidence shows that it's crucial for your health. Your brain is made predominantly of fat, and you need fat to build cell membranes and to protect the sheaths that coat your nerve cells. Fat is a key source of energy, which also helps you to feel full and regulate your blood sugar and hormones. When fat is removed from foods or it's absent from a meal, you end up eating more in order to reach the point where you feel full, because fat helps you to feel satiated. Because of this, an absence of fat can contribute towards obesity – not to mention the fact that low-fat foods are pumped full of sugar and salt to compensate for the flavour that's lost when fat is removed. Fat also enables you to absorb some vitamins and minerals.

Oestrogen, progesterone, DHEA (the 'mother' hormone that other hormones are derived from), cortisol and testosterone are all made from cholesterol from dietary fat, which means that your intake of fat is *essential* for hormone production and function. If you've got a hormonal issue such as low progesterone, low oestrogen, low libido or PMS, then take a minute to look at how much fat you're getting in your diet. Every meal you eat should include a serving of healthy fat. One serving is roughly one to two tablespoons of oil, half an avocado, or a shot glass of nuts and seeds. Sources of healthy fats include:

- Avocados
- Olives
- Eggs
- Nuts and seeds
- Fatty, cold-water fish such as salmon
- Fatty, grass-fed meat
- Extra virgin olive oil, flaxseed oil, walnut oil and avocado oil – use in dressings and to drizzle over meals
- Coconut oil and ghee – use for cooking at higher temperatures. I also love to keep the fat that floats to the top of homemade bone broth when you refrigerate it and use it for sautéing.

Saturated fats are the kind of fats found in butter and other dairy produce, eggs, meat and coconut oil. They're a hot topic, because how good they are for you is debatable. I think it's fair to say that they do have health benefits, but they shouldn't be overused and how good they are for you will largely come down to the quality of the products that you have access to, such as organic butter from grass-fed cows.

Unsaturated fats can be monounsaturated, which is what's in olive oil and avocados, or polyunsaturated (PUFAs), which come from fish, nuts and seeds. Unsaturated fat is the type of fat that's renowned for being really good for your health. Omega-3 fatty acids – the kind of healthy fat that comes from oily fish and nuts and seeds and which most of us are deficient in – are really beneficial as they help to reduce inflammation, period pain, fluid retention, PMS, acne, insulin sensitivity, depression and anxiety, and improve your skin, hair and nails. The Department of Health recommends eating oily fish two to three times per week and you can also take a fish oil supplement, but be warned: some people find that it makes them burp and burping fish oil is not pleasant. Your reaction will vary across brands. I find that BioCare Mega EPA doesn't make me burp at all and I like that they regularly test their fish oil supplements for contamination (fish in the sea accumulate toxins and mercury that you want to avoid ingesting). If you're vegetarian or vegan then you can take omega-3 that's derived from algae instead of taking fish oil.

Try to avoid vegetable oils such as sunflower, corn and canola as they're heavily processed; the heat, chemicals and light that they're exposed to during processing damages them and makes them harmful. They're also high in omega-6 fatty acids, which increase inflammation in the body, so you really want to be limiting them as much as possible or cutting them out altogether. And stay clear of trans fats – they're the type that are found in fried and greasy foods, and appear as 'hydrogenated fat' or 'partially hydrogenated oils' on food labels. They're associated with heart disease, high cholesterol, obesity and Alzheimer's disease, as well as encouraging oestrogen to go down the pathways which increase your cancer risk.

Legumes

Legumes include beans, chickpeas, lentils, peas and peanuts (yup, peanuts aren't technically a nut). They are plant-based sources of protein that are a good source of fibre as well as vitamins and minerals, but they can feed candida, and contain phytic acid and phytates, which may inhibit your ability to absorb nutrients. They also contain a substance called agglutinin which causes inflammation in some people. Soaking, sprouting and fermenting legumes can reduce their amount of phytic acid, phytate and agglutinin, and increase their nutritional value.

Eggs

Eggs have got to be the healthiest fast food out there. They're a nutritional powerhouse and a wonderful source of protein. When I'm working with a client who could do with upping their protein intake – which is most of the people I support – eggs are my favourite recommendation, but you've got to eat the yolk to benefit from their nutritional value. If you're of the belief that eating egg yolks raises your cholesterol and increases your risk of having a heart attack, know that for 75 per cent of the population, dietary cholesterol has very little impact on blood cholesterol. The remaining 25 per cent are referred to as hyper-responders and dietary cholesterol will modestly increase both their LDL ('bad' cholesterol) and HDL ('good' cholesterol), but it doesn't affect the ratio of the two or increase the incidence of heart disease. Buy organic and free-range if you're able to or keep your own chooks.

Meat and fish

Protein provides the building blocks for all the structures in your body, is a major source of energy and keeps your blood sugar steady. Meat and fish are good sources of protein and can also provide important vitamins, minerals and omega-3 fatty acids – but this varies depending on the quality of the produce and how they're cooked.

You are what you eat, but you're also what you eat ate too, and that's definitely the case when it comes to meat and fish. Livestock are routinely given low-dose antibiotics to prevent infection from the appalling conditions they're usually kept in and 80 per cent of antibiotics that are sold are used on them. They're also frequently pumped full of growth hormones, which means that by eating them you're increasing your exposure to hormones too, so it's better to eat organic poultry and meat – especially if you're using their bones to make broth. Organic produce can end up eating up most of your salary, but there are less popular nutrient-dense cuts which are delicious and more affordable.

Larger fish have higher levels of mercury in them and are the ones to be wary of, such as tuna, marlin, swordfish, grouper, king mackerel and shark. Fish that are generally lower in mercury include sardines, anchovies, wild Alaskan salmon, sockeye salmon, crab, Atlantic mackerel, Atlantic pollock, shrimp, crawfish and mussels.

Mackerel, sardines, anchovies, herring and salmon are all great sources of omega-3 fatty acids, but opt for wild salmon where possible because farmed salmon are given antibiotics and are frequently dyed orangey-pink, whereas wild salmon are naturally pink.

Carbohydrates

Most of us could do with eating fewer carbs, but they don't have to be excluded; they're not the devil. In fact, depriving your body of carbs can create stress and mess with your sleep, and during your cycling years it can interrupt ovulation too. Carbs are good for us, but when I say carbs I mean complex carbs, such as brown rice, quinoa, legumes, pulses, and fruit and veg. I'm not saying that you should never eat simple carbs such as white bread and pasta, I'm just recommending that they don't form the majority of what you eat. Wondering just how much complex carbs to eat? A portion the size of a small fist is plenty for most people if they're eating sufficient protein and loading up on non-starchy veg too. Complex carbs are good sources of fibre and most of the population's diet is low in fibre, which is a shame because fibre helps you to feel full, keeps your gut happy, lowers cholesterol levels, balances blood sugar and insulin levels, and helps you to excrete oestrogen when you're done with it.

Unfortunately, most of our diets lack fibre. The recommended intake in the UK was recently increased to 30 grams per day, but only 9 per cent of us achieve that. So how do you get 30 grams of fibre? Porridge with a cup (125 grams) of raspberries or blackberries gets you 12 grams of fibre. Eggs don't contain fibre, but add half an avocado to them and you'll get 5 grams. Add half a cup of black beans and that's another 7 grams. Can't imagine eating black beans for breakfast? It's time for you to look at some 'black bean bowl' recipes and take them for a spin. A salad with spinach leaves or kale as its base, topped with veg such as artichoke, squash, broccoli and beetroot will get you anything from another 10 to 15 grams. Looking for a dinner option? Try a bean and veg stew, and serve it with some pearl barley, quinoa or brown rice and get around 10 grams.

Resistant Starch

Resistant starch is a type of carb that's also a fibre, and that isn't completely broken down and absorbed by the body – it literally resists digestion. Although resistant starches help you to feel full up, you absorb fewer calories. Resistant starch helps to improve the amount of fat we use for energy and because it isn't digested into sugar, your body doesn't need to release a lot of insulin to deal with it. It also adds bulk and water to poo, making it easier to go on the regular, and it keeps your gut bacteria happy too because they can break it down and use it as fuel. Beans and legumes, starchy fruits and vegetables, and whole grains are all sources of resistant starch. And if you cook potatoes or rice and then let them cool, they'll have more resistant starch; one study found that cooling potatoes overnight tripled their resistant starch.

Water

Always start your day with water. It'll rehydrate you and help you to wake up, as well as encouraging your bowels to get going before you have to leave home. Most people could do with increasing their water intake, but just how much to have gets confusing, so I recommend paying attention to your thirst and also to your lips, because they show signs of dehydration quickly. When you reach for your lip balm, consider if you're dehydrated and, if you feel tired during the day, drink some water before you resort to caffeine and sugar, because dehydration also manifests as fatigue. Once you start upping your water intake you'll probably notice that you feel thirstier than you used to. This is normal and is a sign that your body likes you drinking more water. Remember that you do get a lot of water from vegetables (which you're eating more of, right?) as well as soups and other non-caffeinated beverages. If you have a tendency to feel cold, then drink tepid or hot water and herbal teas. Avoid drinking water from the fridge and using ice. Cold water is a shock to the body and is said to dampen your digestive fire in Chinese medicine, therefore room temperature is much better. And don't flood your stomach whilst you're eating as it can weaken your digestive juices. Try to drink water 30 to 60 minutes before a meal instead. If you're worried about your bladder function, then remember that being dehydrated won't help matters and be sure to drink plenty of water early on in the day so that late-in-the-day drinking doesn't have you up in the night.

Endocrine Disruptors

Endocrine disruptors are synthetic substances which disrupt your hormones. They're literally everywhere – you can find them in plastics, pesticides, flame retardants, chemicals and water systems. You're probably breathing them, drinking them, eating them, putting them on your skin and cleaning your kitchen with them. They're even found in the umbilical cords of newborns due to in-utero exposure. Because they're so prevalent, it's easy to get freaked out by them, which of course piles on the stress and we could all do without that. I'm going to give you some straightforward ways to reduce your exposure to them, because the fact that your reproductive years are drawing to a close doesn't mean that you can ignore endocrine disruptors; they impact on obesity, insulin and glucose balance in the body, thyroid function and reproductive cancers.

Endocrine disruptors are similar in structure to the hormones that you produce in your body, such as oestrogen, so they're often described as hormone mimickers, as they mimic them and bind to hormone receptor sites. Hormones work as a lock and key system. Hormonal glands release hormones which travel around your body in your bloodstream until they reach their intended target, at which point they bind to it and cause a reaction. Much like the keys you carry around with you, each of these hormones has a different shape and in the same way a key fits a specific lock, so each hormone will only go into the receptor site that it's intended for and have an effect in the places that it's needed. Endocrine disruptors are sneaky, because they can cause an increase or decrease in hormone levels in three different ways:

1) Fitting in the lock convincingly enough to trick the body into thinking it's a naturally produced hormone. The mimicker can cause a signal that's stronger than the one produced by your natural hormone, which can cause an overproduction or underproduction of hormones, such

as excess oestrogen or an underactive thyroid, or cause a signal at the wrong time. This is a big issue during perimenopause when oestrogen is high and thyroid hormones are often beginning to falter too.

2) Fitting in the lock, but being unable to turn it, so no reaction takes place, but the hole is plugged up, preventing your natural hormones from binding and turning the lock, so the normal hormone signalling fails.
3) Interfering with the way natural hormones and receptors are made.

Endocrine disruptors can cause:

- Early onset of puberty and menstruation.
- Early menopause – 15 chemicals, including phthalates, a chemical that makes plastics soft, and polychlorinated biphenyls (PCBs), which were banned in 1979 but can still be present in older products, have been linked to it.
- Fertility issues.
- Increases in breast, ovarian and prostate cancers.
- Increases in immune and autoimmune diseases, as well as some neurological diseases.
- Reductions in male fertility and a decline in the number of males born.
- Abnormalities in male reproductive organs.

Common endocrine disruptors include:

- Bisphenol A (BPA) is found in a lot of plastics and in countless products that we all use on a daily basis: food containers, water bottles, baby bottles, receipts, the lining of aluminium cans, milk containers, optical lenses, dental sealants, water storage tanks and water pipes. And as a result of its production, around 100 tons of BPA is released into the environment every year, so it's been found in dust particles and drinking water, all of which means we have to limit our exposure to it as much as possible. As levels of BPA in urine increase, measures of fertility decline.
- Phthalates, the compound used to make plastic soft, is found in food packaging, which is hard to avoid these days, but do your best and opt

to use glass containers to store food instead of cling film and plastic Tupperware. Any plastic Tupperware that you do use should be kept out of the dishwasher, freezer and microwaves because hot and cold temperatures cause phthalates to be released. They're also found in Styrofoam cups, baby toys, PVC, vinyl flooring, shower curtains, shampoo, hairspray, perfume and nail polish. Phthalates have been linked to problems with ovulation and fertility, obesity, type 2 diabetes and cancer.

- Pesticides commonly used on fruit and vegetable crops, as well as in your garden, are known endocrine disruptors that can also cause cancer. They'll also be present in any meat or dairy products you eat if the animals consumed feed which was laden with them.
- Surfactants in cleansing products, which means anything that foams, such as facial wash, shower gel and shampoo, are commonly labelled as sulphates. They work by stripping oil away and therefore can cause initial dryness, followed by an overproduction of sebum, because your body thinks it needs to produce more.
- Parabens are found in shampoos, soaps and shower gels, toothpaste, cosmetics and many other personal care products.
- Dioxins, which are known as persistent organic pollutants (POPs), because they take a long time to break down once they're released into the environment. They form as a result of waste incineration (including backyard burning) and burning fuels such as wood, coal and oil, and the chlorine bleaching of pulp and paper. They're highly toxic and can cause cancer, reproductive and developmental problems, and damage to the immune system, as well as screwing with your hormones. You can find them in bleached products such as coffee filters and tampons.
- Solvents in nail polish and nail polish remover.

The list of sources can feel overwhelming, but I find it encouraging and motivating that one study found that using products without phthalates, parabens and phenol brought down levels of substances by 20 to 45 per cent in just three days. You can reduce your exposure by working on a couple of things at a time, starting with the products that you use most frequently and/or liberally, such as the products you use to wash or moisturise with every day. Here are my top tips for limiting your exposure to them:

- Eat organic where possible, prioritising meat and dairy products, and avoiding the Dirty Dozen (see page 270).
- See how your personal care products measure up by looking them up on the EWG's Skin Deep database or on the Think Dirty app and start by replacing those that you use most frequently or liberally, such as body wash or moisturiser.
- Buy BPA-free products.
- Store food and drink in glass or stainless steel containers.
- Avoid canned food and drinks as cans are usually lined with BPA (though some companies like Biona use BPA-free cans).
- Buy food in glass jars instead of cans.
- Don't reheat or freeze food in plastic.
- Keep water bottles out of the sunshine as the heat can cause BPA to leach out into the water.
- Filter the water that you drink.
- Don't take receipts unless you really need them or have them emailed to you, and if your job requires you to handle receipts consider wearing gloves.
- Don't use plastic lids on your takeaway coffee unless you have to as the heat from your coffee can cause any BPA in it to leach out.
- As I write this, we're in the midst of the Covid-19 pandemic, so I say this in the hope that by the time this book is published we're on the other side of things: don't use hand sanitiser or antimicrobial washes. Of course, there are times when it is entirely appropriate to use them, such as during a pandemic or working in an environment where their use is entirely necessary – I'm not talking about those situations. I'm talking about when people use them outside of a global pandemic because they fear regular germs, germs which are usually beneficial for your immune system.
- Avoid having your clothes dry-cleaned or using dryer sheets.
- Use natural household cleaning products and laundry detergent.
- Use unbleached products – coffee filters, tampons, toilet paper. The Environmental Protection Agency (EPA) has determined that just using

bleached coffee filters can result in a lifetime's exposure to dioxin that exceeds acceptable risks.
- When carpeting your home, avoid synthetic carpets and be sure to air your home afterwards as the solvents in the glue used to hold them in place are also xenoestrogens (endocrine disruptors that have oestrogen-like effects).
- Fill your home and workplace with houseplants which cleanse the air and pump it full of oxygen (see the NASA Clean Air Study for a list of suitable plants).

Exercise

There are three types of exercise I think we all need to be doing: strength training, cardiovascular exercise and restorative movement. Many of you will have spent decades opting for (or attempting) cardiovascular exercise such as running, cycling and swimming. It can help you to burn fat and calories, which can support weight loss (no wonder we're conditioned to opt for these types of exercise), as well as lowering your risk of cardiovascular diseases such as high blood pressure and heart attacks. And as we've already established, these are important risks to consider and reduce once we're in perimenopausal territory. But, if you're anything like my client Rachel, it might be time to change how you exercise.

CASE STUDY

Rachel had always been into running. She loved signing up for 10k runs and half-marathons and the training for them gave her an outlet for mental stress, as well as a way to get out of the house and leave the needs of her family members behind her. But Rachel was exhausted, stressed out and not sleeping well, so despite her desire to be able to run longer distances, I suggested that she run less. We discussed ways of supporting her mental wellbeing so that she wasn't reliant upon exercise, but the main thing I suggested was that she spent less time running.

We came up with a plan where she would head out for a short run and then sit in a park or her garden to do some yoga nidra, or just have a nice walk and enjoy being out of the house on her own. Knowing that she had me to coach her through the issues that were causing her to feel stressed, Rachel committed to doing things differently. Sure enough, her brain started chucking up all sorts of issues; issues that she'd been trying to bury by pounding the pavements every day for years and years. But Rachel knew that this was an opportunity for her to take control of her life and to deal with her inner demons, which is exactly what she did. Although she still loved running, Rachel realised that there was a more enjoyable way to run that didn't involve trying to run away from her life.

According to most photos of peri- and postmenopausal women on the internet, strength training involves lifting piddly barbells. Don't get me wrong, starting with them is great and you should always take into account what your body is able to do, but for most of us there's no reason not to lift larger weights. If we're to prevent bone loss, maintain our muscle mass and improve insulin sensitivity, then we need to be doing some strength training several times a week. The male energy of gyms can be off-putting, but finding a CrossFit gym may feel much more comfortable and they will show you what your body is really capable of. Don't be afraid of looking muscley – muscles are strong and sexy.

All of us could do with some restorative movement in our lives and it's something I'm fond of recommending to my clients who are stressed, tired or entirely burnt out. When we talk about exercise, we're usually talking about the very active kind that gets your heart pumping and your skin sweating, and whilst cardio exercise is important, my perimenopausal clients are in need of movement that generates energy, instead of using it up. That's where restorative movement comes in. It's tempting to think that because you're not out of breath and covered in sweat, that you haven't had a workout, but trust me when I say that you'll really feel the effects of movement such as tai qi and qi gong on your muscles the next day.

Restorative Movement

Restorative yoga is not like any yoga class you've been to because you'll hardly move at all – you'll only do a few poses, remaining in each for around 10 to 20 minutes. This may sound torturous, but restorative yoga is floor-based and lots of props such as blankets and bolsters are used to support your body. Rather than using effort to hold a pose, the props support you so that you can stretch passively. This means that you can really relax into the pose and let go. This is a great way of releasing stress and soothing your nervous system. The lights in a class are usually dim and some are even held in candlelight. They're often evening classes too, which makes them a great post-work option so that you can wind down and have a great night's sleep.

Yoga nidra is also referred to as yogic sleep and 30 minutes of yoga nidra is said to equate to two hours of deep sleep, which is why I love recommending it to clients who are frazzled and need a mid-afternoon top-up of energy. It combines guided meditation with yoga to take you through the four main stages of brain wave activity – beta, alpha, theta and delta – so that you reach the place between wakefulness and sleep. All you have to do is sit in a comfortable position or lie down in corpse pose (shavasana) and follow the guided visualisation (see Resources for my favourites). Research into yoga nidra has found that it can improve PMS, anxiety and depression related to the menstrual cycle and blood glucose levels in diabetics, and rage and anxiety related to PTSD in military veterans. If it can work for them, surely it can work for you?

Qi gong (pronounced chee gong) combines slow graceful movement with mental concentration, breathwork and posture to increase and balance your energy. It's part of traditional Chinese medicine, along with acupuncture and herbal medicine, and has been practised for thousands of years. You can do it whilst sitting, standing, lying down or moving, which means it can be done anytime, anywhere, and it's also easy to do. Start with the 8 Brocades of Silk and be amazed at how you feel afterwards. Kirsten, a member of The Flow Collective, decided to give qi gong a go and fell in love with it immediately because of its gentle approach, finding that it calmed her and had a positive effect on her whole body. Kirsten loves doing it before sleep, especially when she hasn't moved much during the day, and it helps her to wind down and leave her day behind.

Tai qi (pronounced tie chee) was originally developed as a martial art in 13th-century China and it involves moving through a series of motions named after animal actions such as 'white crane spreads its wings'. The result of this is that your energy, or qi, builds and flows more smoothly through the body, leaving you feeling energised but serene. It's a low-impact, slow-motion exercise, making it a great option if you're out of shape or you've got health issues that limit what exercise you can undertake. In fact, according to the mounting body of clinical evidence, tai qi can be used to prevent or treat many health problems.

Tai qi improves the strength and flexibility of your upper and lower body as well as your core muscles. It also improves balance and proprioception – your ability to sense the position of your body in space – which is why some research has demonstrated that it can reduce the incidence of falls. I know you're probably not at the age at which falling is a concern (unless you've had too much to drink, that is), but falls are a major health risk and can change your quality of life in a matter of seconds.

Exercise is great for your brain as well as your body. It has an antidepressant effect, improves mood and cognitive function, and can counteract age-related mental deterioration, including dementia and Alzheimer's disease. Exercise can even stimulate the growth of new nerve cells in your brain, which means it's never too late to move your body – even the simplest of exercise plans can make a difference and, if you can exercise outside and/or with others, even better.

EPILOGUE

I have been socialised to be good and polite; rewarded for being compliant and kind; trained to desire praise for being a good girl. And I am utterly ill-equipped to express the rage that I feel. Anger feels dangerous, because I do not know what to do with it. It scares me and I fear what happens next. I am stepping out of the parameters of my being and inhabiting that anger. I am on fire. There is an urgency to my work that is new; that I love and yearn to embrace. But I am stretched and held back by my family, whom I love, but whom I need to be apart from for increasingly long stretches of time so that I can come back to them. Silence and solitude are what I need and crave. And it's relationships with women that I lean into and treasure.

Looking back, it was the desperate and excessive pruning of the tree outside our kitchen window that alerted me to the awareness that I was changing. I was frustrated writing my first book whilst parenting a two-year-old and living in a house that felt as ramshackle as my emotional state. The frantic pruning inflicted upon the tree, and the swearing that accompanied it, was an expression of my fed-upness, of my urge to burn it all to the ground and start again.

Then the shorter cycles began. From 28 on the regular to 24 and 25. My periods started to lengthen, with days of inconvenient trickling. I had night sweats and insomnia in the days before I began to bleed. Impatience, irritability and heightened sensory issues required me to hide from the world and those that I love. I had a softness around my belly that was new and welcome. I had chin hairs that weren't. My hormones were on the move.

I am challenged by anyone's need for me, repelled by any claim on my time or energy. I am ambitious and perhaps self-obsessed, driven by the question of how much time I have left and what I'm going to do with it. There is fury at the years I've squandered and sentimentality at the memories of my youthful naivety. I'm straddling two worlds: 'Who do you think you are?'

and 'Fuck it, let's do this.' I am embracing my peculiarities, moving from self-improvement to self-love. I am standing in the mirror and appreciating everything I bring to the world. I am stepping into my power and owning it like I never have.

I am finding my Perimenopause Power.

APPENDIX

Using the table below, please indicate if you have any of the symptoms listed and the degree to which they are currently bothering you.

SYMPTOMS	Not at all 0	A little 1	Quite a bit 2	Extremely 3
1. Heart beating quickly or strongly				
2. Feeling tense of nervous				
3. Difficulty in sleeping				
4. Excitable				
5. Attacks of anxiety, panic				
6. Difficulty in concentrating				
7. Feeling tired of lacking in energy				
8. Loss of interest in most things				
9. Feeling unhappy or depressed				
10. Crying spells				
11. Irritability				
12. Feeling dizzy or faint				
13. Pressure or tightness in head				
14. Parts of body feel numb or tingling				
15. Headaches				
16. Muscle and joint pains				
17. Loss of feeling in hands or feet				
18. Breathing difficulties				
19. Hot flushes				
20. Sweating at night				
21. Loss of interest in sex				
Total Score				

GLOSSARY

Allopregnanolone (ALLO) A neurosteroid that generally makes people feel calmer, but makes those with PMDD feel anxious and depressed.

Amenorrhoea The absence of periods during the reproductive years.

Androgens A group of hormones traditionally referred to as 'male', but which people of all genders have. Testosterone is an example of an androgen hormone.

Anovulatory cycle A menstrual cycle in which ovulation did not take place and therefore no progesterone was produced by the corpus luteum.

Basal body temperature (BBT) The lowest body temperature reached during rest. It is taken immediately after waking in the morning and, because temperatures are higher after ovulation and throughout the second half of the cycle, it can be used to identify when ovulation has taken place.

Bisphenol A (BPA) An endocrine disruptor which 'mimics' oestrogen. It's present in lots of goods, from water bottles and food containers to the thermal paper receipts are printed on, and it can cause breast cancer and other illnesses and abnormalities.

Body-identical hormone therapy Hormones derived from plant sources that are produced in a laboratory and are identical to the hormones produced by the body. Body-identical hormones are commonly prescribed by GPs and menopause specialists.

Brain-derived neurotrophic factor (BDNF) Low levels of BDNF, caused by low levels of oestrogen in late perimenopause and postmenopause, are responsible for making you forgetful.

Combined hormone therapy Menopausal hormone therapy that combines an oestrogen and a progestogen. If you have a uterus then you must take a progestogen alongside oestrogen to prevent the lining of your uterus from thickening up and causing endometrial hyperplasia.

Compounded bio-identical hormone replacement therapy A type of hormone therapy offered by private clinics that are custom made and unregulated. The British Menopause Society does not recommend them.

Continuous hormone therapy Once your periods have stopped, you can take oestrogen and progestogen every day (rather than following a cyclical pattern).

Corpus luteum Following ovulation, the follicle which contained the egg for that month collapses and forms the corpus luteum, a temporary gland which produces and secretes progesterone in the second half of your cycle.

Cortisol A hormone that's produced by the adrenal glands which regulates a large number of processes in the body, including blood sugar levels and the immune response. It's also released in response to stress.

Cyclical hormone therapy If you have regular periods, you take oestrogen every day but only take the progestogen component towards the end of your cycle. Once your periods become irregular, you take the progestogen component for a set number of days once every three months.

Dehydroepiandrosterone (DHEA) A hormone from which other hormones – notably testosterone and oestrogen – are made. After menopause, it becomes the sole source of oestrogen.

Early menopause When menopause takes place before the age of 45.

Endocrine disruptors Chemicals in food, pesticides, personal care products, plastics and solvents which interfere with how the endocrine system functions.

Endocrine system The hormone-producing glands in your body, such as your pituitary, hypothalamus, thyroid, adrenals and ovaries.

Endometrial hyperplasia Under the influence of oestrogen, the lining of your uterus (endometrium) thickens up and increases your risk of developing uterine cancer. Taking a progestogen alongside oestrogen prevents this from happening, which is why anyone taking menopausal hormone therapy who has a uterus must also take a progestogen to prevent it from becoming too thick.

Endometrium The inner lining of the uterus. In each menstrual cycle it plumps up in preparation for potential implantation of a fertilised egg and is shed during menstruation if conception doesn't take place.

Fertility awareness method (FAM) Fertility awareness is a way to identify fertile and non-fertile times in the menstrual cycle, including the use of BBT charting, and can be used to avoid or achieve pregnancy.

Follicle A fluid-filled sac that contains an immature egg. During ovulation a mature egg is released from its follicle, the follicle then collapses and forms the corpus luteum.

Follicle stimulating hormone (FSH) A hormone produced by your pituitary gland which stimulates the follicles in your ovaries, instructing them to grow and mature.

Follicular phase The first half of the menstrual cycle, beginning when a period starts and ending at ovulation, in which ovarian follicles grow and mature until one releases an egg at ovulation. During this phase the lining of the uterus thickens in preparation for implantation of a fertilised egg.

Genito-urinary syndrome of menopause (GSM) A common condition in perimenopause and during the postmenopausal years, which describes the emergence of genital symptoms (dryness, burning, irritation), sexual symptoms (vaginal dryness, pain during sex) and urinary symptoms (urgency, leakage and urinary tract infections).

Gonadotropin-releasing hormone (GnRH) A hormone released by the hypothalamus gland which stimulates the pituitary gland to release FSH and LH.

Hirsutism Excess hair growth on the face and body, often caused by excess androgens.

Hormone replacement therapy (HRT) Treatments which replace the hormones that decline in midlife. However, as those hormones decline naturally and are not 'missing' and in need of 'replacement', the term menopausal hormone therapy (MHT) is preferred.

Hyperthyroidism When the thyroid gland is overactive and overproduces thyroid hormones.

Hypothalamic amenorrhoea (HA) When periods stop because the hypothalamus gland stops or slows production of GnRH.

Hypothyroidism When the thyroid gland is underactive and doesn't produce enough thyroid hormones.

Hysterectomy The surgical removal of the uterus. When the ovaries and cervix are also removed it is referred to as a total hysterectomy, but when the ovaries and cervix are not removed, it is called a partial hysterectomy.

Luteal phase The second half of your cycle – from ovulation to the start of your period – which is typically 12 to 16 days in length.

Luteinising hormone (LH) A hormone produced by the pituitary gland. The acute rise of LH towards the end of the first half of the cycle triggers ovulation and the development of the corpus luteum.

Menopause The end of your menstruating years, officially reached one year after your last period.

Menopause hormone therapy (MHT) The use of hormones to treat the symptoms of menopause. Also known as hormone replacement therapy (HRT).

Menstrual cycle Starts on the first day of your period and ends when your next period begins.

Menstruation Your period.

Microbiome The community of microorganisms that populate your body, or a specific part of the body – such as the gut and vagina – and which carry out lots of body processes, including manufacturing hormones.

Micronised Made into a very fine powder.

Oestradiol (E2) The main form of oestrogen that we produce during our cycling years, and the type of oestrogen most commonly used in menopausal hormone therapy.

Oestrogen The umbrella term for the three forms of oestrogen: oestradiol, oestrone and oestriol. Oestrogen is responsible for the development and regulation of the female reproductive system, but it's also present in males.

Oestrogen detoxification The ways that you metabolise (process) oestrogen.

Oestrone (E1) Not as strong as oestradiol, but the predominant circulating oestrogen in postmenopause.

Ovulation Occurs when an ovarian follicle releases a mature egg.

Perimenopause The period of time when hormonal changes occur prior to your periods stopping, which can result in 'menopausal symptoms'.

Phthalates They are used to make plastic soft, particularly for food packaging, and are endocrine disruptors.

Polycyclic aromatic hydrocarbons (PAHs) A group of over 100 chemicals classified as persistent organic pollutants, which can damage DNA and cause cancer.

Polycystic ovarian syndrome (PCOS) A condition characterised by irregular periods and enlarged ovaries, which may or may not have cysts on them. High levels of 'male' hormones in your body can lead to hirsutism.

Premature menopause When periods stop before the age of 40.

Premature ovarian insufficiency (POI) A condition in which ovarian function declines prematurely, resulting in irregular or absent cycles which may or may not occur alongside menopausal symptoms such as hot flushes. This is different to early and premature menopause because with POI some ovarian function may remain or return.

Premenopause The time between your first period and perimenopause.

Premenstrual dysphoric disorder (PMDD) A very severe form of PMS that causes mental and physical distress in the week or two preceding menstruation, and which is relieved within a few days of a period starting.

Premenstrual syndrome (PMS) The physical and emotional symptoms that can occur in the week or two preceding menstruation.

Progesterone The hormone made by the ovary after ovulation, which is necessary in order to sustain a pregnancy. You can take 'body-identical' progesterone during perimenopause and postmenopause.

Progestin A synthetic hormone which is similar to but not the same as progesterone.

Progestogen A term which refers to both natural progesterone and synthetic forms of progesterone (progestins).

Prolactin A hormone produced in the pituitary gland. High levels can cause irregular cycles by interfering with ovulation and the normal production of other hormones.

Prolapse When an organ, such as the bladder, rectum or uterus, falls out of its usual position and drops down into the vagina.

Sex hormone binding globulin (SHBG) A protein that's made by your liver which binds to excess hormones, such as oestrogen and testosterone.

Systemic hormone therapy Menopausal hormone therapy that affects you system-wide. This is the type of hormone therapy used to treat symptoms such as hot flushes, sleep issues, cognitive function and joint pain. It can be used in addition to topical (vaginal) oestrogen.

Testosterone A hormone known as an androgen. It's produced in small amounts by the adrenal glands and the ovaries in females and is found in larger amounts in males.

Topical hormone therapy A form of menopausal hormone therapy which is applied to the vulva and vagina to produce a localised effect. This can help with the genito-urinary syndrome of menopause (GSM) but won't have a 'system-wide' effect.

Vagina The internal tube which connects your vulva to your cervix (neck of the uterus).

Very early menopause The beginning of perimenopause in which you notice your cycle becoming slightly shorter and menopausal symptoms such as night sweats, sleep issues, headaches and mood changes around the time of your period starts.

Vulva Your external genitals, including your clitoris and labia. In other words, all the bits you can see.

Withdrawal bleeding The monthly bleeding produced when someone using hormonal birth control such as the pill experiences a drop (or withdrawal) of hormones when they take the placebo pills in their pack, causing their endometrium to shed.

RESOURCES

Further reading

A Mind of Her Own, Dr Kelly Brogan.
Flash Count Diary, Darcey Steinke.
How the Pill Changes Everything, Dr Sarah E. Hill.
Me and My Menopausal Vagina, Jane Lewis.
Menopause, Dr Louise Newsom.
Mind the Gap, Karen Gurney.
Period Repair Manual, Lara Briden.
Sweetening the Pill, Holly Grigg-Spall.
Taking Charge of Your Fertility, Toni Weschler.
The Balance Plan, Angelique Panagos.
The Hormone Cure, Dr Sara Gottfried.
The Hormone Fix, Dr Anna Cabeca.
The Madwoman in the Volvo, Sandra Tsing Loh.
The Pill: Are You Sure It's For You? Jane Bennett and Alexandra Pope.
The Wisdom of Menopause, Dr Christiane Northrup.
The XX Brain, Dr Lisa Mosconi.
Why We Can't Sleep, Ada Calhoun.
Wild Power, Alexandra Pope and Sjanie Hugo-Wurlitzer.

Websites

Bazzmoffat.com for exercise programmes and pelvic floor support.

CoppaFeel.org is a breast cancer awareness charity which promotes early detection of breast cancer by encouraging women and men to regularly check their breasts and chest.

Daisynetwork.org provides information and support for those experiencing POI and premature menopause.

Dameproducts.com for sex toys.

Drannacabeca.com/products/julva for Dr Anna Cabeca's DHEA vaginal cream.

Endowhat.com for an educational and empowering documentary about endometriosis.

Eveappeal.org.uk is a UK charity which raises awareness and funds gynaecological research.

Fpa.org.uk is a sexual health charity which provides information on contraception, STIs and pregnancy choices.

healinghistamine.com has lots of information and tools to heal histamine intolerance.

helloclue.com is a free period tracker.
Hilarylewin.com for menopause workshops and ATMAT treatments.
iapmd.org is the International Association for Premenstrual Disorders.
Imsociety.org is the International Menopause Society.
kindara.com is a free fertility charting app.
Megsmenopause.com is a source of information and advice on all things menopause.
Menopausedoctor.co.uk is menopause expert Dr Louise Newsom's website.
Menopausesupport.co.uk for the #makemenopausematter campaign.
Nancy's Nook Endometriosis Education and Discussion Group can be found at Facebook.com/groups/418136991574617.
Ohnut.co is an intimate wearable that allows users to customise penetration depth and reduce pain.
pms.org.uk is the National Association for Premenstrual Syndrome.
redschool.net for a radical approach to women's leadership, creativity and spiritual life.
Sh-womenstore.com is a female-focussed pleasure and sex shop.
thebms.org.uk is the British Menopause Society.
thehavelockclinic.com is a team of highly specialised doctors and psychologists who treat sexual problems in their clinics and over Skype, as well as through their excellent online therapy workshops, which you can attend anonymously.
Thyroidpharmacist.com for thyroid information.
Yesyesyes.org for natural, pure and certified organic intimate lubricants, moisturisers and washes.

REFERENCES

Chapter 1

'it's estimated that more than 50 million women and those assigned female at birth in the US have now reached the average age of menopause': Howden, L.M. and Meyer, J.A. (2010) *Age and Sex Composition: 2010*, United States Census Bureau.

'By 2050, this figure is expected to quadruple': United States Census Bureau (2015) 90+ in the United States: 2006–2008: https://www.census.gov/library/publications/2011/acs/acs-17.html.

'early perimenopause begins when the length of your cycle varies by seven or more days in consecutive cycles': Soules, M.R *et al* (2001) Executive summary: Stages of Reproductive Aging Workshop (STRAW), *Climacteric*, 4(4), pp. 267–272.

'it places the emphasis on our changing experiences that, better than regular cycles, indicate changes in our hormone levels': Prior, J. C. *Estrogen's Storm Season: Stories of Perimenopause*, (e-book) 2nd ed. Vancouver, BC: CeMCOR (2018).

'CeMCOR states that 'if our experiences have changed, if our hormone levels have changed': Centre for Menstrual Cycle and Ovulation Research website: https://www.cemcor.ca/resources/how-can-i-tell-i-am-perimenopause.

'any three of which can be used to define the start of perimenopause in those with regular, normal-length menstrual cycles': Prior, J. C. (2005) Clearing confusion about perimenopause, *British Columbia Medical Journal*, 47(10), pp. 538–542.

'perimenopause is more often a time when oestrogen remains high': Santoro, N. *et al* (2017) Menstrual cycle hormone changes in women traversing menopause: Study of women's health across the nation, *Journal of Clinical Endocrinology and Metabolism*, 102(7), pp. 2218–2229.

'intact follicles have been found in the ovaries of 70-year-olds': Costoff, A. and Mahesh, V.B. (1975) Primordial follicles with normal oocytes in the ovaries of postmenopausal women, *Journal of the American Geriatrics Society*, 23(5), pp. 193–196.

'at age 52, 4.5 per cent of us will have a period after a year of having none': Treloar, A.E., Boynton, R.E., Behn, B.G. and Brown, B.W. (1967) *Variation of the human menstrual cycle through reproductive life, Int J. Fertil*, Jan–Mar; 12 (1 Pt 2): pp. 77–126, PMID: 5419031.

'it can also exacerbate the genito-urinary syndrome of menopause': Gliniewicz, K. *et al* (2019) Comparison of the vaginal microbiomes of premenopausal and postmenopausal women, *Frontiers in Microbiology*, 10:193.

'hormone therapy, such as taking oestrogen, can increase the number of lactobacilli and acidity of the vagina': Pabich, W.L. *et al* (2003) Prevalence and determinants of vaginal flora alterations in postmenopausal women, *Journal of Infectious Diseases*, 188(7), pp. 1054–1058.

'changes to the junctions between the cells that line the cervix': Gorodeski, G.I. (2000) Effects of menopause and estrogen on cervical epithelial permeability, *Journal of Clinical Endocrinology and Metabolism*, 85(7), pp. 2584–2595.

'reduced blood flow to the cervix': Gorodeski, G.I. (1996) The cervical cycle. In: Adashi, E.Y., Rock, J.A. and Rosenwaks, Z., (eds), *Reproductive Endocrinology, Surgery and Technology*, Lippincott-Raven Publishers, pp. 301–324.

'after menopause it reduces by around 20 per cent': Sokalska, A. and Valentin, L. (2008) Changes in ultrasound morphology of the uterus and ovaries during the menopausal transition and early post-menopause: a 4-year longitudinal study, *Ultrasound in Obstetrics and Gynaecology*, 31(2), pp. 210–217.

'surgeries may disrupt this communication system and lead to alterations in brain functioning': Koebele, S.V. *et al* (2019) Hysterectomy uniquely impacts spatial memory in a rat model: A role for the nonpregnant uterus in cognitive processes, *Endocrinology*, 160(1), pp. 1–19.

'you wanna hang on to them': Fogle, R.H. *et al* (2007) Ovarian androgen production in postmenopausal women, *Journal of Clinical Endocrinology and Metabolism*, 92(8), pp. 3040–3043.

'it produces 75 per cent of your oestrogen and, after menopause, it becomes the sole source of oestrogen': Payne, A.H. and Hales, D.B. (2004) Overview of steroidogenic enzymes in the pathway from cholesterol to active steroid hormones, *Endocrine Review*, 25(6), pp. 947–970.

'follicles grow earlier in the cycle than they used to': Klein, N.A. *et al* (2002) Is the short follicular phase in older women secondary to advanced or accelerated dominant follicle development?, *Journal of Clinical Endocrinology and Metabolism*, 87(12), pp. 5746–5750.

'they also grow more rapidly': Santoro N. *et al.* (2003) Impaired folliculogenesis and ovulation in older reproductive aged women, *Journal of Clinical Endocrinology and Metabolism*, 88(11), pp. 5502–5509.

'only 22.8 per cent of cycles showed evidence of ovulation': Santoro, N. *et al* (2017) Menstrual cycle hormone changes in women traversing menopause: Study of women's health across the nation, *Journal of Clinical Endocrinology and Metabolism*, 102(7), pp. 2218–2229.

'Oestrogen production is maintained at the same level in older women as it is in younger women': Shaw, N.D. *et al* (2015) Compensatory increase in ovarian aromatase in older regularly cycling women, *Journal of Clinical Endocrinology and Metabolism*, 100(9), pp. 3539–3547.

'and can even be higher': Santoro, N. *et al* (1996) Characterization of reproductive hormonal dynamics in the perimenopause, *Journal of Clinical Endocrinology and Metabolism*, 81(4), pp. 1495–1501.

Chapter 2

'in Western countries, up to 88 per cent of us will experience them': Feldman, B.M. *et al* (1985) The prevalence of hot flash and associated variables among perimenopausal women, *Research in Nursing and Health*, 8(3), pp. 261–268; Sievert, L.L. (2013) Subjective and objective measures of hot flashes, *American Journal of Human Biology*, 25(5), pp. 573–580.

'This number does vary and can be as low as 9.5 per cent in Japan': Lock, M. *et al* (1988) Cultural construction of the menopausal syndrome: the Japanese case, *Maturitas*, 10(4), pp. 317–332.

'a more recent study found the rate to be 36.9 per cent': Ishizuka, B. *et al* (2008) Cross-sectional community survey of menopause symptoms among Japanese women, *Maturitas*, 61(3), pp. 260–267.

'though some can last up to an hour': Kronenberg, F. (1990) Hot flashes: epidemiology and physiology, *Annals of the New York Academy of Sciences*, 592, pp. 52–133.

'the average duration was 7.4 years': Avis, N.E. *et al* (2015) Duration of menopausal vasomotor symptoms over the menopause transition, *JAMA Internal Medicine*, 175(4), pp. 531–539.

'At the age of 65, 25 per cent of us will still be experiencing them': Freeman, E.W. *et al* (2014) Risk of long-term hot flashes after natural menopause: evidence from the Penn Ovarian Aging Study cohort, *Menopause*, 21(9), pp. 924–932.

'In one study of women aged 85, around 16 per cent were still experiencing hot flushes and almost 10 per cent of these women were still moderately or very distressed by them': Vikström, J. *et al* (2013) Hot flushes still occur in a population of 85-year-old Swedish women, *Climacteric*, 16(4), pp. 453–459.

'History of taking the oral contraceptive pill': Gallicchio, L. *et al* (2015) Risk factors for hot flashes among women undergoing the menopausal transition: baseline results from the Midlife Women's Health Study, *Menopause*, 22(10), pp. 1098–1107.

'no relationships between the presence of hot flushes and the levels of oestrogens in blood, urine or the vagina': Aksel, S. *et al* (1976) Vasomotor symptoms, serum estrogens and gonadotropin levels in surgical menopause, *American Journal of Obstetrics and Gynecology*, 126(2), pp. 165–169.

'greater frequency and severity of hot flushes when compared to those who had lower levels of anxiety': Freeman, E.W. *et al* (2005) The role of anxiety and hormonal changes in menopausal hot flashes, *Menopause*, 12(3), pp. 258–266.

'in younger women not affected by breast cancer, no increased risk has been found': Kenemans, P. *et al* (2009) Safety and efficacy of tibolone in breast cancer patients with vasomotor symptoms: a doubleblind, randomised, non-inferiority trial, *Lancet Oncology*, 10(2), pp. 135–146.

'reduce the frequency and severity of hot flushes by anywhere from 10 to 64 per cent, depending on the study': Stubbs, C. *et al* (2017) Do SSRIs and SNRIs reduce the frequency and/or severity of hot flashes in menopausal women, *Journal – Oklahoma State Medical Association*, 110(5), pp. 272–274.

'it can reduce the frequency of hot flushes': Pandya, K.J. *et al* (2000) Oral clonidine in postmenopausal patients with breast cancer experiencing tamoxifen-induced hot flashes: a University of Rochester Cancer Center Community Clinical Oncology Program Study, *Annals of Internal Medicine*, 132(10), pp. 788–793.

'gabapentin is as effective as a low-dose oestrogen at improving vasomotor symptoms': Pandya, K.J. *et al* (2005) Gabapentin for hot flashes in 420 women with breast cancer: a randomised double-blind placebo-controlled trial, *Lancet*, 366(9488), pp. 818–824.

'it can also improve sleep quality': Yurcheshen, M.E. *et al* (2009) Effects of gabapentin on sleep in menopausal women with hot flashes as measured by a Pittsburgh sleep quality index factor scoring model, *Journal of Women's Health*, 18(9), pp. 1355–1360.

'does not interact with tamoxifen': Pandya, K.J. *et al* (2005) Gabapentin for hot flashes in 420 women with breast cancer: a randomised double-blind placebo-controlled trial, *Lancet*, 366(9488), pp. 818–824.

'paced respiration reduces frequency of hot flushes by 50 per cent': Freedman, R.R. and Woodward, S. (1992) Behavioral treatment of menopausal hot flushes: evaluation by ambulatory monitoring, *American Journal of Obstetrics and Gynecology*, 167(2), pp. 436–439; Irvin J.H. *et al* (1996) The effects of relaxation response training on menopausal symptoms, *Journal of Psychosomatic Obstetrics and Gynaecology*, 17(4), pp. 202–207.

'CBT is effective at reducing their impact': Mann, E. *et al* (2012) Cognitive behavioural treatment for women who have menopausal symptoms after breast cancer treatment (MENOS 1): a randomised controlled trial, *Lancet Oncology*, 13(3), pp. 309–318.

'supplementing with soy isoflavones for 12 weeks results in a reduction of hot flushes': Aso, T. *et al* (2012) A natural S-equol supplement alleviates hot flushes and other menopausal symptoms in equol nonproducing postmenopausal Japanese women, *Journal of Women's Health*, 21(1), pp. 92–100; Ferrari, A. (2009) Soy extract phytoestrogens with high dose of isoflavones for menopausal symptoms, *Journal of Obstetrics and Gynaecology Research*, 35(6), pp. 1083–1090.

'effective in treating menopausal symptoms such as hot flushes': Frei–Kleiner, S. *et al* (2005) Cimicifuga racemosa dried ethanolic extract in menopausal disorders: a double-blind placebo-controlled clinical trial, *Maturitas*, 51(4), pp. 397–404; Mohammad-Alizadeh-Charandabi, S. *et al* (2013) Efficacy of black cohosh (Cimicifuga racemosa L.) in treating early symptoms of menopause: a randomized clinical trial, *Chinese Medicine*, 8(1), p. 20.

'400 IUs of vitamin E a day for four weeks can reduce hot flushes': Ziaei, S. *et al* (2007) The effect of vitamin E on hot flashes in menopausal women, *Gynecologic and Obstetric Investigation*, 64(4), pp. 204–207.

'pomegranate seed oil can reduce menopausal symptoms': Auerbach, L. *et al* (2012) Pomegranate seed oil in women with menopausal symptoms: a prospective randomized, placebo-controlled, double-blinded trial, *Menopause*, 19(4), pp. 426–432; Huber, R. *et al* (2017) Pomegranate (Punica granatum) seed oil for treating menopausal symptoms: An individually controlled cohort study, *Alternative Therapies in Health and Medicine*, 23(2), pp. 28–34.

'can safely treat menopausal symptoms and reduce the severity of hot flushes': Heger, M. *et al* (2006) Efficacy and safety of a special extract of Rheum rhaponticum (ERr 731) in perimenopausal women with climacteric complaints: a 12-week randomized, double-blind, placebo-controlled trial, *Menopause*, 13(5), pp. 744–759 (published correction appears in *Menopause*, 14(2), p. 339).

'those with oestrogen-dependent cancers should not use it': Vollmer, G. *et al* (2010) Treatment of menopausal symptoms by an extract from the roots of rhapontic rhubarb: the role of estrogen receptors, *Chinese Medicine*, 5:7.

'high levels of these hormones can cause high blood pressure and other heart problems': Nambiar, V. and Chalappurath, D. (2019) Thrombotic tendencies in excess catecholamine states, Intechopen: https://www.intechopen.com/books/biogenic-amines-in-neurotransmission-and-human-disease/thrombotic-tendencies-in-excess-catecholamine-states.

'oestrogen protects against the toxic effects of these hormones': El-Battrawy I. *et al* (2018) Estradiol protection against toxic effects of catecholamine on electrical properties in human-induced pluripotent stem cell derived cardiomyocytes, *International Journal of Cardiology*, 254, pp. 195–202.

'the risk factors for hot flushes, such as increased weight and smoking, are also risk factors for an unfavourable cardiovascular risk profile': Franco, O.H. *et al* (2015) Vasomotor symptoms in women and cardiovascular risk markers: systematic review and meta-analysis, *Maturitas*, 81(3), pp. 353–361.

'it increases in thickness as oestrogen rises': Muizzuddin, N. *et al* (2005) Effect of systemic hormonal cyclicity on skin, *International Journal of Cosmetic Science*, 56(5), pp. 311–321; Eisenbeiss, C. *et al* (1998) The influence of female sex hormones on skin thickness: evaluation using 20 MHz sonography, *British Journal of Dermatology*, 139(3), pp. 462–467.

'the appearance of unwanted facial hair – though this can occur for other reasons too': Hall, G. and Phillips, T.J. (2005) Estrogen and skin: the effects of estrogen, menopause and hormone replacement therapy on the skin, *Journal of the American Academy of Dermatology*, 53(4), pp. 555–572.

'30 per cent of the collagen in your skin is lost in the first five years of postmenopausal life': Brincat, M. *et al* (1987) A study of the decrease of skin collagen content, skin thickness and bone mass in the postmenopausal woman, *Obstetrics and Gynecology*, 70(6), pp. 840–845.

'estimating skin changes could prove to be helpful in estimating bone changes': Aurégan, J.C. *et al* (2018) Correlation between skin and bone parameters in women with postmenopausal osteoporosis: A systematic review, *EFORT Open Reviews*, 3(8), pp. 449–460.

'Between 40 and 54 per cent of us will experience some degree of GSM': DiBonaventura, M. *et al* (2015) The association between vulvovaginal atrophy symptoms and quality of life among postmenopausal women in the United States and Western Europe, *Journal of Women's Health*, 24(9), pp. 713–722.

'only 4 per cent of those experiencing symptoms were able to connect their experience to GSM': Nappi, R.E. and Kokot–Kierepa, M. (2012) Vaginal health: insights, views and attitudes (VIVA) – results from an international survey, *Climacteric*, 15(1), pp. 36–44.

'Only 25 per cent of those with GSM will go to a healthcare practitioner': Palacios, S. (2009) Managing urogenital atrophy, *Maturitas*, 63(4), pp. 315–318.

'prevent important conversations about genital, sexual and urinary health from taking place': Wyeth REVEAL (2009) Revealing vaginal effects at mid-life: surveys of postmenopausal women and healthcare professionals who treat postmenopausal women; Nappi, R.E. and Kokot–Kierepa, M. (2010) Women's voices in the menopause: results from an international survey on vaginal atrophy, *Maturitas*, 67(3), pp. 233–238.

'10 to 15 per cent of those using systemic hormone therapy still experience vulvovaginal dryness': Management of symptomatic vulvovaginal atrophy: 2013 position statement of the North American Menopause Society (2013) *Menopause*, 20(9), pp. 888–904.

'the first non-hormonal treatment for GSM that can be used safely by those who can't use local oestrogen': DeGregorio, M.W. *et al* (2014) Ospemifene: a first-in-class, non-hormonal selective estrogen receptor modulator approved for the treatment of dyspareunia associated with vulvar and vaginal atrophy, *Steroids*, 90:82–93.

'following the surgical removal of the ovaries (which instigates instantaneous menopause) and after natural menopause': Castelo-Branco, C. *et al* (2005) Management of post–menopausal vaginal atrophy and atrophic vaginitis, *Maturitas*, 52, supplement 1, pp. 46–52.

'In people with IC, 75 per cent experience pain with intercourse': Peters, K.M. *et al* (2007) Sexual function and sexual distress in women with interstitial cystitis: a case-control study, *Urology*, 70(3), pp. 543–547.

'90 per cent of women with it report low sexual desire, difficulty with arousal, bladder pain during sex and an urge to urinate during sex': Bogart, L.M. *et al* (2011) Prevalence and correlates of sexual dysfunction among women with bladder pain syndrome/interstitial cystitis, *Urology*, 77(3), pp. 576–580.

'87 per cent of participants with IC had pelvic floor dysfunction': Peters, K.M. *et al* (2007) Prevalence of pelvic floor dysfunction in patients with interstitial cystitis, *Urology*, 70(1), pp. 16–18.

'weaken bladder support and therefore increase the risk of stress incontinence': Robinson, D. and Cardozo, L. (2011) Estrogens and the lower urinary tract, *Neurourology and Urodynamics*, 30(5), pp. 754–757.

'use of oestrogen therapy to treat pure stress incontinence is not recommended': Baber, R.J., Panay, N., Fenton, A. and IMS Writing Group (2016) IMS recommendations on women's midlife health and menopause hormone therapy, *Climacteric*, 19(2), pp. 109–150.

'reduced oestrogen levels can affect the tissues surrounding the urethra': Castelo-Branco, C. *et al* (2005) Management of post-menopausal vaginal atrophy and atrophic vaginitis, *Maturitas*, 52, supplement 1, pp. 46–52.

'Between 40 and 59 a quarter of us will experience it': Nygaard, I. *et al* (2008) Prevalence of symptomatic pelvic floor disorders in US women, *JAMA*, 300(11), pp. 1311–1316.

'By 80 half of us will have pelvic floor issues': Nygaard, I. *et al* (2008) *ibid.*

'with exposure to urine it can jump up to 8.0': Gray, M. (2004) Preventing and managing perineal dermatitis: a shared goal for wound and continence care, *Journal of Wound Ostomy and Continence Nursing* 31(1), pp. S2–S12.

Chapter 3

'The prescription rate for MHT fell by 65–70 per cent in 2002': Kim, N. *et al* (2005) The impact of clinical trials on the use of hormone replacement therapy: a population-based study, *Journal of General Internal Medicine*, 20(11), pp. 1026–1031; Roumie, C.L. *et al.* A three-part intervention to change the use of hormone replacement therapy in response to new evidence, *Annals of Internal Medicine*, 141(2), pp. 118–125.

'they were at 55 per cent greater risk': Karim, R. *et al* (2011) Hip fracture in postmenopausal women after cessation of hormone therapy: results from a prospective study in a large health management organization, *Menopause*, 18(11), pp. 1172–1177.

'I recommend you read an amazing review': Hodis, H.N. and Sarrel, P.M. (2018) Menopausal hormone therapy and breast cancer: what is the evidence from randomized trials? *Climacteric*, 21(6), pp. 521–528.

'reduction in the breast cancer rate of 32 per cent when compared to those taking the placebo': Stefanick, M.L. *et al* (2006) Effects of conjugated equine estrogens on breast cancer and mammography screening in postmenopausal women with hysterectomy, *JAMA*, 295(14), pp. 1647–1657.

'statistically significant reduction of 29 per cent in rate of ductal carcinoma – the most common type of breast cancer': Stefanick, M.L. *et al* (2006) Effects of conjugated equine estrogens on breast cancer and mammography screening in postmenopausal women with hysterectomy, *JAMA*, 295(14), pp. 1647–1657.

'no increased risk of death from cardiovascular disease or cancer was found in those who took hormone therapy': Manson, J.E. *et al* (2017) Menopausal hormone therapy and long-term all-cause and cause-specific mortality: the Women's Health Initiative randomized trials, *JAMA*, 318(10), pp. 927–938.

'those in the placebo arm of the trial *who had previously used hormone therapy* had a decreased risk': Langer, R.D. (2017) The evidence base for HRT: what can we believe? *Climacteric,* 20(2), pp. 91–96.

'Breast cancer risk from using HRT is "twice what was thought"': https://www.theguardian.com/science/2019/aug/29/breast-cancer-risk-from-using-hrt-is-twice-what-was-thought.

'the NHS also points out that around three in every 200 screenings picks up a cancer that wouldn't have otherwise been picked up or become life-threatening': https://www.uhs.nhs.uk/Media/SUHTInternet/Services/BreastImagingUnit/NHS-Breast-Screening---helping-you-decide.pdf.

'one third of non-fatal cardiovascular events occur in women below the age of 60': Baber, R.J., Panay, N., Fenton, A. and IMS Writing Group (2016) IMS recommendations on women's midlife health and menopause hormone therapy, *Climacteric*, 19(2), pp. 109–150.

'It also exerts an anti-inflammatory effect on them': Simoncini, T. *et al* (2004) Genomic and non-genomic effects of estrogens on endothelial cells, *Steroids,* 69(8–9), pp. 537–542.

'heart attack and stroke were *only* seen in the women who had been postmenopausal for 20 or more years': Speroff, L. (2004) A clinician's review of the WHI–related literature, *International Journal of Fertility and Women's Medicine*, 49(6), pp. 252–267.

'HRT significantly *reduced* coronary heart disease in younger women, but not in older women': Salpeter, S.R. *et al* (2006) Brief report: coronary heart disease events associated with hormone therapy in younger and older women: a meta-analysis, *Journal of General Internal Medicine,* 21(4), pp. 363–366 (published correction appears in *Journal of General Internal Medicine*, 23(10), p. 1728).

'supplementing with oestrogen might be useful when it comes to preserving oestrogen receptors and their function during the postmenopausal years': Fu, X.D. and Simoncini, T. (2008) Extra-nuclear signaling of estrogen receptors, *International Union of Biochemistry and Molecular Biology Life*, 60(8), pp. 502–510.

'The current NICE guidance is as follows': https://www.nice.org.uk/guidance/ng23.

'oestrogen reduces the quantity of free radicals generated by mitochondria': Razmara, A. *et al* (2007) Estrogen suppresses brain mitochondrial oxidative stress in female and male rats, *Brain Research*, 1176:71–81.

'glyphosate has also been linked to tens of thousands of cancer cases': https://www.cancerhealth.com/article/bayer-pay-10-billion-settle-roundup-cancer-lawsuits.

'when someone under the age of 40 has had no periods for four months or more': Nelson, L.M. *et al* (1996) Premature ovarian failure. In: Adashi, E.Y., Rock, J.A.

and Rosenwaks, Z., (eds), *Reproductive Endocrinology, Surgery and Technology*, Lippincott-Raven, pp. 1393–410; Woad, K.J. *et al* (2006) The genetic basis of premature ovarian failure, *Australian and New Zealand Journal of Obstetrics and Gynaecology*, 46(3), pp. 242–244.

'Hopefully this figure has reduced since the paper was published in 2002': Alzubaidi, N.H. *et al* (2002) Meeting the needs of young women with secondary amenorrhea and spontaneous premature ovarian failure, *Obstetrics and Gynecology*, 99(5) (Part 1), pp. 720–725.

'5 to 10 per cent of people diagnosed with POI will conceive and have a baby post-diagnosis': Bidet, M. *et al* (2008) Premature ovarian failure: predictability of intermittent ovarian function and response to ovulation induction agents, *Current Opinions in Obstetrics and Gynecology*, 20(4), pp. 416–420; Welt, C.K. (2008) Primary ovarian insufficiency: a more accurate term for premature ovarian failure, *Clinical Endocrinology (Oxford)*, 68(4), pp. 499–509; van Kasteren, Y.M. and Schoemaker, J. (1999) Premature ovarian failure: a systematic review on therapeutic interventions to restore ovarian function and achieve pregnancy, *Human Reproduction Update*, 5(5), pp. 483–492.

'hormone therapy and tibolone are generally not recommended to treat menopausal symptoms such as hot flushes, night sweats and genito-urinary syndrome of menopause': Pinkerton, J.V. and Santen, R.J. (2019) Managing vasomotor symptoms in women after cancer, *Climacteric*, 22(6), pp. 544–552.

'Short-term use of HRT following risk-reducing surgery is not associated with an increased risk of breast cancer': Rebbeck, T.R. *et al* (2005) Effect of short-term hormone replacement therapy on breast cancer risk reduction after bilateral prophylactic oophorectomy in BRCA1 and BRCA2 mutation carriers: the PROSE Study Group, *Journal of Clinical Oncology*, 23(31), pp. 7804–7810.

'in one small study it decreased the risk': Eisen, A. *et al* (2008) Hormone therapy and the risk of breast cancer in BRCA1 mutation carriers, *Journal of the National Cancer Institute*, 100(19), pp. 1361–1367.

'affects at least 1 per cent of women under the age of 40, 0.1 per cent of women under the age of 30 and 0.01 per cent of those under 20': Coulam, C.B. *et al* (1986) Incidence of premature ovarian failure, *Obstetrics and Gynecology*, 67(4), pp. 604–606.

'their periods don't return following pregnancy or when they come off the contraceptive pill': Shelling, A.N. (2010) Premature ovarian failure, *Reproduction*, 140(5), pp. 633–641.

'MHT is widely accepted as an essential treatment strategy for those with POI': de Villiers, T.J. *et al* (2013) Global consensus statement on menopausal hormone therapy, *Climacteric*, 16(2), pp. 203–204.

'Progesterone can also improve hot flushes': Prior, J.C. and Hitchcock, C.L. (2012) Progesterone for hot flush and night sweat treatment – effectiveness for severe vasomotor symptoms and lack of withdrawal rebound, *Gynecological Endocrinology*, 28, Supplement 2, pp. 7–11.

'four separate studies have found no risk or a lower risk of breast cancer with the use of micronised progesterone': Fournier, A. *et al* (2005) Breast cancer risk in relation to different types of hormone replacement therapy in the E3N–EPIC cohort, *International Journal of Cancer*, 114(3), pp. 448–454; Fournier, A. *et al* (2008) Unequal risks for breast cancer associated with different hormone replacement therapies: results from the E3N cohort study, *Breast Cancer Research and Treatment*, 107(1), pp. 103–111 (published correction appears in *Breast Cancer Research and Treatment*, 107(2), pp. 307–308); Espié, M. *et al* (2007) Breast cancer incidence and hormone replacement therapy: results from the MISSION study, prospective phase, *Gynecological Endocrinol*ogy, 23(7), pp. 391–397; Cordina-Duverger, E. *et al* (2013) Risk of breast cancer by type of menopausal hormone therapy: a case-control study among post-menopausal women in France, *PLoS One*, 8(11), p. e78016.

'a full or partial hysterectomy is known to significantly reduce the risk of breast cancer': Press, D.J. *et al* (2011) Breast cancer risk and ovariectomy, hysterectomy and tubal sterilization in the women's contraceptive and reproductive experiences study, *American Journal of Epidemiology*, 173(1), pp. 38–47.

'progesterone/progestogen decreases the risk of endometrial cancer': Manson, J.E. *et al* (2017) Menopausal hormone therapy and long-term all-cause and cause-specific mortality: The Women's Health Initiative randomized trials, *JAMA*, 318(10), pp. 927–938.

'a menopause survey to assess the level of menopause education and training among GPs': https://www.bjfm.co.uk/results-from-the-bjfm-menopause-survey.

Chapter 4

Unless otherwise stated, all the perfect use and typical use rates of the various forms of contraception in this chapter are taken from the NHS contraception guide: https://www.nhs.uk/conditions/contraception/how-effective-contraception.

'one small outdated study which didn't involve microscopic examination of vaginal tissue': Leiblum, S. *et al* (1983) Vaginal atrophy in the postmenopausal woman: the importance of sexual activity and hormones, *JAMA*, 249(16), pp. 2195–2198.

'A more recent study that did look for cellular differences in the vaginal tissue': Hickey, M. *et al* (2017) Non-hormonal treatments for menopausal symptoms, *British Medical Journal*, 359:j5101.

'The unplanned pregnancy rate in those over 40 is 40 per cent': Finer, L.B. (2010) Unintended pregnancy among US adolescents: accounting for sexual activity, *Journal of Adolescent Health*, 47(3), pp. 312–314.

'still estimated to be around 10 per cent chance per year': Baldwin, M.K. and Jensen, J.T. (2013) Contraception during the perimenopause, *Maturitas*, 76(3), pp. 235–242.

'25 per cent of cycles longer than 50 days are ones where ovulation takes place': Fritz, M. and Speroff, L. (2011) *Clinical Gynecologic Endocrinology and Infertility*, 8th edition.

'the current guidance is that contraception should be used for at least two years following your last period': https://patient.info/sexual-health/contraception-methods/contraception-for-the-mature-woman.

'A simpler, safer and more reliable option than female sterilisation': https://sexualhealthdorset.org/contraception/male-sterilisation-vasectomy.

'58 per cent of people using the combined pill take it for non-contraceptive reasons': Jones, R.K. (2011) *Beyond Birth Control: The Overlooked Benefits of Oral Contraceptive Pills*, Guttmacher Institute.

'it can also suppress ovulation in up to 85 per cent of cycles in the first year of use': Kailasam, C. and Cahill, D. (2008) Review of the safety, efficacy and patient acceptability of the levonorgestrel-releasing intrauterine system, *Patient Preference and Adherence*, 2, pp. 293–302.

'There is a small but serious risk of pelvic inflammatory disease': Farley, T.M. *et al* (1992) Intrauterine devices and pelvic inflammatory disease: an international perspective, *Lancet*, 339(8796), pp. 785–788.

'after four months of not taking the pill, levels of SHBG still remained high': Panzer, C. *et al* (2006) Impact of oral contraceptives on sex hormone-binding globulin and androgen levels: a retrospective study in women with sexual dysfunction, *The Journal of Sexual Medicine*, 3(1), pp. 104–113.

'One study of 22 healthy women found that after three months of being on the pill': Battaglia, C. *et al* (2011) Sexual behaviour and oral contraception: a pilot study, *The Journal of Sexual Medicine*, 9(2), pp. 550–557.

'Another small study found that clitoral volume decreases too': Battaglia, C. *et al* (2014) Clitoral vascularization and sexual behavior in young patients treated with drospirenone-ethinyl estradiol or contraceptive vaginal ring: a prospective, randomized, pilot study, *The Journal of Sexual Medicine*, 11(2), pp. 471–480.

'women taking hormonal contraception were more likely to be diagnosed with depression': Skovlund, C.W. *et al* (2016) Association of hormonal contraception with depression, *JAMA Psychiatry*, 73(11), pp. 1154–1162 (published correction appears in *JAMA Psychiatry*, 74(7), p. 764).

'one small study of five men didn't find a single sperm': Zukerman, Z. *et al* (2003) Does preejaculatory penile secretion originating from Cowper's gland contain sperm? *Journal of Assisted Reproduction and Genetics*, 20(4), pp. 157–159.

'a later study of 27 men found that sperm were present in 11 participants' samples': Killick, S.R. *et al* (2011) Sperm content of pre-ejaculatory fluid, *Human Fertility*, 14(1), pp. 48–52.

'With typical use this falls to 76 to 98.2 per cent': Frank-Herrmann, P. *et al* (2007) The effectiveness of a fertility awareness-based method to avoid pregnancy in relation to a couple's sexual behaviour during the fertile time: a prospective longitudinal study. *Human Reproduction*, 22(5), pp. 1310–1319.

'One study of 160 couples where the women were 40 to 55 years old': Fehring, R.J. and Mu, Q. (2014) Cohort efficacy study of natural family planning among perimenopause age women, *Journal of Obstetric, Gynecologic and Neonatal Nursing*, 43(3) pp. 351–358.

Chapter 5

'When you have PMDD, genetic differences mean you process sex hormones differently': Dubey, N. *et al* (2017) The ESC/E(Z) complex, an effector of response to ovarian steroids, manifests an intrinsic difference in cells from women with premenstrual dysphoric disorder, *Molecular Psychiatry*, 22(8), pp. 1172–1184.

'variations in the oestrogen receptor alpha (OSR1) gene and an over-expression of ESC/E(Z) genes': Huo, L. *et al* (2007) Risk for premenstrual dysphoric disorder is associated with genetic variation in ESR1, the estrogen receptor alpha gene, *Biological Psychiatry*, 62(8), pp. 925–933.

'establishes that women with PMDD have an intrinsic difference in their molecular apparatus for response to sex hormones': https://www.nih.gov/news-events/news-releases/sex-hormone-sensitive-gene-complex-linked-premenstrual-mood-disorder.

'There is only one study which looks at autism and menopause': Moseley, R.L. *et al* (2020) 'When my autism broke': a qualitative study spotlighting autistic voices on menopause, *Autism*, 24(6), pp. 1423–1437.

'when progesterone is high in the second half of the cycle': Bäckström, T. *et al* (2014) Allopregnanolone and mood disorders, *Progress in Neurobiology*, 113, pp. 88–94.

'Premenstrual depression, postnatal depression and climacteric depression are related to changes in ovarian hormone levels': Studd, J.W. (2011) A guide to the treatment of depression in women by estrogens, *Climacteric*, 14(6), pp. 637–642.

'Progestogen intolerance produces symptoms': Panay, N. and Studd, J. (1997) Progestogen intolerance and compliance with hormone replacement therapy in menopausal women, *Human Reproduction Update*, 3(2), pp. 159–171.

'substantial systemic absorption of progestogen does happen': Xiao, B. *et al* (2003) Therapeutic effects of the levonorgestrel-releasing intrauterine system in the treatment of idiopathic menorrhagia, *Fertility and Sterility*, 79(4), pp. 963–969.

'the lifetime prevalence of experiencing major depression is 20 per cent': Kessler, R.C. *et al* (1994) Lifetime and 12-month prevalence of DSM-III-R psychiatric disorders in

the United States: results from the National Comorbidity Survey, *Archives of General Psychiatry*, 51(1), pp. 8–19.
'A 2001 study of 10,374 women aged between 40 and 55 found that': Bromberger, J.T. *et al* (2001) Psychologic distress and natural menopause: a multi-ethnic community study, *American Journal of Public Health* 91(9), pp. 1435–1442.
'more likely to be related to demographic factors and health habits': Gallicchio, L. *et al* (2007) Correlates of depressive symptoms among women undergoing the menopausal transition, *Journal of Psychosomatic Research*, 63(3), pp. 263–268.
'events such as divorce or the death of a loved one make you two and a half to five times as likely to experience depressive symptoms': Bromberger, J.T. *et al* (2010) Longitudinal change in reproductive hormones and depressive symptoms across the menopausal transition: results from the Study of Women's Health Across the Nation (SWAN), *Archives of General Psychiatry*, 67(6), pp. 598–607.
'Given the potential side effects of taking antidepressants': Carvalho, A.F. *et al* (2016) The safety, tolerability and risks associated with the use of newer generation antidepressant drugs: a critical review of the literature, *Psychotherapy and Psychosomatics*, 85(5), pp. 270–288.
'demonstrates a strong association between anxiety and hot flushes': Freeman, E.W. *et al* (2007) Symptoms associated with menopausal transition and reproductive hormones in midlife women, *Obstetrics and Gynecology*, 110(2) Part 1, pp. 230–240.
'a high level of social support protects against developing depression by as much as 20 per cent': Bromberger, J.T. *et al* (2010) Longitudinal change in reproductive hormones and depressive symptoms across the menopausal transition: results from the Study of Women's Health Across the Nation (SWAN), *Archives of General Psychiatry*, 67(6), pp. 598–607.
'The NHS website, for example, has some very straightforward, easy-to-follow, exercises': https://www.nhs.uk/conditions/stress-anxiety-depression/ways-relieve-stress.
'was found to be just as effective as taking antidepressants': Blumenthal, J.A. *et al* (1999) Effects of exercise training on older patients with major depression, *Archives of Internal Medicine*, 159(19), pp. 2349–2356.
'resulted in significant reductions in participants' depressive symptoms': Gordon, B.R. *et al* (2018) Association of efficacy of resistance exercise training with depressive symptoms: meta-analysis and meta-regression analysis of randomized clinical trials, *JAMA Psychiatry*, 75(6), pp. 566–576.
'fish oil can improve anxiety and depression': Mocking, R.J. *et al* (2016) Meta-analysis and meta-regression of omega-3 polyunsaturated fatty acid supplementation for major depressive disorder, *Translational Psychiatry*, 6(3), p. e756.
'response to supplementing with iron when you're deficient': Sirdah, M.M. *et al* (2002) Possible ameliorative effect of taurine in the treatment of iron-deficiency anaemia

in female university students of Gaza, Palestine, *European Journal of Haematology*, 69(4), pp. 236–242.

'increases production of GABA, which calms your nervous system': Wu, Q. and Shah, N.P. (2018) Restoration of GABA production machinery in Lactobacillus brevis by accessible carbohydrates, anaerobiosis and early acidification, *Food Microbiology*, 69, pp. 151–158.

'They also make tryptophan more available to your brain': Spring, B. (1984) Recent research on the behavioral effects of tryptophan and carbohydrate, *Nutrition and Health*, 3(1–2), pp. 55–67.

'a diet that's deficient in tryptophan results in poor sleep quality': Bhatti, T. *et al* (1998) Effects of a tryptophan-free amino acid drink challenge on normal human sleep electroencephalogram and mood, *Biological Psychiatry*, 43(1), pp. 52–59.

'magnesium deficiency is common': DiNicolantonio, J.J. *et al* (2018) Subclinical magnesium deficiency: a principal driver of cardiovascular disease and a public health crisis, *Open Heart*, 5(1), p. e000668 (published correction appears in *Open Heart*, 5(1), p. e000668corr1).

'it's as effective as taking fluoxetine (Prozac)': Sanmukhani, J. *et al* (2014) Efficacy and safety of curcumin in major depressive disorder: a randomized controlled trial, *Phytotherapy Research*, 28(4), pp. 579–585.

'more rapid relief from symptoms than when they're taken on their own': Bergman, J. *et al* (2013) Curcumin as an add-on to antidepressive treatment: a randomized, double-blind, placebo-controlled, pilot clinical study, *Clinical Neuropharmacology*, 36(3), pp. 73–77.

'Oestradiol depresses the formation of taurine': Ritz, M.F. *et al* (2002) 17beta-estradiol effect on the extracellular concentration of amino acids in the glutamate excitotoxicity model in the rat. *Neurochemical Research*, 27(12), pp. 1677–1683; Ma, Q. *et al* (2015) Estradiol decreases taurine level by reducing cysteine sulfinic acid decarboxylase via the estrogen receptor–a in female mice liver, *American Journal of Physiology – Gastrointestinal and Liver Physiology*, 308(4), pp. G277–G286.

'plays a major role in the release of neurotransmitters': Wu, J.Y. and Prentice, H. (2010) Role of taurine in the central nervous system, *Journal of Biomedical Science*, 17, Supplement 1, p. S1.

'the activation of GABA receptors in the brain': Ochoa-de la Paz. L. *et al* (2019) Taurine and GABA neurotransmitter receptors, a relationship with therapeutic potential? *Expert Review of Neurotherapeutics*, 19(4), pp. 289–291.

'stimulates bone formation and inhibits bone resorption': Gupta, R.C. and Kim, S.J. (2003) Taurine, analogues and bone: a growing relationship, *Advances in Experimental Medicine and Biology*, 526, pp. 323–328.

'can improve insulin sensitivity': Ito, T. *et al* (2012) The potential usefulness of taurine on diabetes mellitus and its complications, *Amino Acids*, 42(5), pp. 1529–1539.

'it may be useful for those with neurodegenerative diseases': Kuboyama, T. *et al* (2005) Neuritic regeneration and synaptic reconstruction induced by withanolide A, *British Journal of Pharmacology*, 144(7), pp. 961–971.

'It can help with stress of all kinds – physical, chemical and psychological': Cohen, M.M. (2014) Tulsi – Ocimum sanctum: A herb for all reasons, *Journal of Ayurveda and Integrative Medicine*, 5(4), pp. 251–259.

'two compounds that have been shown to stimulate the growth of brain cells': Lai, P.L. *et al* (2013) Neurotrophic properties of the lion's mane medicinal mushroom, Hericium erinaceus (Higher Basidiomycetes) from Malaysia, *International Journal of Medicinal Mushrooms*, 15(6), pp. 539–554.

'prevent the nerve damage associated with Alzheimer's disease': Mori, K. *et al* (2011) Effects of Hericium erinaceus on amyloid β(25–35) peptide-induced learning and memory deficits in mice. *Biomedical Research*, 32(1), pp. 67–72; Chang, H.C. *et al* (2016) Hericium erinaceus inhibits TNFα–i-nduced angiogenesis and ROS generation through suppression of MMP-9/NF-κB signaling and activation of Nrf2-mediated antioxidant genes in human EA.hy926 endothelial cells, *Oxidative Medicine and Cell Longevity*, 8257238.

'reduce depression': Chiu, C.H. *et al* (2018) Erinacine A-enriched Hericium erinaceus mycelium produces antidepressant–like effects through modulating BDNF/PI3K/Akt/GSK–3β signaling in mice, *International Journal of Molecular Sciences*, 19(2), p. 341.

'lower blood sugar levels': Liang, B. *et al* (2013) Antihyperglycemic and antihyperlipidemic activities of aqueous extract of Hericium erinaceus in experimental diabetic rats, *BMC Complementary and Alternative Medicine*, 13, p. 253.

'menopausal women found that eating them reduced feelings of irritation and anxiety': Nagano, M. *et al* (2010) Reduction of depression and anxiety by 4 weeks' Hericium erinaceus intake, *Biomed Research,* 31(4), pp. 231–237.

'influencing the immune system and nerve cell degeneration': Wang, J. *et al* (2017) Emerging roles of *Ganoderma Lucidum* in anti-aging, *Aging and Disease*, 8(6), pp. 691–707.

'forgetfulness was the third most commonly reported symptom': Gold, E.B. *et al* (2000) Relation of demographic and lifestyle factors to symptoms in a multi-racial/ethnic population of women 40–55 years of age, *American Journal of Epidemiology*, 152(5), pp. 463–473.

'BDNF is also involved in depression and is thought to play a role in emotional regulation': Sairanen, M. *et al* (2005) Brain-derived neurotrophic factor and antidepressant drugs have different but coordinated effects on neuronal turnover, proliferation and survival in the adult dentate gyrus, *Journal of Neuroscience*, 25(5), pp. 1089–1094.

'oestrogen hormone therapy increases BDNF and improves mood and depression:' Su, Q. *et al* (2016) Estrogen therapy increases BDNF expression and improves post-stroke depression in ovariectomy-treated rats, *Experimental and Therapeutic Medicine*, 12(3), pp. 1843–1848.

'So does exercise': Liu, P.Z. and Nusslock, R. (2018) Exercise-mediated neurogenesis in the hippocampus via BDNF, *Frontiers in Neuroscience*, 12, p. 52.

'it inhibited their ability to recall information': Newcomer, J.W. *et al* (1999) Decreased memory performance in healthy humans induced by stress-level cortisol treatment, *Archives of General Psychiatry*, 56(6), pp. 527–533.

'those taking oestrogen did not': Sherwin, B.B. (1988) Estrogen and/or androgen replacement therapy and cognitive functioning in surgically menopausal women, *Psychoneuroendocrinology*, 13(4), pp. 345–357.

'The main research being referred to is the Women's Health Initiative Memory Study (WHIMS)': Shumaker, S.A. *et al* (1998) The Women's Health Initiative Memory Study (WHIMS): a trial of the effect of estrogen therapy in preventing and slowing the progression of dementia, *Controlled Clinical Trials*, 19(6), pp. 604–621.

'oestrogen regulates the growth of nerve cells': Cambiasso, M.J. and Carrer, H.F. (2001) Nongenomic mechanism mediates estradiol stimulation of axon growth in male rat hypothalamic neurons in vitro, *Journal of Neuroscience Research*, 66(3), pp. 475–481.

'the damage resulting from blocked arteries in the brain that causes ischemic stroke': Simpkins, J.W. *et al* (1997) Estrogens may reduce mortality and ischemic damage caused by middle cerebral artery occlusion in the female rat, *Journal of Neurosurgery*, 87(5), pp. 724–730.

'potential way of preventing the kind of dementia associated with Alzheimer's disease': Simpkins, J.W. *et al* (1997) Role of estrogen replacement therapy in memory enhancement and the prevention of neuronal loss associated with Alzheimer's disease. *American Journal of Medicine*, 103(3A), pp. 19S–25S; Resnick, S.M. *et al* (1997) Estrogen replacement therapy and longitudinal decline in visual memory: a possible protective effect? *Neurology*, 49(6), pp. 1491–1497.

'why postmenopausal women are more likely then to develop the disease': (2000) Estrogen deprivation leads to death of dopamine cells in the brain. ScienceDaily: www.sciencedaily.com/releases/2000/12/001204072446.htm (source: Yale University).

Chapter 7

'progesterone becomes increasingly absent and reduces the rate of energy consumption during the luteal phase': Webb, P. (1986) 24-hour energy expenditure and the menstrual cycle, *American Journal of Clinical Nutrition*, 44(5), pp. 614–619.

'the scientific way of describing a spare tyre': Peppa, M. *et al* (2013) Body composition determinants of metabolic phenotypes of obesity in nonobese and obese postmenopausal women, *Obesity (Silver Spring)*, 21(9), pp. 1807–1814.

'why the cancer rate is higher amongst those who are diabetic and/or obese': Doyle, S.L. *et al* (2012) Visceral obesity, metabolic syndrome, insulin resistance and cancer, *Proceedings of the Nutrition Society*, 71(1), pp. 181–189.

'underlying cause of insulin resistance and development of type 2 diabetes': Barbagallo, M. and Dominguez, L.J. (2007) Magnesium metabolism in type 2 diabetes mellitus, metabolic syndrome and insulin resistance, *Archives of Biochemistry and Biophysics*, 458(1), pp. 40–47.

'the lower magnesium is, the more insulin resistance there is': Humphries, S. *et al* (1999) Low dietary magnesium is associated with insulin resistance in a sample of young, nondiabetic Black Americans, *American Journal of Hypertension*, 12(8) Part 1, pp. 747–756.

'magnesium improves insulin sensitivity': Morais, J.B.S. *et al* (2017) Effect of magnesium supplementation on insulin resistance in humans: a systematic review, *Nutrition*, 38, pp. 54–60.

'why it's an effective treatment strategy for those with PCOS': Costantino, D. *et al* (2009) Metabolic and hormonal effects of myo-inositol in women with polycystic ovary syndrome: a double-blind trial, *European Review for Medical and Pharmacological Sciences*, 13(2), pp. 105–110.

'support mood changes in the premenstrual phase of the cycle and PMDD': Gianfranco, C. *et al* (2011) Myo-inositol in the treatment of premenstrual dysphoric disorder, *Human Psychopharmacology*, 26(7), pp. 526–530; Cunningham, J. *et al* (2009) Update on research and treatment of premenstrual dysphoric disorder, *Harvard Review of Psychiatry*, 17(2), pp. 120–137.

'positive effects when used in the treatment of metabolic syndrome in postmenopausal women'; Giordano, D. *et al* (2011) Effects of myo-inositol supplementation in postmenopausal women with metabolic syndrome: a perspective, randomized, placebo-controlled study, *Menopause*, 18(1), pp. 102–104.

'A ratio of 40:1 for myo-inositol to D-chiro-inositol is recommended': Nordio, M. *et al* (2019) The 40:1 myo-inositol/D-chiro-inositol plasma ratio is able to restore ovulation in PCOS patients: comparison with other ratios, *European Review for Medical and Pharmacological Sciences*, 23(12), pp. 5512–5521.

'It also improves insulin sensitivity': Eason, R.C. *et al* (2002) Lipoic acid increases glucose uptake by skeletal muscles of obese-diabetic ob/ob mice, *Diabetes Obesity and Metabolism*, 4(1), pp. 29–35.

'and can support weight loss': Li, N. *et al* (2017) Effects of oral α-lipoic acid administration on body weight in overweight or obese subjects: a crossover randomized, double-blind, placebo-controlled trial, *Clinical Endocrinology (Oxford)*, 86(5), pp. 680–687.

'significant improvements to all the components of metabolic syndrome': Gupta Jain, S. *et al* (2017) Effect of oral cinnamon intervention on metabolic profile and body composition of Asian Indians with metabolic syndrome: a randomized double-blind control trial, *Lipids in Health and Disease*, 16(1), p. 113.

'can improve cholesterol levels': Khan, A. *et al* (2003) Cinnamon improves glucose and lipids of people with type 2 diabetes, *Diabetes Care*, 26(12), pp. 3215–3218.

'enhance insulin sensitivity and improve glucose tolerance': Hajimehdipoor, H. *et al* (2008) Identification and quantitative determination of blood lowering sugar amino acid in fenugreek, *Planta Medica*, 74:PH12; Broca, C. *et al* (2004) Insulinotropic agent ID–1101 (4–hydroxyisoleucine) activates insulin signaling in rat, *American Journal of Physiology-Endocrinologyand Metabolism*, 287(3), pp. E463–E471.

'improve cholesterol levels': Shamshad Begum, S. *et al* (2016) A novel extract of fenugreek husk (FenuSMART™) alleviates postmenopausal symptoms and helps to establish the hormonal balance: a randomized, double-blind, placebo-controlled study, *Phytotherapy Research*, 30(11), pp. 1775–1784.

'Berberine has proved to be equal to or superior to metformin at improving insulin resistance': Wei, W. *et al* (2012) A clinical study on the short-term effect of berberine in comparison to metformin on the metabolic characteristics of women with polycystic ovary syndrome, *European Journal of Endocrinology*, 166(1), pp. 99–105.

'Diets that are low in chromium have a negative effect on glucose and insulin': Anderson, R.A. *et al* (1991) Supplemental–chromium effects on glucose, insulin, glucagon and urinary chromium losses in subjects consuming controlled low-chromium diets, *American Journal of Clinical Nutrition*, 54(5), pp. 909–916.

'reduce food cravings and improve eating behaviours, thereby supporting weight loss': Choudhary, D. *et al* (2017) Body weight management in adults under chronic stress through treatment with ashwagandha root extract: a double-blind, randomized, placebo-controlled trial, *Journal of Evidence-Based Complementary Integrative Medicine*, 22(1), pp. 96–106.

'a single night of sleep deprivation doubles cortisol production the following morning': Joo, E.Y. *et al* (2012) Adverse effects of 24 hours of sleep deprivation on cognition and stress hormones, *Journal of Clinical Neurology*, 8(2), pp. 146–150.

'decreases insulin sensitivity by 40 per cent': Spiegel, K. *et al* (2005). Sleep loss: a novel risk factor for insulin resistance and type 2 diabetes, *Journal of Applied Physiology*, 99(5), pp. 2008–2019.

'get less than five to six hours' sleep or more than eight to 10 hours': Ju, S.Y. and Choi, W.S. (2013) Sleep duration and metabolic syndrome in adult populations: a meta-analysis of observational studies, *Nutrition and Diabetes*, 3(5), p. e65.

'shorter sleep duration was associated with an increased risk of metabolic syndrome, but longer sleep duration was not': Xi, B. *et al* (2014) Short sleep duration predicts risk of metabolic syndrome: a systematic review and meta-analysis, *Sleep Medicine Reviews*, 18(4), pp. 293–297.

'When you're sleep-deprived, leptin – the hormone that tells you when you're full – can go down and ghrelin levels can spike': Spiegel, K. *et al* (2004) Brief communication: Sleep curtailment in healthy young men is associated with decreased leptin levels, elevated ghrelin levels, and increased hunger and appetite. *Annals of Internal Medicine*, 141(11), pp. 846–850.

'protein suppresses ghrelin': Blom, W.A. *et al* (2006) Effect of a high-protein breakfast on the postprandial ghrelin response, *American Journal of Clinical Nutrition*, 83(2), pp. 211–220.

'ketosis suppresses the increase in ghrelin that can occur with weight loss': Sumithran, P. *et al* (2013) Ketosis and appetite-mediating nutrients and hormones after weight loss, *European Journal of Clinical Nutrition*, 67(7), pp. 759–764.

'Metabolic syndrome is more common in midlife women than men': Beigh, S.H. and Jain, S. (2012) Prevalence of metabolic syndrome and gender differences, *Bioinformation*, 8(13), pp. 613–616.

'it also affects us more': Rossi, M.C. *et al* (2013) Sex disparities in the quality of diabetes care: biological and cultural factors may play a different role for different outcomes: a cross-sectional observational study from the AMD Annals initiative. *Diabetes Care*, 36(10), pp. 3162–3168.

'E2 has a protective effect on the prevention of diabetes and metabolic syndrome': Pentti, K. *et al* (2009) Hormone therapy protects from diabetes: the Kuopio osteoporosis risk factor and prevention study, *European Journal of Endocrinology*, 160(6), pp. 979–83.

and

Kanaya, A.M. *et al* (2003) Glycemic effects of postmenopausal hormone therapy: the Heart and Estrogen/progestin Replacement Study. A randomized, double-blind, placebo-controlled trial. *Annals of Internal Medicine*, 138(1) pp. 1–9.

and

Margolis, K.L. *et al* (2004) Effect of oestrogen plus progestin on the incidence of diabetes in postmenopausal women: results from the Women's Health Initiative Hormone Trial. *Diabetologia*, 47(7) pp. 1175–1187.

'carries out 90 per cent of thyroid function': Nussey, S. and Witehead, S. (2001) *Endocrinology: An Integrated Approach*, BIOS Scientific Publishers.

'may find their need for thyroid medication and support goes up': Mazer, N.A. (2004) Interaction of estrogen therapy and thyroid hormone replacement in postmenopausal women, *Thyroid*, 14, Supplement 1, pp. S27–S34.

'Progesterone, on the other hand, stimulates thyroid hormone': Sathi, P. *et al* (2013) Progesterone therapy increases free thyroxine levels – data from a randomized placebo-controlled 12-week hot flush trial, *Clinical Endocrinology (Oxford)*, 79(2), pp. 282–287.

'just two hours of use per day can raise TSH and lower T4': Mortavazi, S. *et al* (2009) Alterations in TSH and thyroid hormones following mobile phone use, *Oman Medical Journal*, 24(4), pp. 274–278.

'less than six hours sleep is associated with a reduction in TSH and T4': Kessler, L. *et al* (2010) Changes in serum TSH and free T4 during human sleep restriction, *Sleep*, 33(8), pp. 1115–1118.

'Vitamin D deficiency is associated with an increase in thyroid antibodies in Hashimoto's patients': Unal, A.D. *et al* (2014) Vitamin D deficiency is related to thyroid antibodies in autoimmune thyroiditis, *Central European Journal of Immunology*, 39(4), pp. 493–497. doi:10.5114/ceji.2014.47735

Chapter 8

'oestrogens have a major role to play in the bone turnover process in women (and in men too)': Bilezikian, J.P. *et al* (1998) Increased bone mass as a result of estrogen therapy in a man with aromatase deficiency, *New England Journal of Medicine*, 339(9), pp. 599–603; Falahati-Nini, A. *et al* (2000) Relative contributions of testosterone and estrogen in regulating bone resorption and formation in normal elderly men, *Journal of Clinical Investigation*, 106(12), pp. 1553–1560.

'exceeds the rate at which new bone is being formed, leading to bone loss': Garnero, P. *et al* (1996) Increased bone turnover in late postmenopausal women is a major determinant of osteoporosis, *Journal of Bone and Mineral Research*, 11(3), pp. 337–349.

'you can lose as much as 10 to 20 per cent of your bone mass': Tella, S.H. and Gallagher, J.C. (2014) Prevention and treatment of postmenopausal osteoporosis, *Journal of Steroid Biochemistry and Molecular Biology*, 142, pp. 155–170.

'One in three women over the age of 50 will experience a fracture due to osteoporosis': Kanis, J.A. *et al* (2000) Long-term risk of osteoporotic fracture in Malmö, *Osteoporosis International*, 11(8), pp. 669–674.

'it gets bigger at a rate of 0.4 per cent per year': Ishii, S. *et al* (2013) Trajectories of femoral neck strength in relation to the final menstrual period in a multi–ethnic cohort, *Osteoporosis International*, 24(9), pp. 2471–2481.

'the increase in load outweighs bone strength': Beck, T.J. *et al* (2009) Does obesity really make the femur stronger? BMD, geometry and fracture incidence in the women's health initiative – observational study, *Journal of Bone and Mineral Research*, 24(8), pp. 1369–1379.

'you're 10 to 20 per cent more likely to die than someone else your age who hasn't fractured their hip': Cummings, S.R. and Melton, L.J. (2002) Epidemiology and outcomes of osteoporotic fractures, *Lancet*, 359(9319), pp. 1761–1767.

'Hutterite women have a larger bone size and bone density than other US females': Wosje, K.S. *et al* (2001) Comparison of bone parameters by dual-energy X-ray absorptiometry and peripheral quantitative computed tomography in Hutterite vs. non-Hutterite women aged 35–60 years, *Bone*, 29(2), pp. 192–197.

'that it appears to be the only site it affects': Ma, D. *et al* (2013) Effects of walking on the preservation of bone mineral density in perimenopausal and postmenopausal women: a systematic review and meta-analysis, *Menopause*, 20(11), pp. 1216–1226.

'weight-bearing exercise that includes jumping, such as volleyball, basketball, netball and martial arts, seem to have a greater impact on bone mass density': Kohrt, W.M. *et al* (2004) American College of Sports Medicine position stand: physical activity and bone health, *Medicine and Science in Sports and Exercise*, 36(11), pp. 1985–1996.

'reduce the rate of bone loss of the spine but not result in favourable changes to bone mass density': Nicholson, V.P. *et al* (2015) Low-load very high-repetition resistance training attenuates bone loss at the lumbar spine in active post-menopausal women, *Calcified Tissue International*, 96(6), pp. 490–499.

'women aged 35 to 45 years experienced a significant increase in the bone density of the femoral neck': Heinonen, A. *et al* (1996) Randomised controlled trial of effect of high-impact exercise on selected risk factors for osteoporotic fractures, *Lancet*, 348(9038), pp. 1343–1347.

'prevented the rate of bone loss that was seen in the control "no-exercise" group': Nelson, M.E. *et al* (1994) Effects of high–intensity strength training on multiple risk factors for osteoporotic fractures: a randomized controlled trial, *JAMA*, 272(24), pp. 1909–1914.

'hunched over posture that's common with ageing and osteoporosis': Itoi, E. and Sinaki, M. (1994) Effect of back-strengthening exercise on posture in healthy women 49 to 65 years of age, *Mayo Clinic Proceedings*, 69(11), pp. 1054–1059.

'just as likely to suffer a fracture as those with low calcium intake': Feskanich, D. *et al* (1997) Milk, dietary calcium and bone fractures in women: a 12–year prospective study, *American Journal of Public Health*, 87(6), pp. 992–997.

'annual worldwide sales are several billion dollars': Bolland, M.J. *et al* (2011) Calcium supplements with or without vitamin D and risk of cardiovascular events: reanalysis of the Women's Health Initiative limited access dataset and meta-analysis, *British Medical Journal*, 342:d2040.

'between 1000 and 2000mg calcium per day are associated with a higher risk of fracture': Warensjö, E. *et al* (2011) Dietary calcium intake and risk of fracture and osteoporosis: prospective longitudinal cohort study, *British Medical Journal,* 342:d1473.

'more than 1500mg per day may lead to an increased risk of kidney stones': Wallace, R.B. *et al* (2011) Urinary tract stone occurrence in the Women's Health Initiative (WHI) randomized clinical trial of calcium and vitamin D supplements, *American Journal of Clinical Nutrition*, 94(1), pp. 270–277.

'and cardiovascular disease such as heart attack': Bolland, M.J. *et al* (2011) Calcium supplements with or without vitamin D and risk of cardiovascular events: reanalysis of the Women's Health Initiative limited access dataset and meta-analysis, *British Medical Journal*, 342:d2040.

Chapter 9

'which may take place sooner than if you hadn't had a uterectomy': Moorman, P.G. *et al* (2011) Effect of hysterectomy with ovarian preservation on ovarian function. *Obstetrics and Gynecology,*118(6), pp. 1271–1279.

'14.8 per cent of those who'd had their uterus removed went through menopause within four years': Moorman, P.G. *et al* (2011) *ibid.*

'go through menopause four years earlier': Farquhar, C.M. *et al* (2005) The association of hysterectomy and menopause: a prospective cohort study, *International Journal of Obstetrics and Gynaecology,* 112(7), pp. 956–962.

'Research shows that the sooner you're up and moving following surgery, and eating and drinking again': Simpson, J.C. *et al* (2015) Enhanced recovery from surgery in the UK: an audit of the enhanced recovery partnership programme 2009–2012, *British Journal of Anaesthesia*, 115(4), pp. 560–568.

'patients who are hydrated up until their surgery and who start drinking fluids after their operation report lower pain scores': Hayhurst, C. *et al* (2014) Enteral hydration prior to surgery: the benefits are clear, *Anesthesia and Analgesia*, 118(6), pp. 1163–1164.

'more common if you have a copper IUD': Hubacher, D. *et al* (2009) Side-effects from the copper IUD: do they decrease over time? *Contraception*, 79(5), pp. 356–362.

'use the Depo-Provera shot for contraception': Jacobstein, R. and Polis, C.B. (2014) Progestin-only contraception: injectables and implants, *Best Practice and Research. Clinical Obstetrics and Gynaecology*, 28(6), pp. 795–806.

'von Willebrand disease accounts for around 20 per cent of cases of heavy periods': Edlund, M. *et al* (1996) On the value of menorrhagia as a predictor for coagulation disorders, *American Journal of Hematology*, 53 (4), pp. 234–238; Kadir, R.A. *et al* (1998) Frequency of inherited bleeding disorders in women with menorrhagia, *Lancet*, 351(9101), pp. 485–489.

'they can reduce blood loss (by up to 90 per cent with the Mirena®)': https://www.bmj.com/content/328/7449/1199 (subscription required).

'where the lining of the womb is scraped away or destroyed, results in reduced bleeding 80 to 90 per cent of the time, but comes with a 25 to 50 per cent chance of developing amenorrhoea': Royal Devon and Exeter NHS Foundation Trust (2017) *Endometrial Ablation*: https://www.rdehospital.nhs.uk/documents/patient-information-leaflets/gynaecology/patient-information-leaflet-endometrial-ablation.pdf.

'Supplementing with iron can help to recover from heavy blood loss and prevent further excessive loss': Taymor, M.L. *et al* (1964) The etiological role of chronic iron deficiency in production of menorrhagia, *JAMA*, 187, pp. 323–327.

'shepherd's purse outperforms the NSAID mefenamic acid in reducing blood loss': Naafe, M. *et al* (2018) Effect of hydroalcoholic extracts of Capsella bursa-pastoris on heavy menstrual bleeding: a randomized clinical trial, *Journal of Alternative and Complementary Medicine*, 24(7), pp. 694–700.

'more common in people whose family members have them and in those with an African ancestry': Templeman, C. *et al* (2009) Risk factors for surgically removed fibroids in a large cohort of teachers, *Fertility and Sterility*, 92(4), pp. 1436–1446.

'there's a strong association between alcohol consumption and fibroids': Templeman, C. *et al* (2009) *ibid.*

'there is some evidence that the Mirena® coil is superior to oral progestins when the hyperplasia is atypical': Gallos, I.D. *et al* (2013) LNG-IUS versus oral progestogen treatment for endometrial hyperplasia: a long-term comparative cohort study, *Human Reproduction*, 28(11), pp. 2966–2971.

'only around 5 per cent of breast cancers and 15 per cent of ovarian cancers are due to an inherited gene mutation': https://www.cdc.gov/cancer/breast/young_women/bringyourbrave/hereditary_breast_cancer/index.htm.

'A 2017 study which looked at the risks of breast and ovarian cancer in BRCA1 and BRCA2 mutation carriers': Kuchenbaecker, K.B. *et al* (2017) Risks of breast, ovarian, and contralateral breast cancer for BRCA1 and BRCA2 mutation carriers, *JAMA*, 317(23), pp. 2402–2416.

'The prevalence rates of ovarian cysts in postmenopause is around 14 per cent': Greenlee, R.T. *et al* (2010) Prevalence, incidence and natural history of simple ovarian cysts among women >55 years old in a large cancer screening trial, *American Journal of Obstetrics and Gynecology*, 202(4), pp. 373.e1–373.e3739.

'Up to 15 per cent of us have PCOS': Ding, T. *et al* (2017) The prevalence of polycystic ovary syndrome in reproductive-aged women of different ethnicity: a systematic review and meta-analysis, *Oncotarget*, 8(56), pp. 96351–96358.

'are seen on the ovaries of around 20 per cent of those who do not have PCOS': Lowe, P. *et al* (2005) Incidence of polycystic ovaries and polycystic ovary syndrome amongst women in Melbourne, Australia. *Australian and New Zealand Journal of Obstetrics and Gynaecology*, 45(1), pp. 17–9.

and

Farquhar, C.M. *et al* (1994) The prevalence of polycystic ovaries on ultrasound scanning in a population of randomly selected women. *Australian and New Zealand Journal of Obstetrics and Gynaecology*, 34(1) pp. 67–72.

and

Clayton R.N. *et al* (1992) How common are polycystic ovaries in normal women and what is their significance for the fertility of the population? *Journal of Clinical Endocrinology and Metabolism*, 37(2) pp. 127–134.

'you can have PCOS and not have any cysts on your ovaries': Sheehan, M.T. (2004) Polycystic ovarian syndrome: diagnosis and management. *Clinical Medicine & Research*, 2(1), pp. 13–27.

'more likely to experience increased hirsutism and develop hypothyroidism': Schmidt, J. *et al* (2011) Reproductive hormone levels and anthropometry in postmenopausal women with polycystic ovary syndrome (PCOS): a 21-year follow-up study of women diagnosed with PCOS around 50 years ago and their age-matched controls, *Journal of Clinical Endocrinology and Metabolism*, 96(7), pp. 2178–2185.

'it can also impair insulin resistance after just three months of taking it': Adeniji, A.A. *et al.* (2016) Metabolic effects of a commonly used combined hormonal oral contraceptive in women with and without polycystic ovary syndrome, *Journal of Women's Health*, 25(6), pp. 638–645.

'strength training can improve insulin sensitivity by 24 per cent': Van Der Heijden, G.J. *et al* (2010) Strength exercise improves muscle mass and hepatic insulin sensitivity in obese youth, *Medicine and Science in Sports and Exercise*, 42(11), pp. 1973–1980.

'excision surgery performed by a highly skilled surgeon is the gold standard': Pundir, J. *et al* (2017) Laparoscopic excision versus ablation for endometriosis-associated pain: an updated systematic review and meta-analysis, *Journal of Minimally Invasive Gynecology*, 24(5), pp. 747–756.

'Plus 90 per cent of people with periods experience retrograde menstruation, but the prevalence rate for endo is only 11 per cent': Halme, J. *et al* (1984) Retrograde menstruation in healthy women and in patients with endometriosis, *Obstetrics and Gynecology*, 64(2), pp. 151–154.

'one study found endometriosis in 9 per cent of female foetuses': Signorile, P.G. *et al* (2009) Ectopic endometrium in human foetuses is a common event and sustains the theory of müllerianosis in the pathogenesis of endometriosis, a disease that predisposes to cancer, *Journal of Experimental and Clinical Cancer Research*, 28(1), p. 49.

'Research suggests that the use of CBD oil may be a particularly helpful strategy for people with endo': Bouaziz, J. *et al* (2017) The clinical significance of endocannabinoids in endometriosis pain management, *Cannabis Cannabinoid Research,* 2(1), pp. 72–80.

'Low levels of vitamin D have been linked to endo': Ciavattini, A. *et al* (2017) Ovarian endometriosis and vitamin D serum levels, *Gynecological Endocrinology*, 33(2), pp. 164–167.

'gluten-free diet for one year': Marziali, M. *et al* (2012) Gluten-free diet: a new strategy for management of painful endometriosis related symptoms?, *Minerva Chirurgica*, 67(6), pp. 499–504.

Chapter 10

'researchers found that there was a delay between melatonin secretion and feeling sleepy': Toffol, E. *et al* (2014) Melatonin in perimenopausal and postmenopausal women: associations with mood, sleep, climacteric symptoms, and quality of life. *Menopause*, 21(5) pp. 493–500.

'there's a link between melatonin and ovulation, cycle regularity and progesterone production in the second half of the cycle': Barron, M.L. (2007) Light exposure, melatonin secretion, and menstrual cycle parameters: an integrative review, *Biological Research for Nursing*, 9(1), pp. 49–69 (published correction appears in *Biological Research for Nursing*, 9(3), p.264).

'Taking a warm bath or shower before bed has been shown to elevate BDNF': Haghayegh, S. *et al* (2019) Before-bedtime passive body heating by warm shower or bath to improve sleep: a systematic review and meta-analysis, *Sleep Medicine Reviews*, 46, pp. 124–135.

'the gut microbiome interacts with the genes which regulate your circadian rhythm and sleep patterns': Rosselot, A.E. *et al* (2016) Hong, C.I., Moore, S.R. Rhythm and bugs: circadian clocks, gut microbiota, and enteric infections, *Current Opinion in Gastroenterology*, 32(1), pp. 7–11.

'Blue light in the evening and at night': Chang, A.M. *et al* (2015) Evening use of light-emitting eReaders negatively affects sleep, circadian timing, and next-morning alertness, *Proceedings of the National Academy of Sciences of the United States of America,* 112(4), pp. 1232–1237.

'Research has shown that enjoying the company of women can raise progesterone': Brown, S.L. *et al* (2009) Social closeness increases salivary progesterone in humans, *Hormones and Behavior,* 56(1), pp. 108–111 (published correction appears in *Hormones and Behavior* 56(5), p. 574).

'because oestrogen stimulates the release of histamine': Bonds, R.S. and Midoro-Horiuti, T. (2013) Estrogen effects in allergy and asthma, *Current Opinion in Allergy and Clinical Immunology,* 13(1), pp. 92–99.

'Histamine then stimulates the cells in your ovaries to secrete more oestrogen': Bódis, J. *et al* (1993) The effect of histamine on progesterone and estradiol secretion of human granulosa cells in serum-free culture, *Gynecological Endocrinology*, 7(4), pp. 235–239.

'People who get headaches in relation to the cycle and from painful periods are often histamine intolerant': Maintz, L. and Novak, N. (2007) Histamine and histamine intolerance. *American Journal of Clinical Nutrition*, 85(5), pp. 1185–1196.

'in front of a screen you're likely to eat 25 per cent more calories than you would if you weren't glued to one': Robinson, E, *et al* (2013) Eating attentively: a systematic review and meta-analysis of the effect of food intake memory and awareness on eating, *American Journal of Clinical Nutrition,* 97(4), pp. 728–742.

'one study found that cooling potatoes overnight tripled their resistant starch': Muir, J.G. and O'Dea, K. (1992) Measurement of resistant starch: factors affecting the amount of starch escaping digestion in vitro. *American Journal of Clinical Nutrition,* 56(1), pp. 123–127.

'As levels of BPA in urine increase, measures of fertility decline': Cariati, F. *et al* (2019) Bisphenol a: an emerging threat to male fertility, *Reproductive Biology and Endocrinology*, 17(1), p. 6.

'products without phthalates, parabens and phenol brought down levels of substances by 20 to 45 per cent in just three days': Harley, K.G. *et al* (2016) Reducing phthalate, paraben, and phenol exposure from personal care products in adolescent girls: findings from the HERMOSA intervention study, *Environmental Health Perspectives*, 124(10), pp. 1600–1607.

'Research into yoga nidra has found that it can improve PMS, anxiety and depression': Rani, K. *et al* (2016) Psycho-biological changes with add on yoga nidra in patients with menstrual disorders: a randomized clinical trial, *Journal of Caring Sciences*, 5(1), pp. 1–9.

'tai qi can be used to prevent or treat many health problems': Jahnke. R., *et al* (2010) A comprehensive review of health benefits of qigong and tai chi, *American Journal of Health Promotion*, 24(6):e1–e25.

'some research has demonstrated that it can reduce the incidence of falls': Wolf, S.L. *et al* (2003) Reducing frailty and falls in older persons: an investigation of tai chi and computerized balance training, *Journal of the American Geriatrics Society*, 51(12), pp. 1794–1803.

ACKNOWLEDGEMENTS

I wouldn't have got through this process without my incredible assistant, Bek Botting. Bek, you have shielded me when I needed to hide away from my inbox, checked in on me when you knew I was overwhelmed and cracked me up with your endless on-point GIF selections. You've taken care of so many aspects of my business and I'm astounded at your ability to both read my mind and take care of the stuff that doesn't enter my head. I'm grateful for all you've done and continue to do, and I can't wait for the day when we can actually meet in real life!

Thank you to the members of The Flow Collective – you lot are continually on my mind and you inspire me to up my game again and again and again. Thank you for helping to create such an outstanding community and for always wanting more. Special thanks to those of you who took part in our perimenopause discussion group and who provided some of the quotes in the book.

To my agent, Julia, who asked me to write this book long before I was willing to consider it. Thank you for urging me on at every stage of the wavering process that was this book and for being so supportive when my mum died.

Thank you to the wonderful team at Bloomsbury. I'm delighted to be on this adventure with you again and couldn't be more impressed and thankful for your hard work and belief in me. To Charlotte Croft for being on board with the idea and trusting that I would be able to pull it off during testing times. To Holly Jarrald for your meticulous attention to detail and editing skills – your questions bring out the best in me. Lizzy Ewer and Katherine Macpherson – my powerhouse publicists – you do such a fabulous job of getting my books out there – thank you.

Thank you to Karen Gurney and AJ – that evening we spent at yours was a turning point in this process and I'm grateful for our continued conversations and hang times. Thank you to Baz Moffat for contributing your expertise and to Dr Bella Smith for so generously proofreading the book.

I would not be where I am without the amazing colleagues, teachers and mentors I've had over the years. Christine Hall, I didn't know you for long, but you certainly left your mark, Reina James, Hilary Lewin, Amanda Porter, Louise Crockart, Rosita Arvigo, Diane Macdonald, Alexandra Pope, Sjanie Hugo-Wurlitzer, Nicole Jardim, Jessica Drummond, Carrie Jones, Sarah Gottesdiener, Giusi Pezzotta, Lisa Hendrickson-Jack, Holly Grigg-Spall, Lara Briden, Keris Marsden, Dani Gordon, Angela Heap and, last but not least, Angelique Panagos.

I'm eternally grateful to Brooke Castillo and everyone at the Life Coach School. Brooke, without your teachings and my training with you, my mental health would have been in tatters within the first few chapters. The coaching I've received at the school and the self-coaching you taught me is what made me decide that I could write this in four months during lockdown with a four-year-old at home – my impossible goal. Thank you to Lisa Martinello and everyone in my Friday class, especially Stacy Tuschl, who coached me through my looming deadline. And thank you to Victoria Albina for helping me to realise so much. And, of course, to Stacey Boehman and everyone inside 2k and 200k for spurring me on and challenging my thoughts about what's possible.

To everyone in Fuck You Pay Me; I'm continually blown away by the generosity of our group and inspired by the amazing work you all do. Thanks to everyone in the Rabbit Hole for always being there even when I'm not.

Thanks to Steve Horne for reappearing in my life with *Three Women* and a bar of Green & Blacks, to Meegan and Harriet for all the lols, to Gabby Edlin and Otegha Uwagba for the conversation that made everything okay, to Octavia Bright for the walk and talks and your willingness to go there, to Richard and Craig for the moments of sanity over the garden wall in lockdown, to Anna Jones for being there every step of the way, and to Rebecca Schiller for understanding so much of me and this journey. Kelly Abbott, you are an incredible woman and a force for good in this world, I'm thankful to you for EVERYTHING. Naomi, Natalie, Ryan, William and Hugo, I'm so grateful for our families' friendships, 2020 was a lot and we got through it together. Thank you to Mars Lord who always gets it and is always there, I'm blessed to have you as a friend.

The HUGEST of thanks to Natalie Georgas. Nat, you have brought me back from the brink so many times, been there through the laughter and tears, and endless cups of tea and chocolate. I'm so grateful to you and Frankie for helping me to really realise the beauty of my neurodiversity.

Thanks to Sam, Sandra and wee Jasper. Sam, you're a bloody legend and I'm blessed to have you as a brother. And to Dad, thank you for telling me to listen to Woman's Hour long before I was willing to.

Paul, thank you for knowing that my brain needs me to write. It is quite honestly a testament to our relationship and my love for you that we are still together after ALL THE WHISTLING whilst I wrote this.

To Nelson, my lovely Nelson, I can play with you now.

And to Mum, you didn't get to read this book, but so much of you is in it.

INDEX

Index